Coloring of Food, Drugs, and Cosmetics

FOOD SCIENCE AND TECHNOLOGY

A Series of Monographs, Textbooks, and Reference Books

EDITORIAL BOARD

Owen R. Fennema University of Wisconsin—Madison
Marcus Karel Rutgers University
Gary W. Sanderson Universal Foods Corporation
Steven R. Tannenbaum Massachusetts Institute of Technology
Pieter Walstra Wageningen Agricultural University
John R. Whitaker University of California—Davis

1. Flavor Research: Principles and Techniques, *R. Teranishi, I. Hornstein, P. Issenberg, and E. L. Wick*
2. Principles of Enzymology for the Food Sciences, *John R. Whitaker*
3. Low-Temperature Preservation of Foods and Living Matter, *Owen R. Fennema, William D. Powrie, and Elmer H. Marth*
4. Principles of Food Science
   Part I: Food Chemistry, *edited by Owen R. Fennema*
   Part II: Physical Methods of Food Preservation, *Marcus Karel, Owen R. Fennema, and Daryl B. Lund*
5. Food Emulsions, *edited by Stig E. Friberg*
6. Nutritional and Safety Aspects of Food Processing, *edited by Steven R. Tannenbaum*
7. Flavor Research: Recent Advances, *edited by R. Teranishi, Robert A. Flath, and Hiroshi Sugisawa*
8. Computer-Aided Techniques in Food Technology, *edited by Israel Saguy*
9. Handbook of Tropical Foods, *edited by Harvey T. Chan*
10. Antimicrobials in Foods, *edited by Alfred Larry Branen and P. Michael Davidson*
11. Food Constituents and Food Residues: Their Chromatographic Determination, *edited by James F. Lawrence*
12. Aspartame: Physiology and Biochemistry, *edited by Lewis D. Stegink and L. J. Filer, Jr.*
13. Handbook of Vitamins: Nutritional, Biochemical, and Clinical Aspects, *edited by Lawrence J. Machlin*
14. Starch Conversion Technology, *edited by G. M. A. van Beynum and J. A. Roels*
15. Food Chemistry: Second Edition, Revised and Expanded, *edited by Owen R. Fennema*
16. Sensory Evaluation of Food: Statistical Methods and Procedures, *Michael O'Mahony*
17. Alternative Sweetners, *edited by Lyn O'Brien Nabors and Robert C. Gelardi*
18. Citrus Fruits and Their Products: Analysis and Technology, *S. V. Ting and Russell L. Rouseff*

19. Engineering Properties of Foods, *edited by M. A. Rao and S. S. H. Rizvi*
20. Umami: A Basic Taste, *edited by Yojiro Kawamura and Morley R. Kare*
21. Food Biotechnology, *edited by Dietrich Knorr*
22. Food Texture: Instrumental and Sensory Measurement, *edited by Howard R. Moskowitz*
23. Seafoods and Fish Oils in Human Health and Disease, *John E. Kinsella*
24. Postharvest Physiology of Vegetables, *edited by J. Weichmann*
25. Handbook of Dietary Fiber: An Applied Approach, *Mark L. Dreher*
26. Food Toxicology, Parts A and B, *Jose M. Concon*
27. Modern Carbohydrate Chemistry, *Roger W. Binkley*
28. Trace Minerals in Foods, *edited by Kenneth T. Smith*
29. Protein Quality and the Effects of Processing, *edited by R. Dixon Phillips and John W. Finley*
30. Adulteration of Fruit Juice Beverages, *edited by Steven Nagy, John A. Attaway, and Martha E. Rhodes*
31. Foodborne Bacterial Pathogens, *edited by Michael P. Doyle*
32. Legumes: Chemistry, Technology, and Human Nutrition, *edited by Ruth H. Matthews*
33. Industrialization of Indigenous Fermented Foods, *edited by Keith H. Steinkraus*
34. International Food Regulation Handbook: Policy • Science • Law, *edited by Roger D. Middlekauff and Philippe Shubik*
35. Food Additives, *edited by A. Larry Branen, P. Michael Davidson, and Seppo Salminen*
36. Safety of Irradiated Foods, *J. F. Diehl*
37. Omega-3 Fatty Acids in Health and Disease, *edited by Robert S. Lees and Marcus Karel*
38. Food Emulsions: Second Edition, Revised and Expanded, *edited by Kåre Larsson and Stig E. Friberg*
39. Seafood: Effects of Technology on Nutrition, *George M. Pigott and Barbee W. Tucker*
40. Handbook of Vitamins: Second Edition, Revised and Expanded, *edited by Lawrence J. Machlin*
41. Handbook of Cereal Science and Technology, *Klaus J. Lorenz and Karel Kulp*
42. Food Processing Operations and Scale-Up, *Kenneth J. Valentas, Leon Levine, and J. Peter Clark*
43. Fish Quality Control by Computer Vision, *edited by L. F. Pau and R. Olafsson*
44. Volatile Compounds in Foods and Beverages, *edited by Henk Maarse*
45. Instrumental Methods for Quality Assurance in Foods, *edited by Daniel Y. C. Fung and Richard F. Matthews*
46. Listeria, Listeriosis, and Food Safety, *Elliot T. Ryser and Elmer H. Marth*
47. Acesulfame-K, *edited by D. G. Mayer and F. H. Kemper*
48. Alternative Sweeteners: Second Edition, Revised and Expanded, *edited by Lyn O'Brien Nabors and Robert C. Gelardi*
49. Food Extrusion Science and Technology, *edited by Jozef L. Kokini, Chi-Tang Ho, and Mukund V. Karwe*
50. Surimi Technology, *edited by Tyre C. Lanier and Chong M. Lee*
51. Handbook of Food Engineering, *edited by Dennis R. Heldman and Daryl B. Lund*
52. Food Analysis by HPLC, *edited by Leo M. L. Nollet*
53. Fatty Acids in Foods and Their Health Implications, *edited by Ching Kuang Chow*
54. *Clostridium botulinum*: Ecology and Control in Foods, *edited by Andreas H. W. Hauschild and Karen L. Dodds*

55. Cereals in Breadmaking: A Molecular Colloidal Approach, *Ann-Charlotte Eliasson and Kåre Larsson*
56. Low-Calorie Foods Handbook, *edited by Aaron M. Altschul*
57. Antimicrobials in Foods: Second Edition, Revised and Expanded, *edited by P. Michael Davidson and Alfred Larry Branen*
58. Lactic Acid Bacteria, *edited by Seppo Salminen and Atte von Wright*
59. Rice Science and Technology, *edited by Wayne E. Marshall and James I. Wadsworth*
60. Food Biosensor Analysis, *edited by Gabriele Wagner and George G. Guilbault*
61. Principles of Enzymology for the Food Sciences: Second Edition, *John R. Whitaker*
62. Carbohydrate Polyesters as Fat Substitutes, *edited by Casimir C. Akoh and Barry G. Swanson*
63. Engineering Properties of Foods: Second Edition, Revised and Expanded, *edited by M. A. Rao and S. S. H. Rizvi*
64. Handbook of Brewing, *edited by William A. Hardwick*
65. Analyzing Food for Nutrition Labeling and Hazardous Contaminants, *edited by Ike J. Jeon and William G. Ikins*
66. Ingredient Interactions: Effects on Food Quality, *edited by Anilkumar G. Gaonkar*
67. Food Polysaccharides and Their Applications, *edited by Alistair M. Stephen*
68. Safety of Irradiated Foods: Second Edition, Revised and Expanded, *J. F. Diehl*
69. Nutrition Labeling Handbook, *edited by Ralph Shapiro*
70. Handbook of Fruit Science and Technology: Production, Composition, Storage, and Processing, *edited by D. K. Salunkhe and S. S. Kadam*
71. Food Antioxidants: Technological, Toxicological, and Health Perspectives, *edited by D. L. Madhavi, S. S. Deshpande, and D. K. Salunkhe*
72. Freezing Effects on Food Quality, *edited by Lester E. Jeremiah*
73. Handbook of Indigenous Fermented Foods: Second Edition, Revised and Expanded, *edited by Keith H. Steinkraus*
74. Carbohydrates in Food, *edited by Ann-Charlotte Eliasson*
75. Baked Goods Freshness: Technology, Evaluation, and Inhibition of Staling, *edited by Ronald E. Hebeda and Henry F. Zobel*
76. Food Chemistry: Third Edition, *edited by Owen R. Fennema*
77. Handbook of Food Analysis: Volumes 1 and 2, *edited by Leo M. L. Nollet*
78. Computerized Control Systems in the Food Industry, *edited by Gauri S. Mittal*
79. Techniques for Analyzing Food Aroma, *edited by Ray Marsili*
80. Food Proteins and Their Applications, *edited by Srinivasan Damodaran and Alain Paraf*
81. Food Emulsions: Third Edition, Revised and Expanded, *edited by Stig E. Friberg and Kåre Larsson*
82. Nonthermal Preservation of Foods, *Gustavo V. Barbosa-Cánovas, Usha R. Pothakamury, Enrique Palou, and Barry G. Swanson*
83. Milk and Dairy Product Technology, *Edgar Spreer*
84. Applied Dairy Microbiology, *edited by Elmer H. Marth and James L. Steele*
85. Lactic Acid Bacteria: Microbiology and Functional Aspects, Second Edition, Revised and Expanded, *edited by Seppo Salminen and Atte von Wright*
86. Handbook of Vegetable Science and Technology: Production, Composition, Storage, and Processing, *edited by D. K. Salunkhe and S. S. Kadam*
87. Polysaccharide Association Structures in Food, *edited by Reginald H. Walter*
88. Food Lipids: Chemistry, Nutrition, and Biotechnology, *edited by Casimir C. Akoh and David B. Min*
89. Spice Science and Technology, *Kenji Hirasa and Mitsuo Takemasa*

90. Dairy Technology: Principles of Milk Properties and Processes, *P. Walstra, T. J. Geurts, A. Noomen, A. Jellema, and M. A. J. S. van Boekel*
91. Coloring of Food, Drugs, and Cosmetics, *Gisbert Otterstätter*
92. *Listeria*, Listeriosis, and Food Safety, *edited by Elliot T. Ryser and Elmer H. Marth*

Additional Volumes in Preparation

Complex Carbohydrates in Foods, *edited by Susan Sungsoo Cho, Leon Prosky, and Mark Dreher*

Handbook of Food Preservation, *edited by M. Shafiur Rahman*

Food Safety: Science, International Regulation, and Control, *edited by C. A. van der Heijden, Sanford Miller, Maged Younes, and Lawrence Fishbein*

Coloring of Food, Drugs, and Cosmetics

Gisbert Otterstätter
Dragoco
Holzminden, Germany

translated by
Axel Mixa
Lantana, Florida

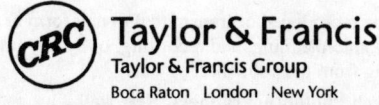

Taylor & Francis
Taylor & Francis Group
Boca Raton London New York

A CRC title, part of the Taylor & Francis imprint, a member of the
Taylor & Francis Group, the academic division of T&F Informa plc.

FIRST INDIAN REPRINT, 2010
ISBN: 0-8247-0215-8

This book was previously published in the original German as *Die Färbung von Lebensmitteln, Arzneimitteln, Kosmetika*, by Gisbert Otterstätter, Behr's Verlag GmbH & Co., Hamburg, Germany © 1995.

Headquarters
Marcel Dekker
270 Madison Avenue, New York, NY 10016
tel: 212-696-9000; fax: 212-685-4540

World Wide Web
http://www.dekker.com

The publisher offers discounts on this book when ordered in bulk quantities. For more information, write to Special Sales/Professional Marketing at the headquarters address above.

Copyright © 1999 Marcel Dekker   All Rights Reserved.

Neither this book nor any part may be reproduced or transmitted in any form or by any means, electronic or mechanical, including photocopying, microfilming, and recording, or by any information storage and retrieval system, without permission in writing from the publisher.

Printed and bound in India by Nutech Photolithographers, New Delhi

FOR SALE IN SOUTH ASIA ONLY

Preface to the English-Language Edition

When coloring food, drugs and cosmetics, marketing and product development personnel are faced with the task of achieving an attractive color. At the same time they must comply with a multitude of national regulations in view of the ever-increasing and intensifying trade relations. This results in various problems. The objective of this book is to give both information on which colorants can be used most profitably for which products as well as additional information on the state of certification in a number of important countries. In addition, analytical methods and activities for quality assurance are described.

Important note: Since the publication of the second German edition in 1995, the commission of the European Union has issued two guidelines that affect food colorants in Europe:

1. The purity requirements of food colorants developed by the EU in 1962–1964 have been modified on a technical basis. New dye specifications (Guideline 95/45/EU) have been developed by using principles from JEFCA and Codex. They have been modernized in the areas of manufacturing methods and analytical methods. In this guideline, each dye is described on the basis of a preset format, indicating its synonyms and defining the dye, followed by a dye classification, Color Index Number (CIN), EINECS number, chemical designation, chemical formula, molecular weight, purity requirements, product description and its features (e.g. appearance of the dye solution, absorption maxima, specific rotation). Important key data for product development personnel can be found in the data sheet section of this book (see Chap. 9). The previous purity standards for European food colorants have been modified for each specific dye and contain only those requirements that are relevant for that dye (e.g. water-insoluble components, byproduct dyes, organic compounds exclusive of the colorants, non-sulfated primary aromatic amines, compounds extracted with ether). What is common for nearly all the dyes is the content of heavy metals:

Arsenic	max. 3 ppm	Lead	max. 10 ppm
Mercury	max. 1 ppm	Cadmium	max. 1 ppm
Total heavy metals	max. 40 ppm		

2. The number of carriers and solvent carriers for food colorants and other food additives has been increased significantly in the EU (Guideline 95/2/EU dd. Feb. 20, 1995, Guideline on food additives other than colorants and sweetening agents). In reality, however, only the solvents and carriers mentioned in Table 11 are used.

As both guidelines are more relevant to the manufacturer than the applying party, and as they are not included in the 2nd edition, these details have been excluded intentionally from the first English edition. It is expected that these will be included in the next German and English editions.

Preface to the English-Language Edition

Because the two German editions of this book have been used since 1988 only in German-speaking countries, I will be very grateful for any feedback and information from readers of this English-Language edition.

Gisbert Otterstätter

Preface to the German Edition

The utilization of coloring materials to make people and the environment appear more beautiful is definitely one of the oldest technical/cultural achievements of mankind. Coloring of food and drugs has become necessary only with the onset of industrialization for several reasons.

In recent times, coloring of food has become the subject of a public discussion, characterized in many cases by insufficient knowledge, insecurity and fear. On the other hand, there exists a very long history of practical knowledge as well as scientific facts and experiences.

It is my endeavor to reorient this discussion objectively and make it more profound by providing factual information on the knowledge of composition, utilization and evaluation of colorants and pigments.

After an introduction to the relationships of coloring reactions, there is a discussion on the basic approval requirements for coloring material in the Federal Republic of Germany, within the European Union (EU) as well as in countries outside the EU. In Chapter 8 (Analysis), the identification of colorants is discussed in detail and an abundance of information on practical implementation can be found.

The second half of this book presents data sheets for the colorants for food, drugs and cosmetics in the EU. They appear in chronological form as per their Color Index Number (CIN). Colorants without the CIN are listed alphabetically by their common name. An extensive list of literature, subdivided into different subjects, makes the access to further sources (primary and secondary) easier.

This book addresses practical professionals in the food, drug and cosmetics industry providing information in a concise form, thus making it useful for everyday applications, such as:

- Application-oriented information
- Simple analytical methods
- Activities for quality assurance
- Information on the approval status of colorants in the most important countries

I am very grateful to Messrs. Dr. Wolfgang Bruhn (Holzminden) and Dr. Dietmar Bücher (Besigheim) for their critical review of the manuscript.

I will greatly appreciate new ideas and information from the reader.

Note Added to the Second Edition

In the EU there have been a series of important changes since 1987 that are relevant to the coloring of foods and drugs. This requires a revision of the first edition, taking into consideration not only the legal changes, but also covering the data sheets for many colorants, increasing their information coverage. Further colorants have been included that are not approved within the EU, but that are in other countries for different purposes.

Gisbert Otterstätter

About the Translator

AXEL MIXA is a food technology consultant based in Norderstedt, Germany. He has wide international experience in both the technical and managerial aspects of dairy product manufacturing and is a member of the Institute of Food Technologists. Mr. Mixa received the M.S. degree (1973) in food technology from the Technical University of Berlin, Germany.

Contents

Preface to the English-Language Edition	iii
Preface to the German Edition	v
About the Translator	vii
Acronyms	xi

1 Basic Definitions — 1
   1.1. Colors and seeing colors — 1
       1.1.1. Fluorescence and optical whiteners — 2
       1.1.2. Interference — 3
   1.2. Additives and subtractive colorant blending — 3
   1.3. Colors and perceptions — 4
   1.4. Color systems — 6
   1.5. Coloring agents, colorants and pigments — 7
   1.6. Systematic of colorants — 11
       1.6.1. The color index — 11
       1.6.2. The EU number — 12

2 Food Coloration — 13
   2.1. Food coloration—why? — 13
   2.2. Technical possibilities — 14
   2.3. Coloring ingredients — 14
   2.4. Legal basis — 15
       2.4.1. European Union — 15
       2.4.2. Countries outside the European Union — 31
       2.4.3. United States — 31

3 Drug Coloration — 37
   3.1. The importance of drug coloration — 37
   3.2. Legal requirements — 37
       3.2.1. European Union/Federal Republic of Germany — 37
       3.2.2. Countries outside the European Union — 38

4 The Coloration of Cosmetic Products — 39
   4.1. The importance of color in cosmetic products — 39
   4.2. Technological possibilities — 39
   4.3. Legal requirements — 39
       4.3.1. European Union/Federal Republic of Germany — 39
       4.3.2. Countries outside the European Union — 45

5 The Coloration of Food, Drugs and Cosmetics in the Public Discussion — 47

6 Product Development — 49
   6.1. Processing indications — 50
       6.1.1. Soluble colorants — 50
       6.1.2. Pigments and coloring paints — 51
       6.1.3. Special preparations — 52
   6.2. Food (a selection) — 52

	6.3. Drugs (a selection)	53
	6.4. Cosmetic products	54
	6.5. Stability tests	59

7 Safety and Quality — 63
- 7.1. Toxicology and dermatology — 63
- 7.2. Quality assurance — 63
- 7.3. Colorimetry and photometry — 64
  - 7.3.1. Principles of a spectral photometer — 64
  - 7.3.2. Evaluation — 67
- 7.4. Measuring color — 68
  - 7.4.1. Basics — 68
  - 7.4.2. Determination — 68
  - 7.4.3. Calculation and evaluation — 70

8 Analysis — 77
- 8.1. Purity requirements — 77
  - 8.1.1. Colorants for food and drugs — 77
  - 8.1.2. Colorants for cosmetic products — 80
- 8.2. Identification of colorants — 80
  - 8.2.1. Water-soluble colorants for food and cosmetics — 80
  - 8.2.2. Oil-soluble food and cosmetic colorants — 84
  - 8.2.3. Aluminum lakes — 85
  - 8.2.4. Pigments — 85
  - 8.2.5. Isolation of the coloring agent in the finished product and its identification — 88

9 Data Sheets of Colorants for Food, Drugs and Cosmetics — 91
- 9.1. Explanations of the data sheets — 91
  - 9.1.1. Names — 91
  - 9.1.2. Chemical name — 92
  - 9.1.3. Color and solubility — 92
  - 9.1.4. Chromatography — 92
  - 9.1.5. Spectral photometry — 92
  - 9.1.6. Major applications — 92
  - 9.1.7. Toxicological and dermatological information — 92
  - 9.1.8. Certification status — 93

10 Literature — 369
- 10.1. General information — 369
- 10.2. Food — 370
- 10.3. Drugs — 371
- 10.4. Cosmetics — 372
- 10.5. Analysis and color determination — 372
- 10.6. Food legislation — 374
  - 10.6.1. Food — 374
  - 10.6.2. Cosmetics — 375

Index — 377

Acronyms

ADI	Acceptable Daily Intake
C.I.	Color Index
CAS	Chemical Abstracts System
CFR	Code of Federal Regulations (USA)
CIE	Commission Internationale de l'Éclairage
COLIPA	Comité de Liaison des Associations Européennes de l'Industrie de la Parfumerie, des Produits Cosmétiques et de Toilette
CTFA	Cosmetic, Toiletry and Fragrance Association
DFG	Deutsche Forschungsgemeinschaft
DSL	Domestic Substances List (Canada)
EBC	European Brewery Convention
ECOIN	European Community Inventory (precursor to EINECS)
EINECS	European Inventory of Existing Commercial Chemical Substances
ELINCS	European List of Notified Chemical Substances
EU	European Union
FAO	Food and Agriculture Organization
FCC	Food Chemical Codex
FDA	Food and Drug Administration
FEMA	Flavors and Extract Manufacturers Association
FFDCA	Federal Food, Drug and Cosmetics Act
GMP	Good Manufacturing Practices
GRAS	Generally Recognized as Safe
IFRA	International Fragrance Association
IFSCC	International Federation of Societies of Cosmetic Chemists
IKW	Industrieverband Körperpflege und Waschmittel e.V.
INCI	International Nomenclature Cosmetic Ingredient
IOFI	International Organization of the Flavor Industry
ISO	International Standards Organization
IUPAC	International Union of Pure and Applied Chemistry
JEFCA	Joint Expert Committee for Food Additives
MITI	Ministry of Trade and Industry (Japan)
MOHW	Ministry of Health and Welfare (Japan)
RIFM	Research Institute for Fragrance Materials
SCF	Scientific Committee for Food
TOSCA	Toxic Substances Control Act (USA)
WHO	World Health Organization

1 Basic Definitions

1.1. Colors and seeing colors

"Die Farben sind die Thaten des Lichts, Thaten und Leiden" (Colors are the acts of light, acts and suffering) – Goethe

In the German language, the word "Farbe" (color) is used both for the human perception as well as for the coloring material itself. The color of a wall is white (visual perception), because it has been painted with a white color (coloring material). In the technical-scientific area, color is used exclusively for the perception by the human eye, not for the coloring ingredient or material.

When sunlight is split by a glass prism (prism trial of Newton), a colored band can be observed; it is the continuous spectrum of the apparently white light as emitted by the sun. In the physical sense, each color of this band—or each spectral color—can be attributed to a defined wavelength[1] (Figure 1).

When sunlight falls onto an apparently colored body, light of a certain wavelength is absorbed because of the molecular structure. Only part of this sunlight spectrum is reflected, that is, the color that we can see. Absorbed and reflected colors are so-called complementary colors; when they are blended, they again result in white light. If the entire light is reflected, then this body appears to be white; if no light is reflected, then it will appear as a black body.

The old proverb "At night, all cats are gray" means two things from a physical point of view:

1. Without light there is no perception of color and
2. The human eye cannot distinguish colors under certain lighting conditions, but can still distinguish between light and dark.

Light that hits the eye, passes through the cornea and the crystalline lens—the optical part of the eye—passes through the glass body and hits the retina. The upper layers of the cornea include the cones and rods, the receptors for light and color. The cones play their role in daylight and color perception, whereas the rods play their part in light-dark perception.

We can safely assume that there are three different types of cones, that react differently to red, green and blue. If all cones are excited in the same way and intensity, then the brain of the observer will give the signal "non-colored", i.e., white. With a simultaneous excitation of blue and red-reacting cones, a *purple* color blend is generated. For the eye, yellow is not a basic color, but a blend of colors. Yellow is created by the simultaneous excitation of red and green-reacting cones.

This concept has to be seen as a model, because stimuli other than the optical variety can cause a color perception in the brain; otherwise how can it be explained that colored pictures can be seen in dreams.

---

[1] The standard unit of measure for wavelength of light is the nanometer (nm). 1 nm = 10^{-9} m = 1 millionth of a millimeter. Compare this to the wavelength of shortwave radiowaves (e.g., 49 meters).

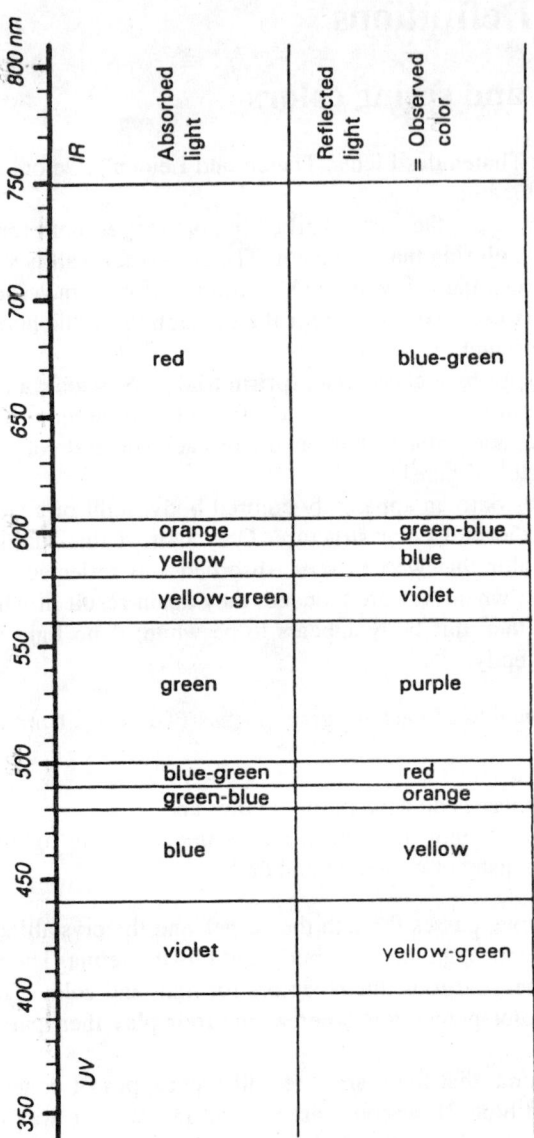

Figure 1 Correlation between wavelength (λ), light absorption and observed color.

1.1.1. Fluorescence and optical whiteners

A special type of color phenomenon is fluorescence. Because of the molecular structure of certain colorants (e.g., xanthen, stilbene), there is not only a selective light absorption in the visible range (which imparts color to a body), but part of the absorbed light energy is returned in the form of light beams with a similar or longer wavelength. For the natural colorant chlorophyll we can observe a red fluorescence in an alcoholic solution, the cosmetic colorants uranine and pyranine show an intensive green fluorescence in water, sulforhodamine shows an intensive red fluorescence.

The optically very interesting fluorescence effects of water-soluble colorants are utilized in the coloration of bathing products. Daylight pigments are used, e.g., in hair spray.

Fluorescent colorants and pigments absorb light in the visual range, and thus have a significant auto-coloration. Optical whiteners absorb light in the non-visible ultraviolet range. They are fluorescent mainly in the blue spectral range, and therefore impart a "whiter" appearance to the body/material.

1.1.2. Interference

A peculiar aspect is the phenomenon of light interference. Interference is the enhancement or suppression of different wavelengths by divergence or refraction in very thin, but optically active layers. Many color phenomena on insects, bird feathers and fishes are based exclusively on light interference.

In cosmetics, pearl pigments are used; their color effect is also based on interference. These are glimmer particles that are coated with titanium dioxide. Incoming light is reflected or absorbed on the boundary layers. Using interference, complementary colors are made visible by interference or transmission, e.g., red/green or blue/yellow; an important aspect is the angle of observation which influences the perception of color. Changing the angle of observation causes color change effects.

1.2. Additive and subtractive colorant blending

Every owner of a TV set knows additive color blending. Using three colors, red, green and violet, any possible color can be created via the human eye in the observer's brain. It only depends on with which intensity the different colors are projected into the eyes that stimulate the cones of the cornea.

When additive color blending is used, all possible colors (including white) can be made by using green, red and violet; when the subtractive color blending is used, the base colors are purple, blue and yellow, which at complete absorption results in the color black (Figure 2).

When subtractive color blending is used, a part of the incoming white light is absorbed (subtracted), therefore it is called subtractive blending. In the narrowest sense, it is considered subtractive blending if one or more filters are positioned in the light passage. Subtractive color blending also exists when incoming light is modified by absorption, e.g., printed paper, a colored body or a colored liquid.

Under normal conditions, additive and subtractive color blending is of no importance, apart from color analysis (see Chapter 7.4). During the development of colored products it is more important to orient oneself on painting lessons received during early schooling. The simplest paint box contains six color pots with blue, yellow, green, red (purple), orange and black colors. Basically, blue, purple and black are sufficient to do paintings (the principle of four-color printing); but painters became comfortable and did not want to manufacture a green color by blending blue and yellow.

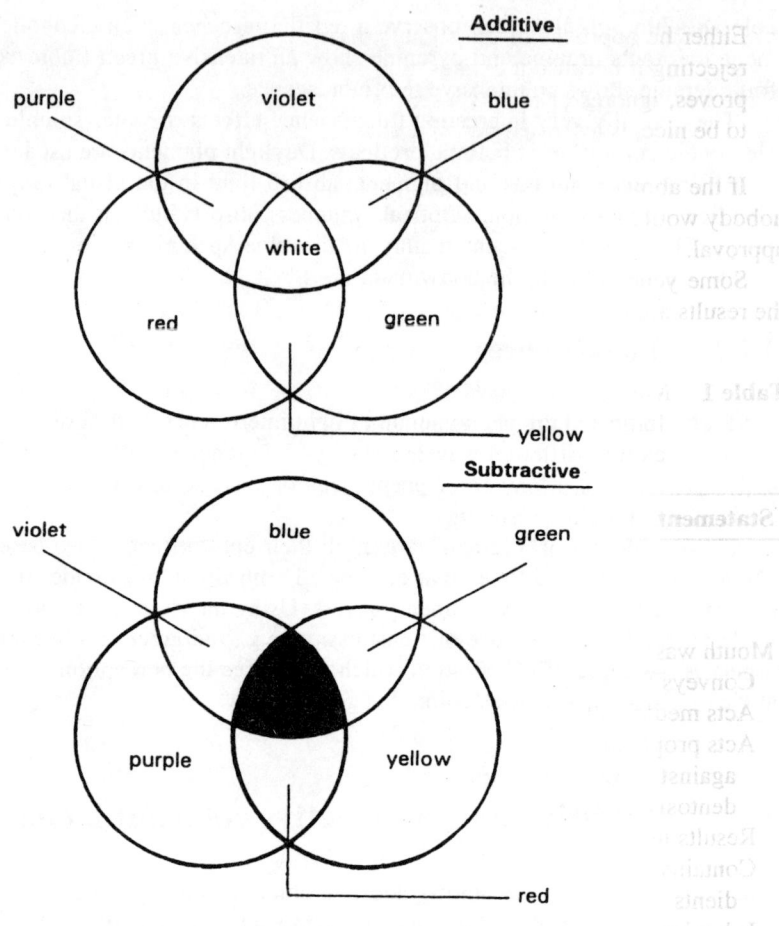

Figure 2 Additive and subtractive color blending.

1.3. Colors and perceptions

In the sixth chapter of his work "Zur Farbenlehre" Johann Wolfgang von Goethe describes the "sensual-moral effect of color":

> "In general, humans enjoy color very much. The eye requires it, as it requires light…"

In his book "Farben—visualsierte Gefühle," Max Lüscher describes extensively, but with less poetry, the stimuli and effects of various colors on human feelings. Among other things he writes:

> "In all cultures, all human beings have the same color perceptions. The sensual perception of a pure red color causes a stimulating incentive. It always stimulates. For this generally valid perception, each person reacts differently with his own feelings.

Basic Definitions

Either he approves of the stimulating perception (because it stimulates him), or he is rejecting it because it excites him. According to the mood of the person, he either approves, ignores or rejects a sensual perception, e.g. a color. A color that he perceives to be nice, is a sensual perception which is approved by his feelings."

If the above statement is transposed onto food and cosmetics, it becomes evident that nobody would buy, voluntarily, a product where color and appearance would not meet his approval.

Some years ago, the importance of color for mouth wash water was researched, and the results are shown in Table 1.

Table 1 Mouth wash, associations between product statements and colors
Indicated are the absolute number of expressions by the test persons (multiple expressions were possible)

Statement	Color					
	Green	Strawberry red	Yellow	Dark red	Colorless	Blue
Mouth wash						
Conveys freshness, cold	14	-	1	1	6	19
Acts medicinally	3	7	-	12	6	10
Acts prophylacticly against caries, paradentosis, bad breath	8	1	2	18	1	5
Results in clean breath	11	1	2	4	11	11
Contains natural ingredients	7	1	3	4	16	4
Is hygienic	4	1	2	4	12	15

(Source: P. Tetweiler, and J.S. Jellinek, Farbe in Mundwässern, DRAGOCO Report 4/5-1982)

These results can be interpreted as follows:

Conveys freshness, cool. Blue and green are predominantly preferred. Here the association of the test persons are oriented toward mountain lakes, cold, young or fresh mint leaves.

Acts medicinally.

Acts prophylactically against caries, etc. In both cases, red is dominant. Red is bitter, sometimes has an unpleasant taste, but is subconsciously oriented toward recuperation.

Results in clean breath. Green, white (colorless) and blue are equally perceived. Associations with mint, menthol, ice, sea breeze are mentioned here; a perception of purity and hygiene.

Contains natural ingredients. White (colorless) was preferred; the relationship to nature is given, because water is a natural ingredient.

Is hygienic. Minor predominance of blue over white (colorless). Blue indicates power, the transposition to, e.g., household cleaning agents with a disinfection effect is very noticeable. White means hygiene.

For the coloration of bathing products, there is a significant preference for the color shades of green, blue and yellow, as the author could determine from his own research (see also Table 2), and as can be seen by walking through the aisles of any supermarket. For this product it is relatively simple to understand the product preferences of a consumer. Blue and green are associated with freshness, cool, cleanliness and nature, yellow is preferred predominantly in egg-shampoos. The colors red, brown and violet are not a factor.

Table 2   Colorants for bathing products, percentages of sales volumes for colorants (own research)

Year	Yellow/orange	Red	Blue	Green	Brown	Violet
1982	27.0	2.7	19.6	46.7	3.2	0.9
1983	27.2	4.2	24.7	38.6	4.0	1.3
1984	19.3	2.8	28.7	44.6	3.7	1.0
1985	22.7	2.0	19.5	52.0	3.4	0.5
1986	14.5	3.1	28.4	49.4	3.5	1.2

1.4. Color systems

An observer with normal vision can recognize and differentiate an immense number of color shades under favorable lighting conditions. It is irrelevant, how many million color shades can be distinguished, as literature information varies on this aspect.

Even when all color shades used by industry are estimated to be about 10,000, it becomes evident that there cannot be a label for each color shade. Even if this would be possible, it does not mean that each observer would perceive the color in the same way. In the past researchers have tried to solve this problem by the creation of color disks and far-ranging color collections (color atlas). Even Goethe was involved in creating color circles when he looked at colors in 1795. Chevreuil tried to systematize colors in 1830 for the French gobelin (tapestry) industry, which were of technical importance, leading to a color atlas with 1442 different and exactly defined color shades. Ostwald worked on colors in 1918 and recorded 680 colors in his color tables. The Swedish "Natural Color System" is established in a similar way and shows 1530 color shades. Dr. Müller's "mobiler Farbkörper" (mobile color object) represents another development based on the Ostwald color system and shows 1093 different color shades. In Germany, the RAL color register is used very often; apart from this, there is the DIN-Farbenkarte (DIN color chart) DIN 6164 with 1001 color samples that are correlated to the RAL color register. In the United States the Munsell color system is most widely used. Color and paint manufacturers work very often with internally established sample cards; further there are color encyclopedia

Basic Definitions

and other sources. Within these color systems color shades can be determined objectively and are characterized, e.g., by the CIE-Lab system (see Section 7.4).

At DRAGOCO we have used for some years now, and with good results, the cost-efficient and internationally applied Pantone® color communication system, which is a color array with 500 different color shades. Under normal conditions this color array can be used as a communication medium in the food, drug and cosmetic industry for marketing, technical development and colorant manufacturer.

1.5. Coloring agents, colorants and pigments

According to DIN 6164 the term colorant is a collective term for all soluble or solubilized coloring agents (e.g., during textile dying), as well as for insoluble pigments that have a color effect in a product because of their distribution. This definition leads to the statement that the term pigment colorant is contradictory and should not be used.

Colorants are differentiated into inorganic and organic products, and further into natural, nature-identical and synthetic colorants (see Table 3). It should be mentioned here, that a colored substance cannot always be used as a colorant. The inorganic potassium permanganate is soluble in water (violet solution), and organic azobenzol is orange, but both forms have no dying properties.

Apart from colorants and pigments there are paint lacquers and water-dispersible pigments; the latter ones play a role in the coloration of soap and aggressive household cleaning products.

Paint lacquers are a group of food colorants that are pseudo-pigments, manufactured by precipitation of water-soluble colorants with aluminum hydroxide. Paint lacquers are nearly insoluble in water and can be processed like pigments. Major applications are in the area of pharmaceutical capsules and decorative cosmetics such as eye makeup and lipstick.

Table 3 System of colorants

Colorants			
Inorganic colorants (pigments)		**Organic colorants** (colorants, their lacquers and pigments)	
Natural	Synthetic*	Natural or nature-identical	Synthetic (artificial)
Chalk	Titanium dioxide	Carotenoids	Azo colorants and pigments
Ochre	Chromium yellow	Carmine	
Umbra	Ultramarine	Chlorophyll	Triaryl methane and
Graphite	Iron oxide	Xanthophyll	Xanthen colorant
Terra di Siena	Aluminum	Anthraquinone	Quinophtalone
others		Indigoide	Phtalocyanin and
		others	others

*By chemical reaction or physical modification of inorganic raw materials.

In the past there was always the question of how the chemical composition of a colorant was linked to its color and its coloring properties.

During the analysis of colored material it was found that certain atomic groups favor the absorption of light of certain wavelengths (selective absorption), and thus impart a color. Such atomic groups are called chromophores. The azo group (—N═N—) is one of the most important chromophore groups. They are the color carrier proper of azo colorants, during their disintegration discoloration occurs, e.g., by reduction agents which split the colorant molecule into two aromatic amines. Another chromophore group is the nitro group(—NO_2), linked to one or more benzene rings (1) systems of numerous conjugated double bonds also cause a colored appearance, as is shown in the example of beta-carotene (2).

(1) C₆H₅—NO_2

(2) [beta-carotene structure]

The absorption of certain wavelengths of white light is caused by the presence of π-electrons in the color molecule. π-electrons are non-localized electrons adhering simultaneously to two atoms, e.g., in beta-carotene. They can be energized fairly easily into higher energy levels and therefore absorb visible light. Energy thus absorbed is reduced by

change into heat
photochemical reactions (for colorants with a low light proof) and/or
emission (e.g., fluorescence phenomena)

The presence of electron dispatching auxochrome groups (—OH, —NH_2) and the electron-attracting antiauxochrome groups (e.g., —NO_2 or ═C═O) to the end of the molecule system increases the color effect. If the insertion of an atomic group causes a color modification in the direction yellow–red–violet–blue, then this effect is called a bathochrome effect; the reverse direction is called a hypsochrome effect. Certain functional groups in the molecule cause the colorant to solubilize in water, e.g., the sulfa-acid group —SO_3, most often in the form of sodium or potassium salts.

On the other hand it is possible to modify a water-soluble colorant into a pigment by the formation of an alkaline salt. By reacting the same base material with different alkaline salts (calcium, barium, strontium or zirconium salt), pigments with very different colors can be produced.

Here we want to mention a small historical diversion. Julius Caesar notes very surprisingly in his book "The Gallic War."

"All Britons are painting themselves with dyer's woad, which causes a blue color, and thus makes their appearance in war more gruesome."

Dyer's woad (*Isaias tinctoria*) and the indigo plant (*Indigofera tinctoria*) belong to agricultural plants known for a long time which can be used for the production of the blue colorant indigo (3).

(3)

Thyric purple, also called Byzantine purple or "the purple of the Elder" is a colorant that is extracted from the purple snail (*Murex brandis*), and is a 6,6'-dibrom-indigo (4). More than 10,000 purple snails are necessary to obtain 1.5 g of this colorant. The Phoenicians developed this colorant, and only the upper classes could avail of these colored textiles.

(4)

Alizarin (5) was of great economic importance in the 18th and 19th century, as this colorant was extracted from the Madder root (German: Krapp plant) and was used mainly for dying uniforms red; today it is manufactured exclusively on a synthetic basis.

(5)

The age of synthetic colorants (dyes) was established in 1771 by Woulffe, who manufactured picric acid (6) by reacting indigo with nitric acid. Picric acid was temporarily used for dying silk (yellow), but it did not have great importance.

(6) 2,4,6-trinitrophenol

In 1856, William Perkin manufactured mauveine by oxidizing aniline (containing toluidine) which is a weak violet colorant used for dying silk; it has low light stability. In the same year, Natanson synthesized Fuchsin (7), a triphenyl-methane colorant.

(7) Fuchsin structure

At the same time, the most profound discovery in the area of synthetic colorants occurred, which still has an impact today; the discovery of the azo compounds by Peter Griess (1858). Five years later, Martius manufactured the first azo colorant—Bismarck Brown (apart from the Bismarck herrings and Bismarck towers one of the least known links to the name of the "Iron Chancellor" Bismarck). Derived from these azo compounds (discovered by Griess), which are characterized by the molecule group —N=N— are numerous food and cosmetic colorants that are used all over the word, e.g., Tartrazine C.I. 19140, Yellow Orange C.I. 15985, Orange II (8) C.I. 15510.

(8) Orange II structure

1.6. Systematic of colorants

1.6.1. The color index

Apart from the classification of coloring agents into colorants and pigments (see Section 1.5) there is also a classification according to other major aspects such as

dying process and application
chemical composition

The color tables of G. Schultz (Leipzig 1931) have been used previously, but are now replaced by the globally utilized "Color Index" which is also known under the name "Color Index number" (acronym C.I.).

Currently the Color Index is contained in eight volumes, describing several thousands of colorants and pigments, and is published by the British Society of Dyers and Colourists in cooperation with the American Association of Textile Chemists and Colorists. In volumes 1–3 of the Color Index (1971), colorants are classified according to the dying process and the area of application:

acid colorants
caustic colorants
basic colorants
dispersion colorants
natural colorants
food colorants (irrespective of the certification status)
leather colorants
direct colorants
sulfur colorants
development colorants
reactive colorants
pigments
solvent colorants
optical whiteners
intermediate products for color development
reduction colorants

Within these groups there is a further differentiation according to their color shades yellow, orange, red, violet, blue, green, brown, black and white (white only for pigments). Therefore each colorant has, independently of the trade names, a clear and concise Color Index name. For example, the food colorant Sunset yellow FCF (Gelborange S, E 110) carries the name C.I. Food Yellow 3. In volume 4 of the Color Index (1971) all coloring agents, whose chemical composition is known, are sorted into 30 groups with an ascending Color Index number. Color Index number C.I. 15985 indicates that it is a monoazo colorant. In volume 4, we find the following information after the five-digit Color Index number:

chemical structure
inventor and information on patent literature
synthesis process, solubility and reaction in acid and base

Volume 5 (1982 or 1987) contains a register of the trade names of these colorants. Chemically identical products, that have different trade names, receive the same Color Index number. It is linked clearly to the chemical composition of the colorant, and is mentioned in all legislative literature whenever it comes to approval or disapproval. However, the Color Index number does not mention the heavy metal content nor does the Color Index number make any statement regarding the purity of the colorant (heavy metals and synthetic byproducts). Volume 6 (1976), 7 (1982) and 8 (1987) of the Color Index are supplements to volumes 1–4.

1.6.2. The EU number

Within the European Union there are several guidelines regarding the approval of food additives in the manufacture of food. Declaration of these food additives is done in the list of ingredients by indicating the generic name and, e.g., the EU number, e.g., acidifier E 330 (citric acid), colorant E 131 (Patent blue) etc.

EU numbers E 100 through 180 have been assigned to food colorants, EU numbers E 200 through 290 have been assigned to preserving agents and EU numbers E 300 through 321 have been assigned to antioxidants (see Bundesanzeiger 22b, December 2, 1982, p. 18, list of EU numbers).

2 Food Coloration

2.1. Food coloration—why ?

Part of the basic experience of mankind is, that certain foods must have a certain color in order to be perceived as tasty or even food-grade. Black citrus candies, green caviar, gray salmon or a violet juice drink cannot even be sold as a joke. Products with these colors would certainly be rejected by consumers. This relationship of human color perception and food-grade quality of food is also explained by the surprising fact, that food colorants are discussed in a public discussion in a very insulated way, and therefore even more critically. Product colors are always the first sensual perception and are very visible. Antioxidants, emulsifiers, chemical preservatives and others remain invisible and are perceived by the consumer only when reading the packaging declaration.

In June 1987 there was an international symposium in Basel, Switzerland, on the subject "Food coloring—why?". A uniform reply to this question could not be expected, and this remains the case today. During discussions, two completely opposite points of reference emerged: on the one hand the emphasis of the industry that coloration of certain food products is necessary from a technological point of view; on the other hand a complete rejection of any food coloration by representatives of consumer organizations. Further, the opinion that only food with a coloring effect, e.g., red beet or those colorants which appear naturally in food, should be used (see Table 4).

Table 4 Naturally occurring food colorants

Food	Colorant
Salad, spinach	Chlorophyll
Carrots	Carotene
Tomatoes	Lycopene
Vegetable, citrus fruits	Beta-Apo-8'-carotenal (C30)
Berries	Anthocyan
Red beet	Betanin
Curcuma spice	Curcumin
Milk, eggs	Riboflavin (vitamin B_2)

The necessity to use food additives (and thus food colorants) is a consequence of a historical development which is characterized by terms such as industrialization, urbanization, changes in nutrition and consumers and production of new types of food. Classical preservation methods like smoke, salt and vinegar were superceded by heat sterilization processes, which because of the thermal stress also leads to significant color loss.

As a principle, food coloration is necessary for reasons of

color modification which has a weaker color intensity than the consumer expects due to its ingredients, e.g., beverages or sauces to achieve a uniform product color, which are manufactured from raw material with changing quality and color intensity

to compensate color loss due to manufacturing processes, e.g., fruit preservation

and then finally in products which by nature are colorless or less appealing such as margarine, candies and dessert products.

Whenever colorants are used, legislative standards and norms, especially the aspect of consumer protection, must be respected (see Section 2.4).

2.2. Technical possibilities

The technical possibilities for food coloring are numerous:

food with coloring properties, e.g., red beet, fruit juice concentrates
natural colorants, which do not exist in food, such as Cochineal-carmine
water-soluble, synthetic (artificial) colorants and their insoluble compounds
inorganic pigments, e.g., iron oxide.

As a consequence of a major bias against "chemistry," natural food colorants are utilized. However this method has its limits, especially when there are taste modifications or when food is light-unstable. Even natural food colorants, irrespective whether they exist in food (e.g., Carotenoids) or not or when they are extracted from other material (e.g., Cochineal-carmine), there are limits such as maximum temperature, pH value, ingredients and light influence; therefore, synthetic (artificial) colorants, paint lacquers and pigments must be used. Which type of colorant is suitable can be seen from Table 5.

Table 5   Application areas of food colorants (selection)

Product	Colorant
Beverages	Water-soluble colorants
Pudding powders and instant products	Water-soluble colorants finely milled
Candies	Water-soluble colorants
Fat products	Fat-soluble colorants, colorants on carriers
Capsules	Paint lacquers or pigments

2.3.   Coloring ingredients

In our time, where "nature = good" and "chemistry = bad," it is the objective of food manufacturers to keep the word "colorant" away from labels. Therefore it is normal during the development of a new food product to obtain the desired color effect with natural colorants. These also have to be mentioned in the list of ingredients, but they are not perceived as being "bad," e.g., "red beet" does not have the notion of being artificial. There is no doubt that colorants have to be mentioned. The most widely used coloring foods are: Red beet, tomato juice, paprika extract, spinach, hibiscus, curcuma spice and extract, Vitamin B_2 (Riboflavin), carrot extract, caramel or caramel sugar (not to be confused with the food colorant caramel E 150).

In some countries of the European Union, sandalwood extract is used for coloring meat. This colorant cannot be labeled as food anymore. The following color shades can be obtained by the above mentioned food products: red, orange, yellow, green, blue-red and brown. Variations of these color shades can be achieved by different dosages, as blending these coloring foods is limited for taste reasons.

In Asia, other coloring products are used as they are considered as coloring food, e.g., gardenia, monassus red (fermented rice), carthamus extracts, safflower, and yellow berries.

2.4. Legal basis

2.4.1. European Union

a) Past

It is not the case, as has been pretended often, that in Germany or in the European Union, any food can be colored with any colorant. Legislation has foreseen three major limitations in Germany (and in the EU in the same spirit):

Legislation has determined which food can be colored.

Legislation has prescribed—beginning with the colorant law of 1887 of the German Reich and since then in many ordinances—which colorants and pigments can be used for defined food products, for placing surface stamps on food, for the coloration of sausage casings and cheese wrappings and for painting egg shells, and with which other material they can be blended by the manufacturer.

The deception paragraph (§17 of the Lebensmittel- und Bedarfsgegenständegesetz) has interdicted, that "approved additives are used, even when declaring them, when they are suitable to deceive the consumer about a reduced value or usability of a food product..."

This "deception paragraph" has been amended by the declaration requirement for food additives and food colorants, and here there is distinction between natural and synthetic colorants. In a symposium in 1954 of Western European scientists on the prophylaxis on cancer a joint statement was made "... that the toxicological evaluation of a colorant must be independent of the fact if the colorant is natural or artificial. The natural origin of a colorant is no guarantee for its innocence, because nature has made the strongest poisons from natural products. However natural substances contained in normal food can probably be assumed to be safe."

This experience has been considered in the years thereafter in corresponding EU guidelines and resulting national ordinances. Therefore, a natural colorant such as chlorophyll must be declared as "colorant chlorophyll" or "colorant E 140." From the point of view of declaration, using a natural colorant therefore has no advantage over using a color-stabilizing synthetic food colorant (at a lower dosage).

October 23, 1962 was the first time that the then European Community (EC) established in a guideline:

which food colorants could be used
which purity standards for food colorants must be met

This guideline has been modified and amended several times.

Besides these EU-standardized guidelines on colorants dated 1962, there are several other guidelines (as of December 1994) enacted in some member states, which permit other colorants for defined food products, that however, cannot be used by the food industries of other countries.

For example, Brown HT E 155 is approved (as of December 1994) in the United Kingdom in the manufacture of sweets, but it is not approved in Germany. As these national approvals are only of national importance, they are not a real problem.

However it is of much greater importance, that there is no common EU guideline: which food can be colored with which colorant.

For example, in Germany the colorant E 104 Chinolingelb (quinolin yellow) is approved for the coloration of desserts or pudding powder, on the other hand, Tartrazine E 102 (which is approved in France) is not permitted for this purpose. Furthermore, in France, quinolin yellow E 102 is not approved for the above mentioned food products.

These inconsistencies led to many court cases appearing before the European Court; further it led to inter-country discrimination as well as the necessity to obtain export permits for importation (actual example in Germany for the import of a beverage powder which contains E 110 Gelborange-yellow orange). Food manufacturers also undertook to manufacture the identical food products for export purposes, also within the community, with different colorants.

This was inconsistent with the spirit of a free exchange of products within the European Union, and there was no justification under the aspect of consumer protection (health aspect).

b) The new EU food colorant guideline

After years of preparation and intensive discussion a new EU guideline was approved on June 30, 1994 regarding the utilization of food colorants and published on September 10, 1994 in the Register of the European Community No. L 237.

The necessity of this guideline is based on the fact that there is still a technological necessity for food coloration and that it is necessary to remove all restriction for a free exchange of goods and unfair competition. This means that consumer protection and health protection must be guaranteed.

Special emphasis was laid on the fact, that non-processed food and certain other food products must be free from food additives, and it was considered necessary, that strict guidelines on the use of additives for baby food must be issued. Further, additional analysis was to be made for the protection of the consumer, looking into effects, including synergistic and cumulative ones, of food colorants. Special emphasis was made on colorants where its innocence was not yet proven, e.g., Amaranth E 123.

Within three years after publication of these guidelines, the member states should have implemented systems which monitor the use and application of food colorants. After five years a report should be established on changes in application and consumption.

c) Demarcation of food colorants/ food with color properties

The EU-guideline 94/36/EU defines colorants as:

> .... products that impart color to food or regenerate color in food; included are natural ingredients/components of food as well as their natural raw material, that are normally not used as food, nor are they used as normal food ingredients.

> Preparations from food and other natural raw material, which are obtained by physical and/or chemical extraction, which permit a selective extraction of their nutrient or aromatic components are considered as colorants in the spirit of this guideline. [Article 1 (2)].

Colorants are not:

> Food in dried or concentrated form and flavors which have flavoring, taste or nutritious properties and have a coloring side-effect, such as paprika, curcuma and saffron

> Colorants of surfaces not destined for consumption such as cheese wrappings and sausage casings. [Article 1 (3)].

For example if betanin has been enriched from red beet, then it is considered as food colorant betanin; it is not the coloring food red beet.
    The same applies to anthocyan extracted from grapes. Here another fact is that grape skin is normally not considered food.
    In both cases the obtained products are considered as colorants in the spirit of Article 1 (2).
    How is it then when, e.g., cherry juice is used which has no flavoring, taste or nutritious effect on the finished product? The addition of food or flavoring substance must be done because of their properties (as per Article 1 (3)), the coloring effect is a by-product. This kind of question is not rhetoric, as food coloring is used in such minimal dosages, that they are not perceived from a taste point of view and they do not have any nutritious effect, its sole purpose is coloring.
    This question was raised in a meeting of the Bund für Lebensmittelrecht und Lebensmittelkunde e.V. in Bonn on November 21 and 22, 1994 and has been discussed extensively. It was the uniform opinion, that a food product, in this case cherry juice, when it is added to another food product, cannot be considered a food additive or colorant, as dosage levels are minimal.
    It would be very much appreciated, if the national authorities would clarify this point when this guideline is implemented as national law.

d) Food colorants

Food colorants approved by the EU are shown in Table 6 (annex I of the guideline). These colorants are considered identical with their aluminum varnish.

Table 6 also contains colorants that were not included in all national colorant lists as well as colorants whose use has been restricted significantly in Germany. Not included are some technologically unimportant carotenoids.

Differentiation of caramels in function of their manufacturing process in E 150a–d serves for summary purposes, as well as for application possibilities in some products:

E 150a simple (caustic) caramel, alcohol-stable, for spirits and sweets
E 150b sulfite lye caramel, alcohol-stable, for spirits
E 150c, Ammonia caramel, for beer, soups and sauces
E 150d, Ammonia sulfite lye caramel, acid stable, for alcohol-free carbonated beverages

e) **Food colorants, which were not approved in all member states of the EU**

Colorants mentioned in Table 6 which were not approved in all member countries:

E 128 Red 2G
E 129 Allura red AC
E 133 Brilliant blue FCF
E 154 Brown FK
E 155 Brown HT

f) **Food colorants, which are permitted for limited use in Germany**

Based on the last major modification of the food additive ordinance of June 13, 1990, the utilization of:

E 102 Tartrazine
E 110 Gelborange (Yellow orange)
E 123 Amaranth
E 127 Erythrosin

was restricted in Germany, especially the use of E 102 Tartrazine, which could only be used in liqueurs and spiced brandies.

g) **Food colorants that are not mentioned in the new EC guideline**

The previously approved carotenoids are of no technological importance:

E 161 Xanthophyll
E 161a Flavoxanthin
E 161c Cryptoxanthin
E 161d Rubixanthin
E 161e Violaxanthin
E 161f Rhodaxanthin

Food Coloration

h) Food

The currently valid and applicable German Zusatzstoff-Verordnung (additive ordinance) contains (like other national ordinances) a positive list of food products which can be colored. The inverse conclusion from this list is, that non-mentioned food products are not permitted to be colored (exceptions are the utilization of Riboflavin, Riboflavin-5'-phosphate, alpha, beta, gamma-carotene and caramel). The new EU guideline is structured differently.

In annex II those food products are mentioned which are not permitted to contain added food colorants (Table 7), unless they are mentioned specifically in the other annexes (III, IV and V). In the first place, in annex II, "non-treated/non-processed food products" are mentioned.

They are defined as such food products,

"which have not been processed at all, which could lead to a significant modification of the natural state of the food product. However, they can be cut, peeled, separated, deboned, minced, deskinned, milled, cleaned, decorated, deep-frozen, frozen, chilled or unpacked." [Article 2 (11)]

Annex III (Table 8) lists those food products, where defined colorants with maximum levels can be added.

Annex IV (see Table 9) lists approved colorants for defined purposes.

Annex V is separated into two parts:

Part 1 (see Table 10a) lists those colorants that can be used in food products of Table 2 to the maximum level (*quantum satis*). Further, these colorants can be used in all other food products to the maximum levels except those mentioned in annex II (Table 7) and annex III (Table 8)

Part 2 (see Table 10b) lists those colorants that can be used in those listed food products with certain maximum levels and specific restrictions.

Food colorants are permitted in combined food products under the following conditions:

"in combined food products that are not mentioned in annex II (Table 7), if the colorant is approved in one of the ingredients of the finished product, or if the food product is destined exclusively for the preparation of a blend of food products and that this combined food product is in accordance with the stipulations of this guideline."

i) Maximum levels/quantum satis

Maximum levels referred to in the same annexes are based on the food product ready to be consumed, which has been prepared according to the instructions, as well as the quantity of the base coloring ingredient in the coloring preparation.[Article 2 (6)]

Example:

In confectionery, the colorant E 104 can be used at a maximum level of 300 mg/kg. The standard colorant E 104 has a purity content of 70%, i.e., this colorant can be used at a maximum level of 428.6 mg/kg, as the quantity restriction is based on the coloring ingredient.

The notation *quantum satis* means that there is no maximum level. However, it is expected that the colorant is used "according to good manufacturing practices and only at those levels in order to achieve the objective." [Article 2 (7)]

j) Colorants for declaration, stamping and egg colorants

For the purposes of food coloration and as a colorant for stamping and egg coloring, the so-called C-colors are currently approved, e.g., methyl violet (C 2) as a meat stamp. Colorants like these will not be approved in the future. The new instruction is:

"For the declaration of food-grade ... and for other declaration purposes, which are prescribed for meat products, the following colorants are approved: E 155 Brown HT; E 133 Brilliant blue FCF and Alizarin Red AC." [Article 2 (8)]

"For the color decoration of egg shells or for stamping purposes on egg shells, only those colorants can be used that are listed in annex I (see Table 6)." [Article 2 (9)]

k) Solvents/carriers

There is no new instruction in the EU guidelines regarding the utilization of solvents and carriers for food colorants. The current instructions remain valid (see Table 11).

l) Special notes

Sales interdiction. Colorants E 123 Amaranth, E 127 Erythrosin, E 128 Red 2G, E 154 Brown FK, E 160b Annatto, E 161g Canthaxanthin, E 173 Aluminum and E 180 Litholrubin cannot be sold directly to a consumer, in contrast to the other colorants of annex I [Article 2 (10)].

This instruction serves for the purpose of special consumer protection, as very low ADI values have been established for these colorants (ADI = Acceptable Daily Intake over the entire life, indication in mg/kg body weight). For Amaranth E 123 the ADI value is 0–0.8 mg/kg (SCF 1983), in contrast to E 129 Allura Red with an ADI value of 0–7.0 mg/kg (SCF 1987), which is a very low value.

Editorial notes. In annex I "List of approved food colorants" the Color Index numbers are missing; they can be found in Table 6 and are noted as *:

E 153	Charcoal	C.I. 77268:1
E 160d	Lycopene	C.I. 75125
E 161b	Lutein	C.I. 75136
E 161g	Canthaxanthin	C.I. 40850
E 173	Aluminum	C.I. 77000
E 174	Silver	C.I. 77820
E 175	Gold	C.I. 77480
E 180	Litholrubin	C.I. 15850:1

Riboflavin (E 101) and Riboflavin-5'-phosphate (previously E 101a) are mentioned under the joint EU number E 101.

m) Transition period

The member states have been asked to establish and publish the necessary instructions until December 1995 to implement the EU guideline 94/36 EU as national law. As of December 31, 1995, trading and utilization of products complying with these guidelines **is permitted**.

Trading and utilization of products which do **not** comply with these guidelines, is not permitted after June 30, 1996. Products distributed and labeled accordingly before this date can be marketed until stocks have been depleted [Article 9 (1)].

n) Summary

Despite some inconsistencies and the sometimes more complicated instructions (compared to the current legislation, e.g., demarcation food colorant to food with coloring properties) and highly varying maximum levels in similar food products, this EU guideline represents a significant progress for the European food industry, as significant trading restrictions have been removed.

Table 6 List of approved colorants

EU number	Common name	C.I. number or description
E 100	Curcumin	75300
E 101	1) Riboflavin	
	2) Riboflavin-5'-phosphate	
E 102	Tartrazine	19140
E 104	Chinolin yellow	47005
E 110	Sunset yellow FCF	15985
	Yellow orange S	
E 120	Cochineal, Carmine acid, Carmine	75470
E 122	Azorubin, Carmoisine	14720
E 123	Amaranth	16185
E 124	Ponceau 4R, Cochineal red A	16255
E 127	Erythrosin	45430
E 128	Red 2G	18050
E 129	Allura red AC	16035
E 131	Patent blue V	42051
E 132	Indigotine, Indigo carmine	73015
E 133	Brilliant blue FCF	42090
E 140	Chlorophyll	75810
	and chlorophyllin	75815
	1) Chlorophyll	
	2) Chlorophyllin	
E 141	Cuprous complex of chlorophyll and chlorophyllin	75815
	1) Chlorophyll	
	2) Chlorophyllin	

(continued)

Table 6 continued

EU number	Common name	C.I. number or description
E 142	Green S	44090
E 150a	Standard caramel	
E 150b	Sulfite lye caramel	
E 150c	Ammonia caramel	
E 150d	Ammonia sulfite caramel	
E 151	Brilliant black BN, Black PN	28440
E 153	Charcoal	77268:1*
E 154	Brown FK	
E 155	Brown HT	20285
E 160a	Carotene	
	1) blend of carotene	75130
	2) beta-carotene	40800
E 160b	Annatto, Bixin, Norbixin	75120
E 160c	Paprika extract Capsanthin, Capsorubin	
E 160d	Lycopene	75125*
E 160e	Beta-apo-8'-carotenal (C 30)	40820
E 160f	Beta-apo-8'-carotenal (C 30) ethyl ester	40825
E 161b	Lutein	75136*
E161gE 162	Canthaxanthin Red beet, betanin	40850*
E 163	Anthocyan	Manufactured by physical methods from fruits and vegetable
E 170	Calcium carbonate	77200
E 171	Titanium dioxide	77891
E 172	Iron oxide and iron hydroxide	77491 77492 77499
E 173	Aluminum	77000*
E 174	Silver	77820*
E 175	Gold	77480*
E 180	Litholrubin RK	15850:1*

Table 7 Foods that are not permitted to contain colorant additives unless they are specifically mentioned in annex III, IV or V*

1. Untreated food
2. Bottled or filled water
3. Milk, partially decreamed or skimmed, pasteurized or sterilized (including sterilization by ultra-high temperature process) (non-flavored)

Table 7 continued

4. Chocolate-flavored milk
5. Fermented milk (non-flavored)
6. Preserved milk according to guideline 76/118/EEC (non-flavored)
7. Buttermilk (non-flavored)
8. Cream and cream powder (non-flavored)
9. Fats and oils of animal or vegetable origin
10. Egg and egg products in the sense of Article 2,2 of the guideline 89/437/EEC
11. Flour and other flour products as well as starch products
12. Bread and similar products
13. Pasta and gnocchi
14. Sugar, including all other mono- and disaccharides
15. Tomato paste and tomato preserves
16. Sauces on tomato basis
17. Fruit juice and fruit nectar according to guideline 75/726/EEC as well as vegetable juices
18. Fruit, vegetable (including potatoes) and mushrooms, preserved or dried; fruit, vegetable (including potatoes) and mushrooms, processed
19. Jam, jelly and chestnut cream according to guideline 79/693/EEC, crème de pruneaux
20. Fish, shell fish and crustacean, meat, poultry, and fowl as well as their preparations, excluding prepared meals which contain these ingredients
21. Cocoa and chocolate ingredients in chocolate products according to guideline 73/241/EEC
22. Roasted coffee; tea; chicory; tea and chicory products; tea, vegetable and fruit infusions as well as blends and ready-to-drink blends of these products.
23. Salt, salt substitutes, spices and spice blends
24. Wine and other products according to the definition in ordinance EEC No. 822/87
25. Spirit, spirit distillate, fruit distillate, Ouzo, Grappa, Tsikoudia from Crete, Tsipouro from Macedonia, Tsipouro from Thessalia, Tsipouro from Tyrnavos, Eau-de-vie de marc, Marque nationale luxembourgeoise, Eau-de-vie de seigle, Marque nationale luxembourgeoise and London Gin according to the definitions in ordinance EEC No. 1576/89
26. Sambuco, Maraschino according to the definition in ordinance EEC No. 1180/91
27. Sangria, Clarea and Zurra according to the definition in ordinance EEC No. 1601/91
28. Vinegar
29. Baby and toddler food according to the definition in guideline 89/398/EEC as well as for sick babies and small children
30. Honey
31. Malt and malt-ripened products
32. Ripening and non-ripening cheese (non-flavored)
33. Butter from sheep and goat milk

* Terms used in annex II do not influence or restrict the principle of transmission in those cases where products contain ingredients with colorants which per se are approved.

Table 8 Food which can contain only defined colorants

Food		Permitted colorant	Maximum level
Malt bread	E 150a	Standard caramel	Quantum satis
	E 150b	Sulfite lye caramel	
	E 150c	Ammonia caramel	
	E 150d	Ammonia sulfite caramel	
Beer, Cider	E 150a	Standard caramel	Quantum satis
	E 150b	Sulfite lye caramel	
	E 150c	Ammonia caramel	
	E 150d	Ammonia sulfite caramel	
Butter (including butter with a reduced fat content and butter fat)	E 160a	Carotene	Quantum satis
Margarine, margarine with reduced fat content, other fat emulsions and moisture-free fats	E 100	Curcumin	Quantum satis
	E 160a	Carotene	Quantum satis
	E 160b	Annatto, Bixin, Norbixin	10 mg/kg
Sage-Derby cheese	E 140	Chlorophyll, chlorophyllin	Quantum satis
	E 141	Cuprous complex of chlorophyll and chlorophyllin	
Ripening orange-colored, yellow and pearl-white cheese; non-flavored processed cheese	E 160a	Carotene	Quantum satis
	E 160c	Paprika extract	
	E 160b	Annatto, Bixin, Norbixin	15 mg/kg
Red Leicester cheese	E 160b	Annatto, Bixin, Norbixin	50 mg/kg
Mimolette cheese	E 160b	Annatto, Bixin, Norbixin	35 mg/kg
Morbier cheese	E 153	Charcoal	Quantum satis
Red-veined cheese	E 120	Cochineal, Carmine acid, Carmine	125 mg/kg
	E 163	Anthocyan	Quantum satis
Vinegar	E 150a	Standard caramel	Quantum satis
	E 150b	Sulfite lye caramel	
	E 150c	Ammonia caramel	
	E 150d	Ammonia sulfite caramel	
Whisky, whiskey, cereal-based spirits (with the exclusion of Korn or Kornbrand or eau-de-vie de seigle, Marque luxembourgeoise), Rum, Brandy, Trester, Trester-brand (except Tsikoudia, Tsipouro and eau-de-vie de marc, Marque luxembour-	E 150a	Standard caramel	Quantum satis
	E 150b	Sulfite lye caramel	
	E 150c	Ammonia caramel	
	E 150d	Ammonia sulfite caramel	

Table 8 continued

Food	Permitted colorant		Maximum level
geoise), Grappa invecchiata and Bagaceira velha according to ordinance EEC No. 1576/89			
Flavored wine-like produts (excluding Bitter soda) and flavored wine according to ordinance EEC No. 1601/91	E 150a E 150b E 150c E 150d	Standard caramel Sulfite lye caramel Ammonia caramel Ammonia sulfite caramel	Quantum satis
Americano	E 150a E 150b E 150c E 150d E 163 E 100 E 101 E 102 E 104 E 120 E 122 E 123 E 124	Standard caramel Sulfite lye caramel Ammonia caramel Ammonia sulfite caramel Anthocyan Curcumin 1) Riboflavin 2) Riboflavin-5'-phosphate Tartrazine Chinolin yellow Cochineal, Carmine acid, Carmine Azorubin, Carmoisine Amaranth Ponceau 4R	Quantum satis 100 mg/l (individual or as a blend)
Bitter Soda and Bitter Vino according to ordinance EEC No. 1601/91	E 150a E 150b E 150c E 150d E 100 E 101 E 102 E 104 E 110 E 120 E 122 E 123 E 124 E 129	Standard caramel Sulfite lye caramel Ammonia caramel Ammonia sulfite caramel Curcumin 3) Riboflavin 4) Riboflavin-5'-phosphate Tartrazine Chinolin yellow Sunset yellow FCF Cochineal, Carmine acid, Carmine Azorubin, Carmoisine Amaranth Ponceau 4R Allura Red AC	Quantum satis 100 mg/l (individual or as a blend)
Liquor vines and quality liquor from defined regions	E 150a E 150b E 150c E 150d	Standard caramel Sulfite lye caramel Ammonia caramel Ammonia sulfite caramel	Quantum satis

(continued)

Table 8 continued

Food		Permitted colorant	Maximum level
Vegetable soaked in vinegar, brine or oil (excluding olives)	E 101	1) Riboflavin	Quantum satis
	E 140	2) Riboflavin-5'-phosphate	
	E 141	Chlorophyll and chlorphyllin Cuprous complex of chlorophyll and chlorophyllin	
	E 150a	Standard caramel	
	E 150b	Sulfite lye caramel	
	E 150c	Ammonia caramel	
	E 150d	Ammonia sulfite caramel	
Vegetable soaked in vinegar, brine or oil (excluding olives)	E 160a	Carotene 1) carotene blends 2) beta-carotene	Quantum satis
	E 162	Red beet, betanin	
	E 163	Anthocyan ammonia caramel	
Extruded, puffed breakfast cereals flavored with/without fruit	E 150c	Carotene	Quantum satis
	E 160a	Annatto, Bixin, Norbixin	25 mg/kg
	E 160b	Paprika extract, Capsanthin,	Quantum satis
	E 160c	Capsorubin	
Breakfast cereals flavored with fruit	E 120	Cochineal, Carmine acid, Carmine	200 mg/kg (individual or as a total sum)
	E 162	Beet red, betanin	
	E 163	Anthocyan	
Jams, jellies and marmalades according to guideline 79/693/EEC and similar fruit preparations including low-calorie products	E 100	Curcumin	Quantum satis
	E 140	Chlorophyll and chlorophyllin	
	E 141	Cuprous complex of chlorophyll and chlorophyllin	
	E 150a	Standard caramel	
	E 150b	Sulfite lye caramel	
	E 150c	Ammonia caramel	
	E 150d	Ammonia sulfite caramel	
	E 160a	Carotene 1) blend of carotene 2) beta-carotene	
	E 160c	Paprika extract, Capsanthin, Capsorubin	
	E 162	Beet red, betanin	
	E 163	Anthocyan	
Jams, jellies and marmalades according to guideline 79/693/EEC and similar fruit preparations including low-calorie products	E 104	Chinolin yellow	100 mg/kg (individual or as a total sum)
	E 110	Sunset yellow	
	E 120	Cochineal, Carmine acid, Carmine	
	E 124	Ponceau 4R, Cochineal	
	E 142	Green S	
	E 160d	Lycopene	
	E 161b	Lutein	

Food Coloration

Table 8   continued

Food	Permitted colorant		Maximum level
Sausage, paté and paté dishes	E 100	Curcumin	20 mg/kg
	E 120	Cochineal, Carmine acid, Carmine	100 mg/kg
	E 150a	Standard caramel	Quantum satis
	E 150b	Sulfite lye caramel	
	E 150c	Ammonia caramel	
	E 150d	Ammonia sulfite caramel	
	E 160a	Carotene	20 mg/kg
	E 160c	Paprika extract, Capsanthin, Capsorubin	10 mg/kg
	E 162	Beet red, betanin	Quantum satis
Luncheon meat	E 129	Allura Red AC	25 mg/kg
Breakfast sausage with a cereal content of minimum 6%	E 129	Allura Red AC	25 mg/kg
Minced meat with a vegetable and/or cereal content of minimum 4%	E 120	Cochineal, Carmine acid, Carmine	100 mg/kg
	E 150a	Standard caramel	Quantum satis
	E 150b	Sulfite lye caramel	
	E 150c	Ammonia caramel	
	E 150d	Ammonia sulfite caramel	
Chorizo sausage	E 120	Cochineal, Carmine acid, Carmine	200 mg/kg
Salchichon	E 124	Ponceau 4R, Cochineal red A	250 mg/kg
Sobrasada	E 110	Sunset yellow FCF	135 mg/kg
	E 124	Ponceau 4R, Cochineal red A	200 mg/kg
Pasturmas (edible coating)	E 100	Curcumin	Quantum satis
	E 101	1) Riboflavin 2) Riboflavin-5'-phosphate	
	E 120	Cochineal, Carmine acid, Carmine	
Potato flakes	E 100	Curcumin	Quantum satis
Processed mushy and Garden Peas	E 102	Tartrazine	100 mg/kg
	E 133	Brilliant blue	20 mg/kg
	E 142	Green S	10 mg/kg

Table 9   Colorants used only for defined purposes

Colorant	Name	Purpose	Maximum level
E 123	Amaranth	Apéritif, spirits including products with an alcohol content of less than 15%	30 mg/l
		Fish rye	30 mg/kg
E 127	Erythrosin	Cocktail cherries and candied cherries, Bigarreaux cherries	200 mg/kg
		Kaiser cherries in syrup/in fruit cocktails	150 mg/kg

(continued)

Table 9 continued

Colorant	Name	Purpose	Maximum level
E 128	Red 2G	Breakfast sausage with a cereal content of minimum 6%	20 mg/kg
		Minced meat with a vegetable and/or cereal content of minimum 4%	
E 154	Brown FK	Kippers	20 mg/kg
E 161g	Canthaxanthin	Saucisses de Strassbourg	15 mg/kg
E 173	Aluminum	Coatings and sweets for decoration of cakes and bakery products	Quantum satis
E 174	Silver	Coatings of sweets	Quantum satis
		Decorations of pralines	
		Liquors	
E 175	Gold	Coatings of sweets	Quantum satis
		Decorations of pralines	
		Liquors	
E 180	Lithorubin BK	For cheese rind, destined for consumption	Quantum satis
E 160b	Annatto, Bixin, Norbixin	Margarine, fat-reduced margarine and other fat emulsions and moisture-free fats	10 mg/kg
		Decorations and coatings	20 mg/kg
		Bakery products	10 mg/kg
		Ice cream	20 mg/kg
E 160b	Annatto, Bixin, Norbixin	Liquors including all beverages with added alcohol with less than 15% alcohol content	10 mg/kg
		Flavored processed cheese	15 mg/kg
		Ripening orange-colored, yellow and pearl-white cheese	15 mg/kg
		Non-flavored processed cheese	
		Dessert products	10 mg/kg
		Snacks: salted and dried snack products on the basis of potatoes, cereals or starch	
		- extruded and expanded salted snack products	20 mg/kg
		- other salted snack products as well as salted snack products based on nuts and hazelnuts	10 mg/kg
		Smoked fish	10 mg/kg
		Edible cheese rind and sausage casings	20 mg/kg
		Red Leicester cheese	50 mg/kg
		Mimolette cheese	35 mg/kg
		Extruded, puffed and/or fruit-flavored breakfast cereal products	25 mg/kg

Food Coloration

Table 10a Approved colorants in food which are not listed in annex II and III (Tables 7 and 8) part 1

E 101	1) Riboflavin
	2) Riboflavin-5'-phosphate
E 140	Chlorophyll and chlorophyllin
E 141	Cuprous complex of chlorophyll and chlorophyllin
E 150a	Standard caramel
E 150b	Sulfite lye caramel
E 150c	Ammonia caramel
E 150d	Ammonia sulfite caramel
E 153	Charcoal
E 160a	Carotene
E 160c	Paprika extract, Capsanthin, Capsorubin
E 162	Beet red, betanin
E 163	Anthocyan
E 170	Calcium carbonate
E 171	Titanium dioxide
E 172	Iron oxide and iron hydroxide

Table 10 b Approved colorants in food which are not listed in annex II and III (Tables 7 and 8) part 2 (restricted use)

E 100	Curcumin
E 102	Tartrazine
E 104	Quinolin yellow
E 110	Sunset yellow FCF, Yellow orange S
E 120	Cochineal, Carmine acid, Carmine
E 122	Azorubin, Carmoisine
E 124	Ponceau 4R, Cochineal red A
E 129	Allura red AC
E 131	Patent blue V
E 132	Indigotin, Indigo carmine
E 133	Brilliant blue FCF
E 142	Green S
E 151	Brilliant black BN, Black PN
E 155	Brown HT
E 160d	Lycopene
E 160e	Beta-apo-8'-carotenal (C 30)
E 160f	Beta-apo-8'-carotene acid (C 30) ethyl ester
E 161b	Lutein

(continued)

Table 10b continued

Food	Maximum level
Non-alcoholic flavored beverages	100 mg/l
Candied fruit and vegetable, Mostardia di frutta	200 mg/kg
Red fruit preserves	200 mg/kg
Sweets	300 mg/kg
Decorations and coatings	500 mg/kg
Pastry (breakfast pastry, cookies, cakes and waffles)	200 mg/kg
Ice cream	150 mg/kg
Flavored processed cheese	100 mg/kg
Dessert products including milk-based products	150 mg/kg
Sauces, spices (e.g., curry powder, Tandoori), pickles, appetizers, chutney and picallili	500 mg/kg
Mustard	300 mg/kg
Patés from fish and crustacean	100 mg/kg
Precooked crustacean	250 mg/kg
Salmon imitate	500 mg/kg
Surimi	500 mg/kg
Fish rye	300 mg/kg
Smoked fish	100 mg/kg
Snacks: salted and dried snacks on the basis of potatoes, cereals or starch:	
-extruded and expanded salted snack products	200 mg/kg
-other salted snack products as well as salted snack products on the basis of nuts and hazelnuts	100 mg/kg
Edible cheese rind and sausage casings	Quantum satis
Complete preparations which can be used as meals or daily rations for an overweight person	50 mg/kg
Complete preparations or nutritional supplements which are consumed under medical control	50 mg/kg
Nutritional supplements/dietetic supplements in liquid form	100 mg/kg
Nutritional supplements/dietetic supplements in solid form	300 mg/kg
Soups	50 mg/kg
Meat and fish substitutes on the basis of vegetable protein	100 mg/kg
Spirits (including products with an alcohol content of less than 15% with the exception of spirits mentioned in annex II and III)	200 mg/kg
Flavored wine, flavored wine-containing beverages and flavored wine-containing cocktails according to ordinance EEC No. 1601/91 with the exception of those products mentioned in annex II and III	200 mg/kg
Fruit wines (non-foamy or foamy) Apple and pear cider (except Cider bouchée) Flavored fruit wines, apple and pear cider	200 mg/kg

Table 11 Solvents and carriers for colorants*

Product	EEC number	Utilization
Alginate		
Ammonium alginate	E 403	
Potassium alginate	E 402	
Sodium alginate	E 401	
Bees wax	—	
Glycerin	E 422	For blending with products of Table 6
Sodium carbonate	—	
Sodium hydrogen carbonate	—	
Paraffin	—	For cheese coatings
Magnesium stearate	—	As a fluidizing agent during filling of colorant powders used for coloring or painting of egg shells
Ethyl cellulose	—	For lacquering of painted or colored egg shells as well as stamping color for eggs and cheese coatings
Benzyl alcohol	—	
Kolophonium	—	
Kopal	—	
Lactic acid ethyl ester	—	
Shellac	—	
6-Palmitoyl-L-ascorbic acid	E 304	For blending of products such as E 160 (Carotenoids) and E 161 (Xanthophyll)
Carrageenan	E 414	
Gum arabic	E 414	

* Further, it is admissible to blend colorants with sugar, lactose starch and others.

2.4.2. Countries outside the European Union

In the past century, utilization of synthetically manufactured dyes were used for the coloration of food, only those products were used that were available on a local basis. During a transitional period, when food coloring was put on a legally defined basis, various countries published their own individual lists of permitted food colorants. Harmonizing these lists has now been achieved in the EU, but not in countries outside the EU. The same applies for the coloration of cosmetics and drugs. Significant differences to the guidelines of the EU can be found e.g., in the U.S., Japan and Norway. This creates a great problem for exporters of colored foods, drugs and cosmetics, as there are not only national differences for dyes, but also for, e.g., food additives. Under certain circumstances it might become necessary to use different colorants for different countries as they are subject to different limitations. For further details national laws and guidelines must be consulted.

2.4.3. United States

The Code of Federal Regulations, title 21, parts 1 to 99 (CFR 21) contains the approved colorants for use in food, drugs and cosmetics. Their use is controlled by the Food and

Drug Administration (FDA), an organization of the U.S. Department of Health, Education and Welfare, according to the Federal Food, Drug and Cosmetic Act dd. 25.6.1938. The CFR can be ordered from:

U.S. Government Printing Office, Superintendent of Documents,
Mail Stop: SSOP, Washington, DC 20402-9328.

For each colorant the CFR contains:

- specifications (minimum colorant content, purity requirement)
- restrictions for application
- labeling requirements and obligatory warning information as well as
- if the colorant needs an FDA approval certificate (see below) or if it can be used without certification

In the EU, the basic differences regarding colorants are:

- For all colorants, purity requirements are different for the time being (e.g., maximum lead content is 10 ppm in the U.S., and 20 ppm in the EU) and the approved colorants must have a higher purity than in the EU.
- Colorants are classified into two groups (see Table 12) such as:
  - Colorants requiring an FDA certificate for further processing (all artificial colorants) and
  - Colorants which can be used without a certificate

Manufacturers are controlled on compliance with the good manufacturing practice (GMP) guidelines during production.

The certificate is obtained upon request and subsequent analysis in a laboratory of the FDA, referring to the relevant batch. Each batch must be controlled. The certificate is granted in case of compliance, and contains a control number, a so-called lot number. It consists of two characters and 4 numbers, e.g., AH0628. Since all colored food, drugs and cosmetics, which are imported into the U.S., must comply with CFR 21, U.S. authorities require the lot number of the colorant used.

**Table 12 Colorants for food, drugs and/or cosmetics in the U.S.
(source: Code of Federal Regulations 21 / CFR 21, April 1, 1993)**

A. Colorants (utilization requires FDA certificate)

Designation	See data sheet (Chap. 9) (§ CFR 21)	Food	Drugs	Cosmetics
FD&C Blue No.1	C.I.42090	§74.101	§74.1101	§74.2101
FD&C Blue No.2	C.I.73015	§74.102	§74.1102	–
FD&C Green No.3	C.I.42053	§74.203	§74.1203	§74.2203

Food Coloration

Table 12 continued

Designation	See data sheet (Chap. 9) (§ CFR 21)	Food	Drugs	Cosmetics
FD&C Red No.3	C.I.45430	§74.303	§74.1303	–
FD&C Red No.4	C.I.14700	–	§74.1304	§74.2304
FD&C Red No.40	C.I.16035	§74.340	§74.1340	§74.2340
FD&C Yellow No.5	C.I.19140	§74.705	§74.1705	§74.2705
FD&C Yellow No.6	C.I.15985	§74.706	§74.1706	§74.2706
D&C Blue No.4	C.I.42090	–	§74.1104	§74.2104
D&C Blue No.9	C.I.69825	–	§74.1109	–
D&C Brown No.1	C.I.20170	–	–	§74.2151
D&C Green No.5	C.I.61570	–	§74.1205	§74.2205
D&C Green No.6	C.I.61565	–	§74.1206	§74.2206
D&C Green No. 8	C.I.59040	–	§74.1208	§74.2208
D&C Orange No.4	C.I.15510	–	§74.1254	§74.2254
D&C Orange No.5	C.I.45370:1	–	§74.1255	§74.2255
D&C Orange No.10	C.I.45425:1	–	§74.1260	§74.2260
D&C Orange No.11	C.I.45425	–	§74.1261	§74.2261
D&C Red No.6	C.I.15850	–	§74.1306	§74.2306
D&C Red No.7	C.I.15850:1	–	§74.1307	§74.2307
D&C Red No.17	C.I.26100	–	§74.1317	§74.2317
D&C Red No.21	C.I.45380:2	–	§74.1321	§74.2321
D&C Red No.22	C.I.45380	–	§74.1322	§74.2322
D&C Red No.27	C.I.45410:1	–	§74.1327	§74.2327
D&C Red No.28	C.I.45410	–	§74.1328	§74.2328
D&C Red No.30	C.I.73360	–	§74.1330	§74.2330
D&C Red No.31	C.I.15800:1	–	§74.1331	§74.2331
D&C Red No.33	C.I.17200	–	§74.1333	§74.2333
D&C Red No.34	C.I.15880:1	–	§74.1334	§74.2334
D&C Red No.36	C.I.12085	–	§74.1336	§74.2336
D&C Red No.39	C.I.13058	–	§74.1339	–
D&C Violet No.2	C.I.60725	–	§74.1602	§74.2602
Ext.D&C Violet No.2	C.I.60730	–	–	§74.2602a
D&C Yellow No.7	C.I.45350:1	–	§74.1707	§74.2707
Ext.D&C Yellow No.7	C.I.10316	–	§74.1707a	§74.2707a
D&C Yellow No.8	C.I.45350	–	§74.1708	§74.2708
D&C Yellow No. 10	C.I.47005	–	§74.1710	§74.2710
D&C Yellow No.11	C.I.47000	–	§74.1711	§74.2711
Orange B	C.I.19235	§74.250	–	–
Citrus Red No.2	C.I.12156	§74.302	–	–

(continued)

Table 12 continued

B. Colorants (for which no FDA certificate is required)

Designation	See data sheet (Chap. 9) (§ CFR 21)	Food	Drugs	Cosmetics
Alumina (dried aluminum hydroxide)	C.I.77002	–	§73.1010	–
Aluminum powder	C.I.77000	–	§73.1645	§73.2645
Annatto	C.I.75120	–	–	§73.2030
Annatto extract	C.I.75120	§73.30	§73.1030	–
ß-Apo-8'-carotenal	C.I.40820	§73.90		
Bismuth citrate	Bismut citrate	–	–	§73.2110
Bismuth oxichloride	Bismut oxichloride	–	§73.1162	§73.2162
Bronze powder	C.I.77400	–	§73.1646	§73.2646
Calcium carbonate	C.I.77220	–	§73.1070	–
Canthaxanthin	C.I.40850	§73.75	§73.1075	–
Caramel	Caramel	§73.85	§73.1085	§73.2085
Carmine	C.I.75470	–	–	§73.2087
ß-Carotene	C.I.75130	§73.95	§73.1095	§73.2095
Carrot oil	#	§73.300	–	–
Chlorophyllin copper complex, see Potassium				
Chromium-cobalt-aluminum oxide	#	–	§73.1015	–
Chromium hydroxide green	C.I.77289	–	§73.1326	§73.2326
Chromium oxide greens	C.I.77288	–	§73.1327	§73.2327
Cochineal extract, carmine	C.I.75470	§73.100	§73.1100	–
Copper powder	C.I.77400	–	§73.1647	§73.2647
Corn endosperm oil	#	§73.315	–	–
Dehydrated beets, beet powder	Beet red	§73.40	–	–
Dihydroxyacetone	Dihydroxy acetone	–	§73.1150	§73.2150
Disodium EDTA-copper	Disodium...	–	–	§73.2120
Dried algae meal	#	§73.275	–	–
Ferric ammonium citrate	#	–	§73.1025	–
Ferric ammonium ferrocyanide	C.I.77520	–	§73.1298	§73.2298
Ferric ferrocyanide	C.I.77510	–	§73.1299	§73.2299

Food Coloration

Table 12 continued

Designation	See data sheet (Chap. 9) (§ CFR 21)	Food	Drugs	Cosmetics
Ferrous gluconate	Ferrous gluconate	§73.160	–	–
Fruit juice	#	§73.250	–	–
Grape color extract	#	§73.169	–	–
Grape skin extract, (enocianina)	Anthocyan	§73.170	–	–
Guaiazulene	Guaiazulen	–	–	§73.2180
Guanine	C.I.75170	–	§73.1329	§73.2329
Henna	C.I.75480	–	–	§73.2190
Lead acetate	#	–	–	§73.2396
Logwood extract	#	–	§73.1410	–
Manganese violet	C.I.77742	–	–	§73.2775
Mica	C.I.77019	–	§73.1496	§73.2496
Paprika	#	§73.340	–	–
Paprika oleoresin	#	§73.345	–	–
Potassium sodium copper chlorophyllin	C.I.75810	–	§73.1125	§73.2125
Pyrogallol	#	–	§73.1375	–
Pyrophyllite	Pyrophyllite	–	§73.1400	§73.2400
Riboflavin	Lactofavin	§73.450	–	–
Saffron	#	§73.500	–	–
Synthetic iron oxide	C.I.77491/2/9	§73.200	§73.1200	§73.2250
Talc	C.I.77718	–	§73.1550	–
Toasted partially defatted cooked cottonseed flour	#	§73.140	–	–
Tagetes (Aztec marigold) extract	#	§73.295	–	–
Titanium dioxide	C.I.77891	§73.575	§73.1575	§73.2575
Turmeric	C.I.75300	§73.600	–	–
Turmeric oleoresin	#	§73.615	–	–
Ultramarine blue	C.I.77007	§73.50		
Ultramarine	C.I.77007	–	–	§73.2725
Vegetable juice	#	§73.260		
Zinc oxide	C.I.77947	–	§73.1991	§73.2991

In the EU these colorants are considered as coloring food or they are used exclusively in the U.S. Therefore chapter 9 does not contain data sheets for these compounds. More information can be obtained from the relevant section of CFR 21 (Code of Federal Regulations 21)

3 Drug Coloration

3.1. The importance of drug coloration

Drugs are normally used when a patient needs them for his recovery. The purpose of coloration is not to entice the consumer into consumption. The sole purpose of coloring drugs is a safety aspect, an absolute pharmaceutical necessity. It is a regrettable fact that numerous fatal accidents happen when children have access to drugs, stored in a careless way, and perceive them to be candies and sweets.

The manufacturer of drugs must guarantee by far-ranging safety activities, that the product cannot be confused with another one either during manufacturing and packaging as well as with the patient at a later stage. This is especially true in hospitals, where numerous prescriptions are handed out, that the possibility for a re-identification is given. For a clear identification of drugs there are different possibilities:

- Size and shape can vary within limits.
- Tablets or capsules can be packed uncolored into labeled push-through packaging material. For clinics and hospitals this type of packaging is less suitable. Vision-restricted patients can get into difficulties with the sometimes foreign-appearing names. It is another bad habit of patients to carry several drugs in a small pill box, as this does not permit identification later on.
- The drug can carry printed information. Here colors must be used, although this is of no help to vision-restricted patients.

The coloration of a solid drug is undoubtedly the best method to exclude a confusion, and contribute to the safety of drugs. This is the reason, why a list of pharmaceuticals has been established (see literature sources, Section 10.3), where solid drugs are listed systematically in the form of their shape (dragee, tablet, soft capsule, hard capsule), outer appearance (round, oval, oblong, square), color, multicolored, classification and dimension.

3.2. Legal requirements

3.2.1. European Union/Federal Republic of Germany

Until a few years ago, the coloration of drugs was not standardized, neither in Germany nor in other countries. It was the task of the Bundesgesundheitsamt (Federal Health Authority) to check new drugs during the certification phase, which colorant could be used without any side-effects. It was common practice to use food colorants.

In the EU guidelines dated December 12, 1977 (78/25/EEC) on the harmonization of legal instructions for the member states on components which can be added to drugs for the purpose of coloration, it is stated: "It is the experience, that there should be no health reason to approve colorants in drugs, when they are used in food products."

For drugs, that are destined only for external application (e.g., for medical baths), there was a deviation from this standard, and cosmetic colorants were used. Since August

25, 1982, the utilization of colorants, pigments and paint lacquers has been legislated in the Arzneimittelfarbstoff-Verordnung (AMFarbV). It is stated specifically in §1, section 1:

"For the manufacture of drugs according to §2, section 1 of the Arzneimittelgesetz, which are destined for commercialization in a member state of the European Community, only those ingredients and materials can be used which are listed for the purpose of coloring..."

This list of approved colorants as per the Arzneimittelfarbstoff-Verordnung is identical to the list of approved food colorants; however, it does not contain (as per December 1994) the colorants E 128, E 133, E 154 and E 155,

This means a very early harmonization of the regulations, which has not been achieved for food colorants within the EU countries.[1]

The Arzneimittelfarbstoff-Verordnung does not distinguish between drugs for external or internal application. It also does not apply to dental material. This observation leads to an interesting fact, that a medical bath can contain food colorants, a cosmetic foam bath can contain only cosmetic colorants of application group 3[2] This will not influence the consumer/patient; however, this will influence the development of drugs for external applications for reasons of possible light stability problems.

According to the Arzneimittel-Warnhinweisverordnung of the Federal Republic of Germany, dated December 21, 1984, §1, section 1, 2 and §2, section 3, drugs which contain the food colorant Tartrazine[3] E 102: "... can be commercialized only when a warning note 'contains Tartrazine, read through the enclosed information' has been attached to it."

This instruction is applied also for other drugs that are destined for external application. Therefore Tartrazine is rarely used in the pharmaceutical industry. It can be replaced, albeit at very high costs, by Chinolin yellow E 104 and Yellow orange E 110.

3.2.2. Countries outside the European Union

Each individual country has its own legislation for the coloration of food as well as drugs. However, it cannot be assumed that the nationally approved food colorants are approved for pharmaceutical products. For the coloration of drugs in the U.S. we refer to Section 2.4.3.

---

[1] The new French Pharmacopeia uses special specifications for food colorants.
[2] See also (Table 14 in Chapter 4).
[3] Tartrazine is considered to cause allergies in certain persons in connection with certain drugs, functional ingredients or certain preservatives when taken orally (see also "Tartrazine, die gelbe Gefahr" Arzneimitteltelegramm 8/84 and Whitehill, I.: Human idiosyncratic responses to food colors, FFIPP, March 1980)

4 The Coloration of Cosmetic Products

4.1. The importance of color in cosmetic products

Color plays a dominant role in decorative cosmetics. Lipstick, eye shade, mascara powder, shading cream and makeup are of no value without color. Other products are offered to the consumer whose purpose is not solely to cover or to color. In order to market a product successfully, the color must be harmonized with the product claims, as has been shown in the example of the mouth wash water (Table 1). Soap with a sandalwood scent should not be colored blue. Color plays a major role in uncolored bathing products which are totally unattractive. The purchasing decision is the result of color and packaging of a product. Some years ago, a shampoo with a bright green fluorescing color and an apple flavor was a major success in the market. It can be safely assumed that apart from an effective TV commercial, the brilliant green color of the product was one, if not the major reason for this success.

4.2. Technological possibilities

For the coloration of cosmetic products there are water-soluble colorants as well as insoluble lacquers available in the market plus a number of fat-soluble colorants and finally pigments and their water-dispersible derivatives. The list of EU-approved cosmetic colorants includes, logically, all food colorants. Which colorant group can be used most profitably for the coloration of cosmetic products can be seen from Table 13.

Table 13 Applications of cosmetic colorants

Cosmetic product	Colorant
Shampoo, foam bath, shower gel	Water-soluble colorants
Soap	Water-soluble colorants, pigments, water-dispersible pigments
Eye makeup	Pigments, paint lacquers
Shading cream	Pigments (in the majority iron oxide and titanium dioxide)
Lipstick	Organic pigments, eosin, paint lacquers

4.3. Legal requirements

4.3.1. European Union/Federal Republic of Germany

Although utilization of cosmetic colorants is as old as mankind, a legislative basis has been established only very recently. The "Farbengesetz" (law on colorants) was published in Germany on July 5, 1987, which regulates the use of colorants for food, drugs and auxiliary material for the first time. In §3 of the Farbengestz, cosmetic products were mentioned. The utilization of harmful colorants was of course forbidden. At that time there was, e.g., lead carbonate, which was used as a common cosmetic product during the Renaissance. For other colorants there was also the possibility of a health risk. It was therefore a basic necessity to test cosmetic colorants on their toxicological and dermatological properties. This task was accepted by the Farbstoff-Kommission of the Deutsche Forschungsgemeinschaft (DFG), which published their communication §3 with a complete list of all colorants and pigments used in cosmetics in 1952. Listed were 180 colorants; it was amended several times, considering the latest results from dermatology and toxicology, and was republished in 1977 by the Farbstoff-Kommission of the DFG in the form of the Red Ringbook Kosmetische Färbemittel.

Shortly before, on July 26, 1976, a similar guideline was published by the commission of the European Community. It listed 314 colorants that were subjected to certain application restrictions in many cases.

Apart from some special colorants, this EC guideline listed only the purity requirements for colorants which were simultaneously used as food colorants or were used in the past as such (see also Section 8.1.2). The EC guideline contained the instruction, that certain colorants were not permitted after a transition period as long as (which was not mentioned in the guideline) toxicological and dermatological data would not be available.

In December 1977, this EC guideline was modified in Germany into an ordinance (Kosmetik-Verordnung KVO). The EC-mentioned transition periods were modified (in a typical German manner) into concrete interdiction dates.

The utilization of colorants for hair dying and hair shades were not mentioned in the Kosmetik-Verordnung, and they are still not governed by legislation as of today.

The Kosmetik-Verordnung contains numerous editorial and technical deficiencies; a total of eight amendments (transition of the interdiction date, editorial mistakes, addition and deletion of various colorants) made the paper so complex, that a completely revised Kosmetik-Verordnung was published in the Bundesanzeiger in 1985.

After the interdiction date was moved to July 31, 1986 (as published in the 10th Änderungsverordnung dated December 31, 1985), the Commission of the European Community approved the seventh guideline on cosmetic products on February 28, 1986. In comparison to the guideline of 1976, there was a drastic reduction of approved colorants (to 159 colorants) and—surprisingly as in 1976—a classification of the colorants into application groups. This EC guideline was published as the 11th Verordnung zur Änderung der Kosmetik-Verordnung (11th amendment of the amendment of the cosmetic ordinance) in the Bundesgesetzblatt of the Federal Republic of Germany and was modified further on March 24, 1986 by eleven more amendments. This latest amendment interdicted the use of various colorants, e.g. C.I. 45170, 12075, 42460 and 42535. Annex 3 to §3 contains the finally approved colorants and pigments for cosmetic products, classified by ascending C.I. numbers. Part B contains colorants, which can be used within time limits, and are later either forbidden or reclassified into other application groups. For each colorant there is a indication of the application group.

Application group 1: These colorants can be used in the manufacture of all cosmetic products.

Application group 2: These colorants cannot be used in the manufacture of cosmetic products that can touch the mucous membrane of the eye, especially those cosmetics and products for removing makeup.

Application group 3: These colorants cannot be used in the manufacture of cosmetic products that can get in touch with mucous membranes.

Application group 4: These products can only be used in the manufacture of cosmetic products that are in contact with the skin for a very short time.

Application group 5: These colorants can only be used in the manufacture of nail lacquer (BGBl. No. 22, 18.3.1987, p.1032). This application group was valid only for C.I. Solvent Yellow, whose approval was limited until March 31, 1992.

For some colorants, there are maximum levels in the finished product. The purity requirements of the "old" Kosmetik-Verordnung remain in effect. In Table 14, the current status is described. Colorants in this table are sorted, in contrast to the EC guideline or Kosmetik-Verordnung, not as per the ascending Color Index number, but based on color shades. For each colorant, solubility and major application areas are indicated. Additional details are found in the data sheets (see Section 9.2).

The application importance of the listed colorants is very different, many of them are not synthesized and cannot be purchased. The real important colorants, are marked with an *.

4.3.1.1. Declaration of colorants in cosmetic products

The declaration of colorants in cosmetic products is governed by the guideline 93/35/EC of the European Community, dated June 14, 1993 in article 6, section 6, 1g. It reads as follows:

"Colorants can be listed in an unsorted sequence after other components according to the numbers of the Color Index..."

For decorative cosmetics that are marketed as part of range of color nuances (shades), it is permitted to list all colorants of this range, as long as the words "may contain" are indicated."

By declaring the Color Index number, it can be avoided that the manufacturer of cosmetic products can assume, that the colorants with CTFA or INCI names are automatically suitable for the manufacture of products that are exported to the United States of America. This is the case because of peculiarities of U.S. law. An additional fact is, that no CTFA names are attached to most of the European cosmetic colorants, as they are unknown in the U.S.

Table 14 Colorants which are approved for cosmetics

Color shade		C.I. No.	Solubility			Application group				Major applications, remarks
			Water	Oil	Pigment	1	2	3	4	
Blue	*	42045	X					X		Bathing products
	*	42051	X			X				Bathing products, Toothpaste (gel)
		42080	X						X	Bathing products
	*	42090	X			X				Bathing products, Toothpaste (gel)
		42735	X					X		Bathing products

(continued)

Table 14 continued

Color shade		C.I. No.	Solubility			Application Group				Major applications, remarks
			Water	Oil	Pigment	1	2	3	4	
Blue		44045	X					X		
(con't)	*	61585	X						X	Soap, bathing products
		62045	X						X	
		69800			X	X				
		69825			X	X				
		73000			X	X				
		73015	X			X				
		74100							X	
	*	74160			X	X				Soap
		74180	X						X	
	*	77007			X	X				Decorative cosmetics, soap
		77510			X	X				
		Bromthymol yellow	X						X	
Brown		12010		X				X		
		12480			X					
		77400			X	X				
		77480			X	X				
		Caramel	X			X				
Yellow		10316	X				X			Soap
	*	11680			X			X		Soap
	*	11710			X			X		Soap
		12700	X						X	
	*	13015	X				X			Bathing products
		18690	X						X	
		18820	X						X	
		18965	X				X			
	*	19140	X				X			Bathing products
		20040			X				X	
		21100			X				X	
		21108			X				X	
		21230		X				X		
	*	45430	X				X			Fluorescent, bathing products
		47000		X					X	
	*	47005	X				X			Soap, bathing products
		75100	X				X			
		75125		X			X			
		75135		X			X			
		75300					X			Soluble in ethanol
	*	77492			X	X				Decorative cosmetics, soap

The Coloration of Cosmetic Products

Table 14 continued

Color shade		C.I. No.	Solubility			Application group				Major applications, remarks
			Water	Oil	Pigment	1	2	3	4	
Yellow (con't)		Lactoflavin	X			X				
Green		10016			X				X	Soap
		10020	X					X		Soap
		42035	X			X				
		42100	X						X	
		42170	X						X	
		44090	X			X				
	*	59040	X					X		Fluorescent, soap, bathing products
	*	61565		X		X				Fatty products
	*	61570	X			X				Soap, bathing products
	*	74260			X		X			Soap
		75810	X	X		X				
		77288			X	X				
		77289			X	X				
		77346			X	X				
	*	Bromkresol green	X						X	Bathing products
Orange		11725			X				X	
	*	11920		X		X				Transparent soap
		14270	X			X				Fatty products
	*	15510	X		X					Bathing products
		15980	X			X				Not available commercially
	*	15985	X			X				Bathing products
		16230	X					X		
		20170	X					X		
		40215	X						X	
		40800		X		X				
		40820		X		X				
		40825		X		X				
		40850		X		X				
		45370				X				Soluble in ethanol
		45396	X			X				Lipstick
		71105		X				X		
		75120		X		X				
		75130		X		X				
		77489			X	X				
		Capsanthin		X		X				
Red	*	12085			X	X				Lipstick
		12120			X					

(continued)

Table 14 continued

Color shade		C.I. No.	Solubility			Application group				Major applications, remarks
			Water	Oil	Pigment	1	2	3	4	
Red (con't)	*	12150		X		X				Fatty products
		12370			X				X	
		12420			X				X	
	*	12490			X	X				Lipstick, soap
		14700	X			X				
		14720	X			X				
		14815	X			X				Mouth wash
		15525			X	X				
		15580			X	X				
		15620	X						X	
	*	15630			X	X				Lipstick
		15800			X			X		
	*	15850			X	X				Lipstick
	*	15865			X	X				Lipstick
	*	15880			X	X				Lipstick
		16035	X			X				Bathing products
		16185	X			X				
	*	16255	X			X				Bathing products
		16290	X			X				
		17200	X			X				
		18050	X					X		
		18130	X						X	
		18736	X						X	
		24790	X						X	
		27290	X						X	
		45100	X						X	Bathing products, fluorescent
		45220	X						X	
		45380	X				X			Lipstick
		45405	X							
		45410	X				X			
		45425	X				X			
		45430	X				X			
		58000			X	X				Lipstick
		73360			X	X				Toothpaste
		73915			X				X	
		75470	X			X				
		77015			X	X				
		77491			X	X				Decorative cosmetics
		77745			X	X				
		Beet red	X			X				
		Anthocyan	X			X				
		Acid red 195						X	X	

(continued)

Table 14 continued

Color shade	C.I. No.	Solubility			Application group				Major applications, remarks
		Water	Oil	Pigment	1	2	3	4	
Black	20470	X							
	27755	X			X				
	28440	X			X				
	50420	X					X		
	77266			X	X				Decorative cosmetics
	77267			X	X				
	77268:1			X	X				Decorative cosmetics
	77499			X	X				Soap
Violet	42510	X					X		
	42520	X						X	
	45190	X						X	
	50325	X						X	
	51319			X				X	Soap
	60724			X				X	
	60725				X				Fatty products
	60730	X					X		
	73385			X	X				
	73900							X	
	77742			X	X				Decorative cosmetics
White	75170			X	X				
	77000			X	X				
	77002			X	X				
	77004			X	X				
	77120			X	X				
	77163			X	X				
	77220			X	X				
	77231			X	X				
	77713				X				
	77820				X				
	77891				X				
	77947				X				
	Al, Zn, Mg, Ca-stearate				X				Decorative cosmetics, soap

4.3.2. Countries outside the European Union

In contrast to food coloration, coloration of cosmetic products is strictly controlled in the European Union and countries such as the United States, Japan, Australia, Argentina, Brazil, Mexico, Philippines, Thailand, Venezuela and Poland. Other countries orient themselves on the guidelines of the European Union or on the regulations of the U.S. (e.g., the Central American countries). This is done either by publication of nearly identical colorant lists in the national legislative publications or is in consent with the EU or U.S.-approved colorants without indicating the details in their respective national legislative publications. For individual colorants, details can be found in the data sheets (see Section 9.2). For cosmetic colorants in the U.S., the statements made in Section 2.4.3 apply.

5 The Coloration of Food, Drugs and Cosmetics in the Public Discussion

For a long time, the coloration of food with synthetic colorants was a recurring issue at irregular times, both for experts as well as for the general public. In many cases, this discussion includes an overview on the necessity and profit of food colorants.

Coloring drugs or cosmetics is rarely mentioned in these discussions, primarily for reasons of safety; secondly, decorative cosmetics are very old and are inconceivable without colorants.

Food coloration and its colorants, as they are permitted by law, are evaluated by different persons: trained technical-scientific experts as well as consumers (which react with fear and anxiety, most often due to insufficient knowledge and experience), specifically within the context of a discussion on the necessity and risks of chemistry and nuclear energy.

In many public discussions, e.g., in television but also in private talks, an insufficient knowledge on the basis of chemistry can be observed. Nature and natural products are always perceived to be good, chemistry is seen as negative. Even the prefix "bio" is sufficient to convert a product into a good one.

Chemistry is neither good nor bad; it is the science of materials and their transformation. Chemical reactions such as the breathing process, the citric acid cycle in the human organism, the isomerization of vision pigments are all based on the same principles as they exist during the synthesis of a colorant, the functionality of a drug component or the reactions during cooking and braising of food. Woehler's synthesis of urea in 1828—the transformation of ammonia cyanide into urea by heat treatment—was early proof that it is possible for mankind to manufacture natural components. The synthesis of Indigo, Alizarin and beta-Carotene should be mentioned in the first place.

From the experience that the results of technical-scientific research, especially in the 20th century, were not always to the benefit of mankind, it is no surprise, that consumers are very skeptical, even mistrustful, vis-à-vis industrially manufactured products. On the other hand there is the observation that serious information is not considered, horror stories are accepted without doubt. Such an observation could be made in Germany since 1985. The Bund für Lebensmitelrecht und Lebensmittelkunde has made a publication "Additives in food—an information," that reads as follows:

"Distribution of fake lists"

Flyers should create fear and insecurity, where additives should be listed with their E-numbers as well as health assessments such as "suspicious, dangerous" and "causes cancer." They are distributed in canteens, schools and kindergarten and are even passed on between friends and families according to the snowball system.

These lists are fake. The assessment of additives is wrong and cannot be maintained on a scientific basis. The most gross example is the assessment of E 330 Citric Acid, causing cancer. Citric acid is essential in the human metabolism and exists naturally in fruits.

The origin of such statements is supposed to be the hospital at Villejuif, Chaumont or Chauny (in France), but they have distanced themselves from this pamphlet and are not responsible for this supposed consumer information. It is not known who supports this very directed campaign.

Even the Bundesgesundheitsministerium (Federal Health Ministry), the Working Group of Consumers and others have publicly warned about this campaign:

These lists are fake. The assessment in these lists, that attach harmful properties to these substances, have no basis at all." (Bundeshesundheitsministerium)

The concern of the consumer about his health is abused by a list that has been forged in an excellent way and is distributed anonymously in order to create confusion and anxiety. All food colorants approved in Germany and the EU have been tested very carefully and are certified only when they have no harmful effects on health. This attempt to put fear and anxiety into the consumer's mind is irresponsible. Apparently, consumer concern about health was to be abused in such a way as to make some food products doubtful and to attack the food industry.
(Working Group of Consumers)

An interesting question about the quantities (in kilogram) of synthetic colorants are consumed on an annual basis in Germany has been researched by the Mineralfarbenverband (Association of manufacturers of mineral colors) in June 1985 by circulating a questionnaire among its members. The result is, that in 1984, based on 100 pure colorants, about 456 metric tons of colorants were manufactured. Two-thirds of this quantity was exported, the remaining 154 metric tons went into domestic consumption, of which only 7 metric tons were used by products destined for consumption. Transforming this quantity into a per capita basis and considering the fact, that food colorants were imported from Italy and the United Kingdom and other countries, there is a per capita consumption of 1.5 gram of food colorants. If this number is linked to the toxicological risk of colorants (see Chapter 7), the statement is justified that there is no risk to the consumer due to food colorants.

There is a much higher risk, characterized by the words "too much, too fatty, too sweet and too much alcohol," as can be confirmed by every general practitioner. For some people the argument is insufficient, the reason being that the eye also participates in eating and therefore coloring certain food is a necessity (basic food is excluded). However, it is a valid question in view of the toxicological risk (minimal annual consumption quantity and declaration of food colorants), if the ideal of a healthy, additive-free nutrition should be extended in such a way, that there should be no coloration of food in general. It should be noted finally, that the colors around us are, including those in food, an expression of joy.

6 Product Development

The reader may ask himself, why coloration of such diverse products (such as food, drugs and cosmetics) should be dealt with.

The reason is very simple, when research is done on common factors for approved food colorants, colorants for drugs (whose coloration is deemed necessary) and the usually colored cosmetics during their manufacture, and when coloration is looked at in the overall context of product development. It is therefore recommended to read through all of this chapter, and not look only at a single area of application.

Apart from products of decorative cosmetics, colorants play (from the point of view of quantity as well as value) a minor role in the finished product. There are other common factors such as:

All foods, drugs and cosmetics are mixtures of materials, consisting of one or more components. Each colorant or blend of colorants is exposed to three key factors, which can lead to a discoloration under the most adverse conditions: light, heat and the interaction between the components of the finished product. For example, when we look at the formula of a simple foam bath (see Table 15), and when we consider, that the perfume (essence) by itself consists of more than 50 components and that the other ingredients also consist of several components, it is very much evident, that it is nearly impossible to determine the real culprit during a storage test, why a color change has taken place.

In a joint trial performed in 1993 by the Working Group on Colorants of the Deutsche Gesellschaft für wissenschaftliche und angewandte Kosmetik e.V. (DGK) with water from different sources it could be clearly shown, that the quality of water used during production has a decisive influence on light stability.

Therefore it can be assumed as a rule, that: the coloration of a product, irrespective of whether it is a food, drug or cosmetic, is the last step during formula development. A later change of the formula must be avoided whenever possible.

Table 15 Foam bath formula

Functional ingredients	60.0%
Foam stabilizer	3.0%
Refattening substances	3.0%
Salt	1.5%
Essence	2.0%
Water*	30.5%

* Colorant dissolved in water, dosage level about 200 g/ton finished product

If for cost reasons, a raw material is substituted with another from a different manufacturer (apparently identical), then this called a hidden formula change. This is not the case in products, which cannot be identified in chemical terms, as they are blends of isomers, for products that can be synthesized in different ways, and therefore contain traces of their precursors. Instabilities are observed in the finished product, as soon as the substitution takes place.

Before development commences, a check must be performed,

which kind of colorant should be preferably used (see Tables 5 and 16) and

which legal requirements must be observed in the relevant countries (basically the approval status of the colorant, application limitations, maximum levels of the colorant in the finished product).

If the last aspect is disregarded, it can happen very easily, that a product was developed for the EU, and this product cannot be sold outside the EU due to the colorant mix, even though it is stable. For example, the food colorants Patent blue V (E 131, C.I. 42051) or the cosmetic colorant Food Yellow 2 (C.I. 13015) are **not** approved outside the EU for food, drugs or cosmetics.

Table 16 Type of colorant/application (examples)

Type of colorant	Food	Drugs	Cosmetics
Water-soluble colorant	Beverages, sauces, pudding powder, instant products, candies, artificial ice cream, pollack	Juices, creams	Bathing products, creams
Oil-soluble Colorant	Margarine, fat-containing filler	Oil	Oil, soap
Pigment	Candies, capsules	Capsules	Toothpaste, makeup, powder, lipstick, soap
Lacquer		Capsules	Eye makeup, lipstick
Special preparation	Fat-containing filler		Soap

Basic technical problems are described, when two aspects as well as the aspect of stability of the used colorant are checked before using them in the development of food, drugs and cosmetics. In general there are no problems in utilizing the colorants during manufacturing.

Special issues regarding application or processing can be discussed directly between the producer, colorant supplier and equipment supplier. In many cases an exchange of ideas in seminars, congresses or expositions can be of help.

6.1. Processing indications

6.1.1. Soluble colorants

Color solutions made from water-soluble colorants in general are always transparent and show no cloudiness in a dilution. The same applies for oil-soluble colorants, dissolved in oil or various organic solvents. For colorant blend it must be kept in mind, that the appearance of the powder in general is not the same as the appearance of the solution, and that there can be variations between the individual production batches. Brown powders

Product Development

can result in green or red solutions; dark metallic powders can give a fluorescent pink solution. However, there are some surprises.

In a normal consignment, only the color shade and the color intensity of a solution (with a predefined concentration) have to conform to the standard.

When soluble colorants are processed, irrespective of whether they are water or oil-soluble, about 30–50 g of colorant powder are dissolved in 1 liter of hot water (for oil-soluble colorants oil or organic solvents are used). The solubility of the colorants can be very different; literature indicates, e.g., for Tartrazine (E 102, C.I. 19140) there is a solubility of 60 g/l in water of 20°C, and 130 g/l at 90°C; for Patent blue V (E 131, C.I. 42051) there is a solubility of 20 g/l at 20°C, and 100 g/l at 90°C. It is therefore recommended to operate in a concentration range, where there is no risk of crystallization. The consequences could be technical problems such as the blocking of pipelines and valves as well as color shade changes. This is especially the case when color blends are used, consisting of several components with different solubility, e.g., a green color made with Tartrazine and Patent blue (see above), the components must be dissolved completely. In cases of working on the extreme edge of solubility, the entire colorant solution must be checked by filtration.

A special application problem is the coloration of products with an alcohol content of more than 70%. On the one hand the light stability of water-soluble food and cosmetic colorants is significantly reduced in alcohol compared to water, on the other hand, the alcohol content influences the solubility. Dissolving the colorants and then coloring the alcohol-containing product with this stock solution is not recommended. A different, but slightly more complicated procedure is recommended, if a well-trained production staff is available.

A completely saturated alcoholic stock solution is made for each colorant at room temperature. If the objective is a brown color, then yellow, red and blue components are solubilized. These solutions are then filtered. By blending parts of these stock solutions the desired color can be obtained in the finished product. Possible defects with this procedure are: if the water content of the alcoholic solution varies and if the room temperature is different from batch to batch, then stock solutions are obtained, which have different concentrations. The color setting in the finished product is not obtained by a fixed formula, but must be adjusted from batch to batch.

This sometimes-laborious procedure is not necessary when water-soluble colorants are used. Procedures are fixed during formula development (colorant, concentration, and quantity). The aspect of color stability is discussed in Section 6.5.

6.1.2. Pigments and coloring paints

Pigments (e.g., Ultramarine blue C.I. 77007) are colorants that do not dissolve in the product to be colored, but will achieve the color effect when the colorant has been distributed evenly in the product. Although manufactured in a different way (see Section 1.5) color of the lacquers is based on the same principles. Pigments and lacquers are processed with standard technologies.

When coloring a product with pigments or lacquers (e.g., capsule, powder or lipstick) it is very important, that the colorant particles are uniformly distributed in the finished product, and that localized agglomerations of pigments or lacquers are broken up and that there is a complete development of the color effect. Depending on the finished product there are numerous technical devices available and installations such as blending, mixing, kneading machines, roller mills and others.

6.1.3. Special preparations

6.1.3.1. Water soluble pigments

The basic chemical composition of water-dispersible pigments has been described in Section 1.5. They can be used in the same way as water-soluble colorants and are used mainly in the production of soap. In contrast to water-soluble colorants, these stock solutions (correct "dispersions") are not clear but have a noticeable opaqueness, which becomes evident as a function of the concentration.

6.1.3.2. Special fat pigments

In the area of cosmetics there are numerous approved fat-soluble colorants; in the area of food colorants there are significantly less (Chlorophyll, Annatto, beta-Carotene and others). This is the reason why many color shades (e.g., red, blue, brown) cannot be achieved in the finished product. This deficiency can be overcome only in a few cases for liquid fatty products in the food and pharmaceutical industry; it can be solved in pasty and highly viscous finished products.

Fat-containing fillers, creams, suppositories and others can be colored in principle by pigments and/or lacquers; however, for pigments the choice of color shades is very limited. Another obstacle is the high price of lacquers.

This is a potential area for the application of special fat pigments, which is a preparation of water-soluble food colorants on the basis of cornstarch. As all water-soluble colorants can be modified in such a way into special fat pigments, the number of color shades becomes indefinite.

Special fat pigments are added dry into the fat-containing product and are distributed evenly. The required amounts are in the area of 0.5 to 3.0%. They are not suitable for the coloration of low-viscous fat products, e.g., oil, because they would form a deposit in the finished product.

6.2. Food (a selection)

If the coloration of a certain food appears to be necessary from a technological point of view, then the desired effect can be achieved with the approved colorants, pigments or lacquers. However, it has become standard procedure in the food industry (due to the anti-colorant campaign), if the color effect cannot be achieved with a coloring food ingredient.

Spray-dried spinach is suitable for the coloration of artificial ice cream (dosage level about 1%), green noodles and soup stock in dried form.

Red beet powder can be used for the coloration of ice cream, beverage powder, pudding (dosage level about 0.2%) as well as hibiscus flavor, which also can be used for the coloration of instantized hibiscus tea powder (dosage level about 200 g/100 l of tea).

Vacuum-dried blends of coloring food ingredients such as red beet powder and paprika can be used for the coloration of sauces, e.g., for fish preserves (dosage level about 200–500 g/100 kg sauce) because of their relatively good heat stability.

Product Development

Carrot extract, beta-Carotene (pro-vitamin A) in its oil-soluble and water-dispersible form and Riboflavin (vitamin B_2) and Curcuma (dosage level about 50 g/100 kg) are well suited to achieve a yellow color effect.

§17 of the Lebensmittel- und Bedarfsgegenständegesetz (food law) must be considered from the point of "deception" when it comes to using coloring food ingredients. It is not permitted, to add Curcuma to pasta products in order to create the impression of a higher egg content. In the list of ingredients it must be mentioned if coloring foods have been added (see also Article 1 §6 of the Lebensmittelkennzeichnungs-Verordnung, food labeling ordinance dated December 22, 1981).

If the coloring used for food ingredients show that they are not color stable or do not achieve the desired color shades, which cannot be obtained with coloring food ingredients, then food colorants as mentioned in Table 6 could be an alternative.

Most of the food products, where coloration is permitted, can be colored with water-soluble colorants. The colorant or blend of colorants is dissolved in water as described in Section 6.1.1. During processing the following distinctions are made:

Food products which are colored completely, and where the stock solution is added directly in order to achieve the desired color shade, e.g., ice cream and beverages.
Food products which are colored only on the surface, such as candies.
Food products which are colored by immersion in a colorant solution, such as fish rye products ("artificial" caviar), pollack and entire fruits (e.g., cherries in fruit preserves
Powder food products, where the colorant is added in dry form and the coloration becomes visible only during the preparation of the product in milk or water, e.g., cream products, puddings and carbonated drinks.

Utilization of fat-soluble food colorants is limited to the coloration of fat-containing fillers and utilization in margarine and some cheese products.

Paint lacquers, pigments and special fat preparations are used mainly in the manufacture of sugar coatings, capsules, marchpane (for color effects in fat-containing fillers). For the coloration of capsules (candies or pharmaceutical products) a discoloration of the sugar coating is sometimes observed. Normally they are due to the influences of the core of the product. This phenomena can be prevented by the application of one or more insulating layers before applying the color layer.

6.3. Drugs (a selection)

In the coloration of drugs there is a clear overlap with the coloration of food products and cosmetic products, also from the point of view of legislation. From the point of view of how color is applied it is not important, whether it is a liqueur with herbs or a liquid drug, a medical or cosmetic bathing product, a cosmetic or pharmaceutical cream. There are some differences in the food and cosmetic group: for capsules and for medical bathing products.

In order to color capsules, it is not sufficient to only blend the powdery capsule mass before pressing with the colorant powder. This process would yield a very non-appealing if not uncolored product. Coloration would become evident only when the tablet is dissolved in water; the purpose of coloration, identification, would not be achieved as intended.

Therefore coloration of the powdered tablet mass is done by spraying a colorant or part or the entire mass in a special blending device equipped with heating devices. After spraying of the powder, the added moisture can be removed by heating. If no blender with heating facility is available, then only a part (e.g., 10%) of the mass is sprayed with a colorant. The colored product is dried in a cabinet drier and is then blended with the balance of the product.

In the confectionery industry, candies are normally colored with water-soluble colorants, if no iron oxide pigments are available to obtain a yellow or brown color or if no titanium dioxide is available for a white color. When consuming candies, the tongue of the consumer appears colored. This effect can be considered acceptable for candies, but it is not for high-priced drugs. For the coloration of capsules, the above mentioned pigments are one alternative; another alternative is lacquers. Lacquers are used in the manufacture of gelatin capsules and for suppositories.

Coloration of medical bathing products is done in the same way as cosmetic bathing products from a technical point of view. The choice of colorants is limited compared to those used for cosmetics. In Germany, the Arzneimittelfarbstoff-Verordnung (Ordinance on colorants in drugs) must be respected; only food colorants can be used. The same is valid for other pharmaceutical products, which have a cosmetic pendant, e.g., creams, oils for skin treatment, mouth wash water and lip care products.

6.4. Cosmetic products

Coloration of cosmetic products, especially decorative cosmetics, has been performed over a long period of time, compared to coloring certain foods and drugs. Numerous products exist in the market place. Their manufacture is described extensively by G.A. Nowak (Die kosmeti-schen Präparate, see literature sources). If a water- or oil-soluble colorant is more suited for a cosmetic product, whether a pigment or lacquer should be used, is the result of the cosmetic formula and its application in many cases.

a) **Shampoo, foam bath, shower gel, liquid soap**

For the coloration of this product category, basically all water-soluble food and cosmetic colorants of application group 1-4 of the current Kosmetik-Verordnung (cosmetic ordinance) or EU guideline can be used (for foam baths, colorants of application group 1-3 can be used). Specifically suited are:

colour	name	C.I. number
blue	Patent blue types	C.I.42045
		C.I. 42051
		C.I.42090
	Acid blue 80	C.I. 61585
yellow	C.I. Food Yellow 2	C.I. 13015
	Tartrazine	C.I. 19140
	C.I. Acid Yellow 73 (Uranin)	C.I.45350 (fluorescent)
	C.I. Food Yellow 13 (Chinolin yellow)	C.I. 47005
green	D&C Green No. 5 (Alizarin cyanin green)	C.I. 61570
	C.I. Solvent Green 7 (Pyranin)	C.I. 59040 (fluorescent)
orange	C.I. Acid Orange 7 (Orange II)	C.I.15510
	C.I. Food Yellow 3 (Yellow orange)	C.I. 15985

Product Development

pink	Ponceau 4R	C.I. 16255
	C.I. Acid Red 52 (Sulforhodamin B)	C.I. 45100

Brown can be obtained by a combination of red, yellow (or orange) and blue colorants
Violet can be obtained by a blend of red and blue

Fluorescent effects can be obtained by the addition of Uranin or Pyranin. All colorants mentioned above can be blended with each other, or are offered by colorant manufacturers as blends. Processing of these colorants is done by making a stock solution first (see 6.1.1) and then by the addition of water until the desired color intensity is achieved.

b) Bathing salt, bathing tablets

Coloration of these products is done similarly for all other water-soluble food and cosmetic colorants or water-dispersible pigments of application groups 1-3 of the current Kosmetik-Verordnung or EU guideline. The light stability of the used colorant depends very much on the moisture content of the product and the used essence. Commercially available products are colored red with Erythrosin (C.I. 45430); blue with Patent blue V (C.I. 42090) or Indigotin (C.I. 73015); green with Alizarin cyanin green (C.I. 61570); yellow with Chinolin yellow (C.I. 47005) or Uranin (C.I. 45350)(fluorescent). Processing of these colorants has been described in Section 6.3.

c) Oil and cream baths

Products of this kind, that may contain water, can also be colored with water-soluble food or cosmetic colorants. Products without moisture content can be colored with oil-soluble cosmetic colorants.

blue	C.I. Solvent Violet 13 (Irisol)	C.I. 60725
yellow	C.I. Solvent Yellow 29 (Ceres yellow GRN)	C.I. 21230
turquoise	D&C Green No.6 (Alizarin cyanin green fat-soluble)	C.I. 61565
orange	C.I. Solvent Orange 3 (Sudan orange)	C.I. 11920
red	C.I. Solvent Red 1 (Sudan red G)	C.I. 12150

All mentioned colorants can be blended with each other. During processing the colorants are solubilized in the oil portion (e.g., soybean oil) of the bathing product.

d) Soap

For the coloration of toilet soap both water and oil-soluble colorants as well as pigments and their water-dispersible preparations of application groups 1-4 can be used. As the light stability of the soluble colorants is fairly limited in soap, pigments and their preparations (in the form of a pigment dough) are normally preferred.
Specifically suited are the following colorants and their blends:

blue	C.I. Acid Blue 80 (Acid blue 80)	C.I. 61585
	C.I. Pigment Blue 15 (Phtalocyanin blue)	C.I. 74160
	C.I. Pigment Blue 29 (Ultramarine blue)	C.I. 77007

yellow	C.I. Acid Yellow 1 (Naphtol yellow)	C.I. 10316
	C.I. Pigment Yellow 1 (Hansa yellow)	C.I. 11680 & 11710
	C.I. Pigment Yellow 83 (Graphtol yellow RCL)	C.I. 21108
	C.I. Food Yellow 13 (Chinolin yellow)	
	C.I. Pigment Yellow 42,43 (Iron oxide yellow)	C.I. 47005
		C.I. 77492
green	C.I. Pigment Green 8 (Pigment green B)	C.I. 10006
	C.I. Acid Green 1 (Green PLX)	C.I. 10020
	C.I. Solvent Green 7 (Pyranin)	C.I. 59040
	D&C Green No. 5 (Alizarin cyanin green)	C.I. 61570
	C.I. Pigment Green 7 (Phtalocyanin green)	C.I. 74260
orange	C.I. solvent Orange 3 (Sudan orange G)	C.I. 11920
red	C.I. Pigment Red 5 (Permanent carmine FB)	C.I. 12490
	C.I. Pigment Red 101,102 (Iron oxide red)	
		C.I. 77491
black	C.I. Pigment Black 11 (Iron oxide black)	C.I.. 77499
violet	C.I. Pigment Violet 23 (Sandarin violet BL)	C.I. 51319
	C.I. Pigment Blue 29 (Ultramarine violet)	
		C.I. 77007
white	C.I. Pigment White 6 (Titanium dioxide)	C.I. 77891

Glycerin-based soap (transparent soap) can be colored only with soluble colorant in order to maintain transparency. If a minimal opaqueness is accepted, then water dispersible pigments can be used, but not pigments without dispersing agents.

Dosage of the water-soluble colorants and dispersible pigments in soap is in the range of 0.01–0.05%; if pigments are used, then the range is 0.1–0.5% in order to achieve an attractive color. If stock solutions are used during the processing of water-soluble and water-dispersible pigments, then it becomes necessary to dissolve fat soluble colorants in mineral oils or lanolin, before incorporating them into the soap mass.

Pigments are added together with soap flakes into the perfume essence. An optimal distribution is necessary (kneading, roller mill). An insufficient distribution of the pigments leads to dots and streaks in the finished soap cake.

e) Oil-in-water emulsion (e.g., O/W cream)

Products of this kind are colored with water-soluble food or cosmetic colorant of application group 1-3 (for a longer residence time on the skin) in a minimal dosage (e.g., 0.2% in a 1% solution). The colorant solution is added to the aqueous phase before emulsification.

f) Water-in-oil emulsion (e.g., W/O cream), oil

These products are colored with fat-soluble colorants of the cosmetic application group 1-3, and the colorants are dissolved in oil and are added to the oil-phase of the cream before emulsification in very small amounts (e.g., 1% of a 1% solution). Oil can be colored directly.

Product Development

g) Shading cream, makeup

For the coloration of shading cream and makeup, in many cases blends of Iron oxide yellow (C.I. 77492), Iron oxide red (C.I. 77491), Iron oxide black (C.I. 77499) and Titanium dioxide (C.I. 77891) are used. If these products are of the O/W emulsions, then the pigments of the aqueous phase are added at the required level and are thoroughly dispersed (e.g., by using an Ultra-Turrax blender). Dosage levels depend on the amount of Titanium dioxide and are in the range of 2 to 8%. Thereafter emulsification of the fat phase takes place. For special effects, mother of pearl pigments can be used.

h) Eye makeup

For the coloration of eye makeup, (lid shade, mascara, eyebrow stick), most often pigments of the cosmetic application group 1 are used, including mother of pearl pigments. In some cases, aluminum lakes of food colorants are used.

Pigments such as Ultramarine blue (C.I. 77007), Prussian blue (C.I. 77510), Iron oxide yellow (C.I. 77492), Iron oxide red (C.I. 77491), Iron oxide black (C.I. 77499) and Carbon black (C.I. 77266 or 77268:1) as well as Ultramarine violet (C.I. 77007) and Manganese violet (C.I. 77742) are used in many cases. Sometimes the aluminum lakes of Indigotin (C.I. 73015) or Chinolin yellow (C.I. 47005) are used. All mentioned colorants can be blended with each other, with Titanium dioxide and with mother of pearl pigments of the type Titanium dioxide/Mica. Dosage of pigments in mascara is 5%, in lid shade up to 30%.

i) Lipstick

Lipstick can be colored with two different kind of colorants:

- Eosin colorants, which color the lips in an intensive and long-term manner, and
- With pigments which complement the covering layer, and which impart coloration to the lipstick

In recent years this has become standard practice, to color lipstick only with pigments or lakes.

When using Eosin colorants, it is necessary that the basic material of lipstick contain the appropriate Eosin solvent (e.g., castor oil, polyethylene glycol, oleyl-alcohol, isopropyl myristate). Eosin colorants are dissolved in them before adding to the mass, whereas pigments are mixed into the warm, high-viscosity and finished lipstick base mass and dispersed optimally (e.g., by using a roller mill).

Fashion dictates changing colors. Additions of Eosin vary between 0.1–2%, pigments vary between 1–10%, when pigment paste is used the content varies up to 24%; pastel shades can be achieved by adding Titanium dioxide (C.I. 77891). By varying the percentages of Eosin, pigments and Titanium dioxide color nuances can be obtained, which impart the typical fashionable color shade to the lipstick.

j) Mouth and tooth care products

Coloring toothpaste (and gels) is done with food colorants, although the current Kosmetik-Verordnung or EU guidelines would also permit other colorants of the cosmetic application groups 1 and 2.

Our own research of various brands has shown, that the actual number of colorants is fairly limited. We have identified food colorants such as Patent blue V (E 131, C.I. 42051), Patent blue AE (C.I. 42090), Indanthren brilliant pink (C.I. 73360, C.I. Vat red 1) and Phtalocyanin green (C.I. 74260, C.I. Direct Blue 86).

For the coloration of toothpaste only soluble colorants can be used, in order not to reduce the transparency of the gel.

For the coloration of mouth wash water, only soluble colorants or blends thereof are used, e.g., Azorubin (E 122, C.I. 14720 C.I. Food Red 3) or Amaranth (E 123, C.I. 16185 C.I. Food Red 6). An attractive red color can be obtained by a blend of Ponceau 4R (E 124 C.I. 16255 C.I. Food red 7) with Amaranth (E 123, C.I. 16815) at equal percentages and adding 1% of a 1% stock solution to mouth wash water.

In mouth wash water, that is not distributed in Germany, we identified a cosmetic colorant (which is not a food colorant), i.e., Alizarin cyan green (C.I. 61570 D&C Green No. 5).

k) Hair dying and coloration products

The provisions of the current Kosmetik-Verordnung are not applicable for "cosmetic materials, that are to be used for hair dying and coloration." Cosmetic colorants approved by the EU can be used technically only to a limited extent for hair dying and coloration.

For hair coloration two different types of colorants are used: (1) oxidation hair dyes, which dye the hair permanently and (2), direct effect colorants, which dye the hair only on the exterior; they can be washed out (semi-permanent dying).

Oxidation dyes are based on the principle, that a precursor product penetrates into the hair and reacts there with added hydrogen peroxide (therefore the name oxidation colorant). Here no colorants are used, as the color process takes place in the hair. Direct effect colorants, most often based on cationic colorants, cannot penetrate into hair because of their molecular structure, these adhere only on the exterior, and can therefore be removed very easily.

The following colorants have been proven to be very effective in the group of direct effect colorants: C-ext. Red 64 (C.I. 12245), C-ext. Brown 5 (C.I. 12250) C-ext. Brown 6 (C.I. 12251), C-ext. Yellow 25 (C.I. 12719) and C-ext. Blue 17 (C.I. 56059) (see also data sheets in Section 9.2). Other colorants are contained in a recommended list of the European Cosmetic Association (COLIPA), Brussels. The above mentioned colorants are cationic. When developing formulas it must be considered, that only cationic or amphotere tensides are to be used; when using anionic tensides, undesirable precipitations can be observed. Colorants can be used in a pH range of 3 to 9.5; a high pH value is favorable for dying and washing. Maximum color intensity is obtained after a contact time of 20 minutes. The recommended dosage depends on the application and color shade and is on a level of 0.05–0.5%. A detailed description on the formulation of hair dying products can be found in G.A. Nowak, Die kosmetischen Präparate, Chapter XIII.

l) Nail polish

The manufacture of nail polish is less a question of the colorant used, but more of the technical requirements on the polish and the manufacturing technology. When transparent polish is manufactured, soluble cosmetic colorants such as Sudan red G (C.I. 12150, C.I. Solvent Red 1) are used. Cream polish contains organic colored pigments and mother of pearl pigments. See also G.A. Nowak, Die kosmetischen Präparate, Chapter XVII.

6.5. Stability tests

An absolute stability of a colorant does not exist. It always depends on the type and composition of the material to be colored (dyed) and the test conditions. This applies to food, drugs and cosmetics. In lieu of textile fibers (on which most of the common water-soluble colorants have been tested), other substrates are used, e.g., sugar, fruit acids, fats, oils, salts and flavors for food items; functional and auxiliary materials for drugs; active ingredients, emulsifiers, cosmetic agents and perfumes/essences for cosmetic products. Other factors are temperature during manufacture and storage of the finished product. The cotton standard (DIN 54004) cannot be used for the purpose of classification of light stability for food and cosmetic products.

In order to conduct a light stability test within a short time, UV light is used in many places at a very high light intensity. Unfortunately this is done not only to obtain an overview of which colorant can be used, but also to extrapolate from the test period on the light stability in a showcase or in a bathroom. The question is shelf life when, in which month of the year and where? UV light tests are subjected to this kind of light, and in my opinion this color stability is overestimated for food, drugs and cosmetics by many experts.

The short-wave absorption limit of the atmosphere varies because of the varying ozone level (it varies during the year and even during the day) and is found at a wavelength of 287 to 305 nm. Food, drugs and cosmetics are stored (with few exceptions) in storage rooms. Here the most effective protection takes over, which is the window glass. If the product is filled into a glass bottle, then there is the added effect of the packaging material. UV light at a wavelength of less than 300 nm is absorbed completely by glass; even at 330 nm there is still a noticeable absorption. It is therefore not realistic nor close to everyday conditions to select test parameters which correspond to conditions outdoors, in the mountains, seaside or near the equator where sales conditions do not correspond to the test parameters, or when products are sold under an open sky.

We have observed, that we could obtain usable results by comparing a freshly colored sample, to a sample that has been exposed to sunlight behind a glass window and a sample stored at 35–40°C in a heated cabinet. It is interesting to note, that samples from exposure in a northerly window in many cases show a stronger decoloration than samples from a Southerly window.

In test protocols the azimuth and exposure should be noted. Other parameters are: start and end times of the test and the approximate period of sunshine during the test. The test can be performed under identical conditions except for the light factor (use artificial light) in order to simulate conditions in a supermarket.

The minimum test period should be 2–4 weeks. Basically the following test results can be obtained:

1. The colorant is destroyed even during coloration of the product or changes its tone—an effect that can be observed very often when working with triphenyl colorants (e.g., Patent blue V E 131; when acidifying with citric acid, color changes from blue to green).
2. The product is discolored within 2–4 weeks when exposed to light or heat.

In cases of 1 or 2 the colorant cannot be used.

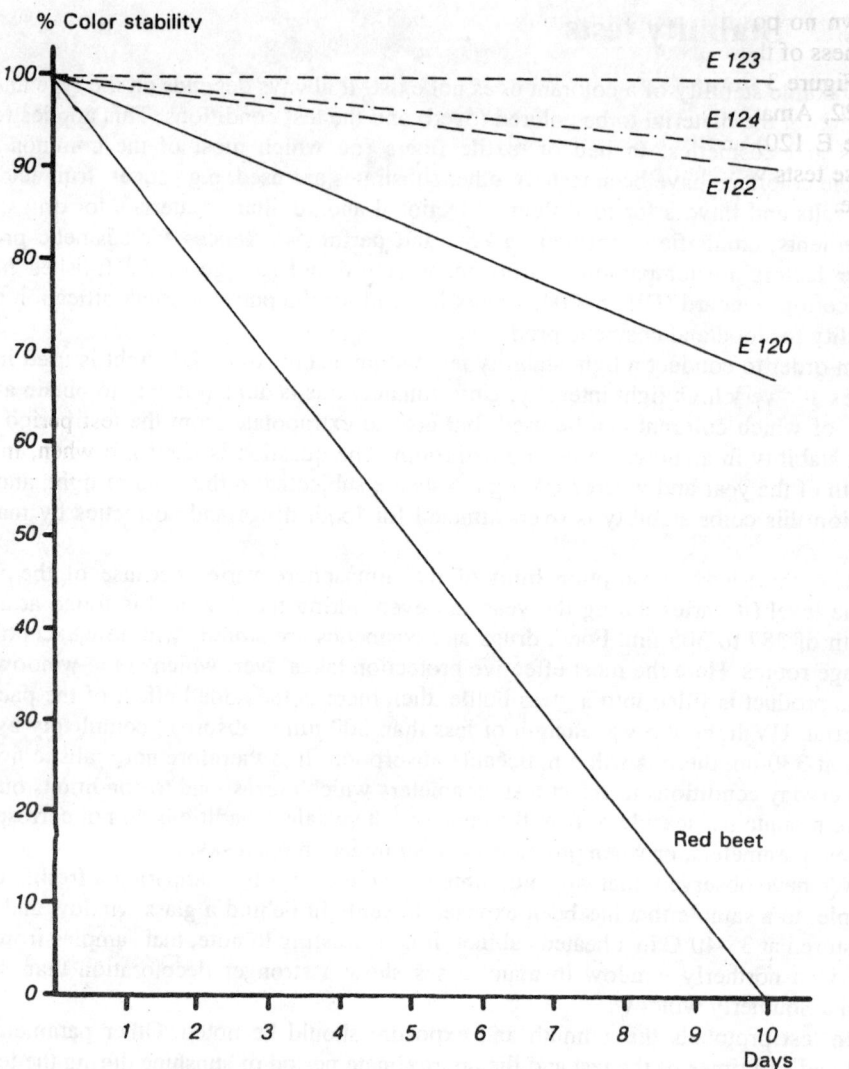

Figure 3 Light stability in water.

3. The freshly colored sample and the heat-treated sample are identical, the light-treated sample (either window or room sample) shows a weaker color; i.e., the colorant is resistant to chemical reactions; it is only influenced by the oxygen content.
4. If the samples are still color-identical after four weeks, then we have obtained an ideal result. A formula change must be avoided at all costs, as it can lead to a totally different result.

The color stability of water-soluble colorants is significantly lower in alcohol-containing products than in water. In many cases, attempts are made to improve color stability with UV light absorbing material (protective filters). Our own research has shown no positive results regarding the use of UV light absorbing material. The effectiveness of these absorbers must be tested on specific products.

Figure 3 shows the color stability of three synthetic water-soluble colorants (Azorubin E 122, Amaranth E 123 and Ponceau 4R E 124), of a natural colorant (Cochineal Carmine E 120) and of a coloring food product (Red beet) in water as a function of time. These tests were performed in May 1986 behind a southerly window with moderate sunshine.

7 Safety and Quality

7.1. Toxicology and dermatology

The reader may ask, why the term "ecology" is not mentioned in this heading. The reason is very simple. The data on food and cosmetic colorants clearly show, there is absolutely no reason for concern or anxiety from a toxicological, dermatological or ecological point of view (see also data sheets in Section 9.2). Further colorants used in the food, pharmaceutical or cosmetic industry enter the wastewater system at extremely low concentrations, when used properly.

Since 1949, a working group (Farbstoff-Kommission of the Deutsche Forschungs Gemeinschaft) in Germany has worked jointly with various organizations of the European Union, other countries and the World Health Organization on aspects of toxicology, dermatology and analytical procedures for colorants in food, drugs and cosmetics. In 1978 and 1980 this body issued ringbooks ("Farbstoffe in Lebensmitteln" – Colorants in foods; "Untersuchungsmethoden zur Prüfung der Reinheit von Lebensmittelfarbstoffen" –Analytical methods for the determination of purity in food colorants) and thus represent the state of the art. However, and this should be noted positively, the ADI values mentioned in the 1978 edition have been increased for several of these colorants. The ADI value (acceptable daily intake) is a value which indicates how many milligrams per kilogram bodyweight of a food additive can be ingested over an entire lifetime without any harmful effects.

The ADI value has been determined in such a way that in feeding trials with animals the maximum harmless dose has been determined which has no adverse effects over one's entire lifetime. The percentage of this level has been set as the ADI value. This considers transfer effects between animals and human beings, and other factors such as special protection for children, old and sick persons. Other nutritional factors are also considered. The long and global experience of toxicology has shown, that this safety system works.

The toxicological and dermatological experiences of the Farbstoff-Kommission and other competent institutions have been collected over a long period of time. Summaries are made in numerous publications (see Chapter 10). It can be said that hardly any other group of food additives has been researched as intensively as food colorants. Cosmetic colorants have also been researched extensively. Dermatological and toxicological data can be found in the data sheets for each colorant. Even the remotest suspicion of a potential risk or harm has been a reason in the past to prohibit a given colorant. Currently used colorants for food, drugs and cosmetics can be considered safe.

7.2. Quality assurance

When a colored product is launched in the market place, it is important to keep the color constant and not vary it too much. Often, the consumer perceives a color change to be a quality change. Production is controlled in many cases by a simple comparative test (compared to a standard reference sample). If this test is performed visually or even when using a color determination device, then subjective visual characteristics are part of the test result (even when ideal testing conditions are available). An observer with a normal color visualizing capability can distinguish between an immense number of colors; therefore there is a low probability, that sample and standard are perceived to be identical in color. At the moment, quality assurance is faced with the question, whether the product is still acceptable from the point of view of color, or whether it is beyond the acceptable range. The decision depends on the opinion of the observer; it is subjective.

In order to put the quality control of colored items on an objective and reproducible basis, there are two basic principles:

> VIS spectral photometry in the visual range for soluble colorants, transparent and other dilutable colorants, e.g., for beverages, liquid drugs, bathing products etc.; this method determines the transmission of light through a sample.
>
> Determination of remission, i.e., the determination of the reflected light by spectral or triple-range method; this method can be used for pigments and insoluble or non-transparent products.

These physical methods can be used in those cases, when it is not possible to maintain a color standard over a longer period of time.

Color determination with the spectral photometer is common for soluble products over a long period of time; color determination of insoluble products became common only when the programmable computer entered our life (due to the complexity of mathematical procedures).

Quality assurance of colored products begins with the control of purchased raw materials. If deviations in intensity or color are observed, then formula adjustments can be made. To adjust the color defect in the finished product is far more difficult and requires a long experience in order to remain within color standards. A reliable supplier and a good raw material control are the basic requirements for a smooth operation without shutdown periods due to upgrading activities.

7.3. Colorimetry and photometry

Colorimetry is the determination of the color intensity of a solution by comparing it with the color of a standard solution of known concentration. The procedure can be such, that either the thickness of the color layer of one of the solutions is varied until color equality is achieved (colorimeter according to Dubosq) or dilution series are made and the solutions are compared at the same layer thickness. The basic requirement in the application of colorimetric methods is, that color intensity of a solution changes in a proportional manner to its concentration (Lambert-Beer law).

In colorimetry the total light absorption of a solution in the visual range is covered (light absorption in the range of 350–750 nm). The comparison of color intensity can be done visually or by photoelectric means. Reproducibility is limited when comparing visually, as different observers have different subjective perceptions on color equality. The previously used Dubosq colorimeter has been replaced by recording spectral photometers.

7.3.1. Principles of a spectral photometer

A spectral photometer consist of six basic elements: light source, monochromator, cuvette with the colored solution (sample or reference), receiver, amplifier and indicator (recorder) (see Figure 4).

Safety and Quality

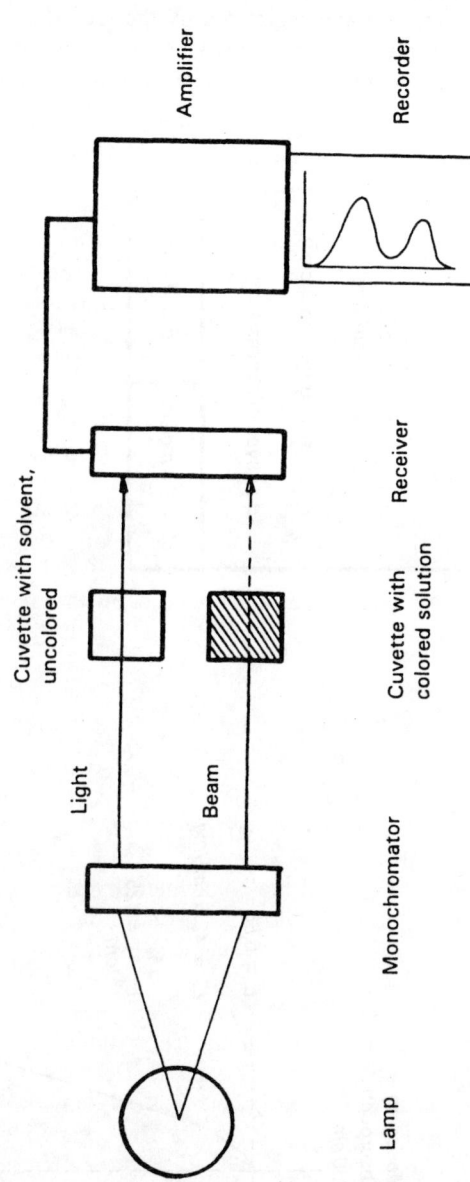

Figure 4 Principle of a dual-beam spectral photometer.

A cuvette with the colored sample solution is positioned alternately with the reference (uncolored solvent) in the light path of monochromatic light (wavelength 350 to 750 nm).

The law of Lambert-Beer says, that light absorption is proportional to the number of absorbing molecules or concentration. The conclusion is, that the non-colored solvent does not absorb light over the entire wavelength range of visual light. Its transmission T is 100%, its absorption (or extinction) E is 0%. The colored solution absorbs light at a product-specific wavelength, as a function of its concentration c of the colorant and the layer thickness d of the solution that is equal to the inner diameter of the cuvette.

Differences in the transmission between solvent and sample are measured photo-electrically, and are amplified and registered by the recorder as a function of the wavelength. Figure 5 shows such a curve; it shows not only the transmission, but extinction E of the analyzed solution. The mathematical relationships are shown in Section 7.3.2.

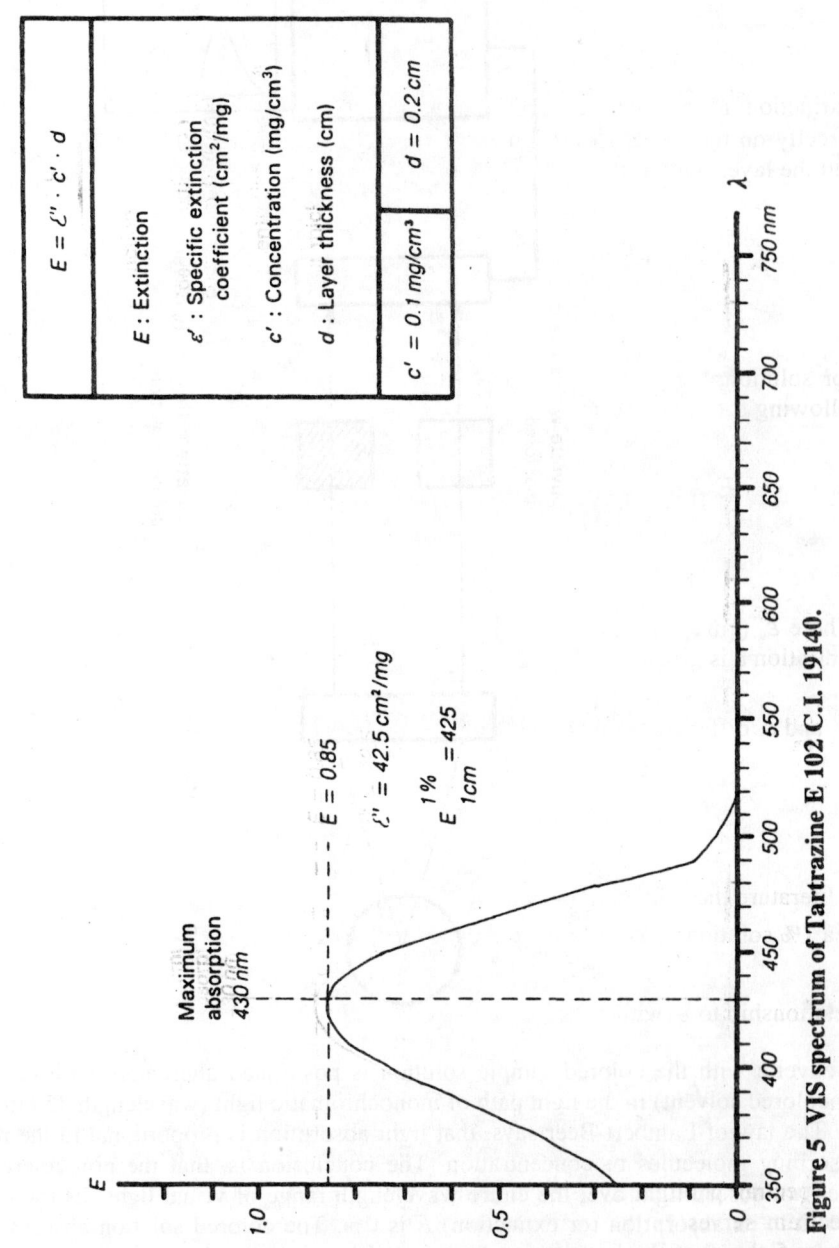

Figure 5 VIS spectrum of Tartrazine E 102 C.I. 19140.

7.3.2. Evaluation

Transmission T is defined as the ratio of intensity of monochromatic light before the solution I_o to the intensity of light after the solution I:

$$T = \frac{I}{I_o}$$

Extinction E at a defined wavelength $E\lambda$ is the logarithm of extinction. It depends directly on the molar extinction coefficient ε of the colorant, its concentration c (Mol/l) and the layer thickness d.

$$E\lambda = \log \frac{I}{I_o} = \varepsilon \cdot c \cdot d$$

For solutions where the molar concentration is unknown, e.g., blends of colorants, the following formula is used:

$$E'\lambda = \log \frac{I}{I_o} = \varepsilon \cdot c \cdot d$$

Where ε' (cm2/cm) is the specific extinction coefficient of the colorant blend and concentration c is given in (mg/cm^3).

ε and ε' differ by the factor molecular weight M:

$$\varepsilon = \varepsilon' \cdot M$$

In literature the following indication is found very often $E_{1cm}^{1\%}$. This indicates extinction of a 1% solution at a cuvette thickness of 1 cm.

Relationship to ε (without the derivations):

$$E_{1cm}^{1\%} = \varepsilon' \cdot 10(\text{cm}^2) \cdot c(g^{-1})$$

Spectral photometry is well suited for analysis in the visual range; the obtained spectrum serves as the analytical protocol and direct indication of the color intensity. Figure 5 shows such a sample spectrum with its calculations.

7.4. Measuring color

7.4.1. Basics

The basic principles on how humans perceive color have been described in Section 1.1. To combine the sensory perceptions of man with physical results has been the objective of numerous scientists.

The mathematical tricks that were necessary to combine color TV and color measurement, have been used in normal analytical practice as well as in a specific colorimetric dictionary. The International Commission on Lighting (CIE: Commission International de l'Éclairage) has developed a system that is based on experience that any color can be created by the additive blending of three primary colors: red, green and violet (principle of color TV). As the colors of an object depend on the spectral composition of light which is used, CIE has established four standard types of light that are used in color determination:

> Standard light type A is used when lighting conditions are required which simulate a normal light bulb
> Standard light type B corresponds direct sunlight
> Standard light type C corresponds to average daylight
> Standard light type D65 contains the normal UV percentage of daylight

It is self-evident that the used standard light type as well as the visual area of the observer are indicated in the test results.

If the primary colors red, green and violet are given equal value, then each color (created with these colors) can be defined by them. For this purpose the term *Standard Color Value* is used. The standard color values X, Y and Z represent the percentage of red, green and violet primary colors, which are the result of additive color blending and when this color is described in numerical terms.

7.4.2. Determination

Color determination is described on the basis of the relatively triple-beam process. The precision of this method is sufficient for normal analysis in the food, pharmaceutical and cosmetic industry, whereas in the paint and lacquer industry a spectral process must be used in order to cover the so-called metameric effects and conduct computer-based color calculations (metamer: conditionally equal, e.g., identical in daylight, significant differences in artificial light and vice versa).

A triple-beam color measuring device consists of a sensor (which contains the entire optical part as well as a photo element), the norm spectral filters X, Y and Z (which adjust the sensor to the spectral sensitivity of the color and light-dark receptors of the eye) as well as a digital indicator (which indicates the corresponding remission of the sample) (see Figure 6).

Before the analysis, the device is calibrated with a white body. A body is considered white when the entire incoming light is reflected); normally Barium sulfate is used as a white standard and a remission level of 99% is attributed to it. After installation of the corresponding normal spectral filters in the sensor, a value of 98 is set on the indicator of

Safety and Quality

the device with Barium sulfate used as a reference sample. If the white reference sample is replaced by another colored sample, the corresponding remission levels (R_x, R_y, R_z) are indicated.

The optical principle, that a result is achieved, is relatively simple. Both the white color standard as well as the sample are lighted by a halogen lamp at an angle of 0°, i.e., perpendicular from the top. Light, reflected in a diffuse manner, is analyzed at 45°, after passing the corresponding normal spectral filters and hitting the silicon photo element, is transformed, amplified and indicated digitally. The process is comparable to the function of a photometer.

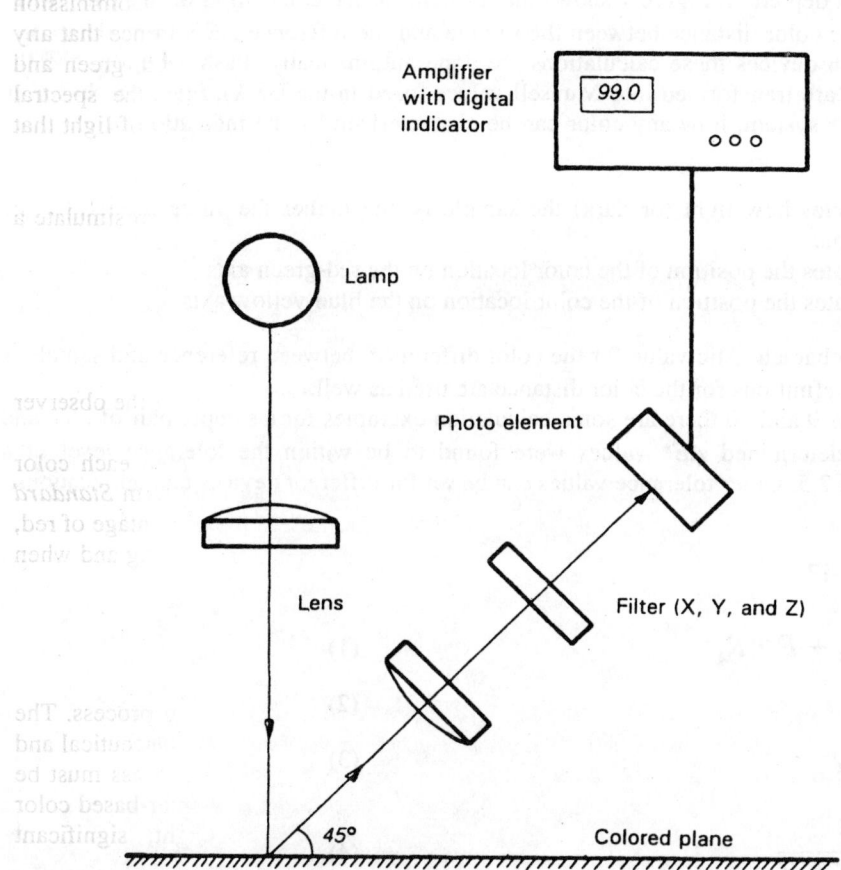

Fig. 6 Principle of a triple-beam colorimeter.

Currently there are several devices commercially available, also with other measuring configurations, or with automatic filter change or integrated calculating devices. Basically plan areas can be measured as well as paste, powders and granules (using special devices). The measurement of transparent liquids is possible with a special cuvette device, where the thickness can be set in a reproducible way. The preparation of the sample and the reproducibility of the preparation are decisive for the test result.

7.4.3. Calculation and evaluation

In many textbooks, the color triangle is depicted in the form of a shoe sole, which is mathematically correct; but it has the disadvantage that it does not correspond with the perceptions. The human eye perceives mathematical equal distances between two color locations not always as being equidistant. In the blue-violet area even the smallest distanced variances can be perceived, whereas in the green area far larger distance differences are not differentiated. CIE therefore issued a color distance formula in 1976 (CIELAB, DIN 6174), where the distances of the color differences are nearly identical in the graphical depiction. Figure 7 shows the formula for the calculation of the Lab* value as well as the color distance between the sample and the reference ΔE^*. In modern color determination devices these calculations are done automatically. Push a button, and the Lab* values are transformed into Munsell values (used in the USA). Figure 8 shows, in the CIE Lab* system, how any color can be characterized by the indication of the three values of L:

  L* indicates how light (or dark) the sample is; the higher the value the lighter the sample
  A* indicates the position of the color location on the red-green axis
  B* indicates the position of the color location on the blue-yellow axis

Another characteristic value for the color difference between reference and sample is ΔE^*. Other definitions for the color distance are used as well.

In Figures 9 and 10 there are some calculation examples for a sample pair of blue and green. The determined ΔE^* values were found to be within the tolerance level of a maximum of 2.5. Other tolerance values can be set for different devices and applications.

Equations 1–13

$$X = A \cdot R_x + B \cdot R_z \quad (1)$$

$$Y = R_y \quad (2)$$

$$Z = C \cdot R_z \quad (3)$$

$$x = \frac{X}{X + Y + Z} \quad (4)$$

$$y = \frac{Y}{X + Y + Z} \quad (5)$$

$$z = \frac{Z}{X + Y + Z} \quad (6)$$

$$L^* = 116 \sqrt[3]{Y / Y_w} - 16 \quad (7)$$

Safety and Quality

$$a^* = 500(\sqrt[3]{X/X_w} - \sqrt[3]{Y/Y_w}) \qquad (8)$$

$$b^* = 200(\sqrt[3]{Y/Y_w} - \sqrt[3]{Z/Z_w}) \qquad (9)$$

$$\Delta L^* = L^* \text{ sample} - L^* \text{ standard} \qquad (10)$$

$$\Delta a^* = a^* \text{ sample} - a^* \text{ standard} \qquad (11)$$

$$\Delta b^* = b^* \text{ sample} - b^* \text{ standard} \qquad (12)$$

$$\Delta E^* = \sqrt{(\Delta L)^2 + (\Delta a^*)^2 + (\Delta b^*)^2} \qquad (13)$$

Value for standard white	Filter factor	For standard light	
		C	D65
X_x = 97.28	A	0.7832	0.77
Y_w = 100	B	0.1972	0.18
Z_w = 116.14	C	1.181	1.089

Figure 7 Calculation of Lab* and color distance formula ΔE^*.

Figure 11 shows a very simple test method for pigments; although it does not conform with the test methods for checking pigments, but it can be used for laboratories that are not equipped to test colorants.

For color comparison and color testing there are numerous DIN norms (color determination: DIN 5033, part 1 to 9; color comparison: DIN 6173 part 1 & 2; as well as DIN 53204, 53218, 53235 part 1& 2, 55985). Seminars on color metrics are conducted regularly by the Bundesanstalt für Materialprüfung (BAM) working group 5.4 color metrics, Unter den Eichen 87, D 12205 Berlin or by the supplier of color measuring devices.

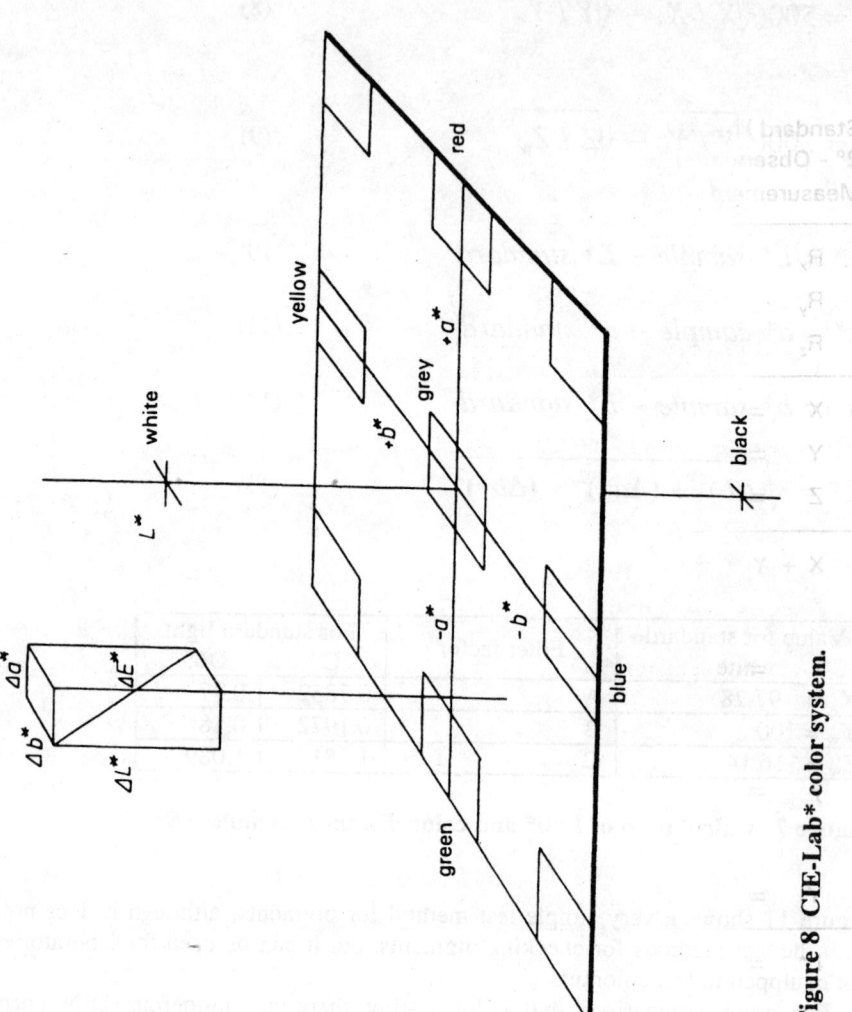

Figure 8 CIE-Lab* color system.

Safety and Quality

Standard light type C
2° - Observation

Measurement of Baryt white standard (99%)		Sample	Standard
R_x	=	42.8	42.5
R_y	=	50.1	49.0
R_z	=	83.0	82.0
$X = 0.7832 \cdot R_x + 0.1972 \cdot R_z$	=	49.9	49.5
$Y = R_y$	=	50.1	49.0
$Z = 1.181 \cdot R_z$	=	98.0	96.8
$X + Y + Z$	=	198.0	195.3
$x = \dfrac{X}{X + Y + Z}$	=	0.2519	0.2532
$y = \dfrac{Y}{X + Y + Z}$	=	0.2530	0.2509
$Y = R_y$	=	50.1	49.0
$L^* = 116 \sqrt[3]{Y/Y_w} - 16$	=	76.1	75.5
$a^* = 500 (\sqrt[3]{X/X_w} - \sqrt[3]{Y/Y_w})$	=	3.1	4.9
$b^* = 200 (\sqrt[3]{Y/Y_w} - \sqrt[3]{Z/Z_w})$	=	-30.2	-30.6
$\Delta E^* = \sqrt{(\Delta L^*)^2 + (\Delta a^*)^2 + (\Delta b^*)^2}$	=	1.9	
X_w, Y_w, Z_w: Value for standard white $X_w = 97.28 / Y_w = 100 / Z_w = 116.14$			

Figure 9 Calculation example for blue.

Standard light type C
2° - Observation

Measurement of Baryt white standard (99%)		Sample	Standard
R_x	=	74.0	73.8
R_y	=	62.5	62.2
R_z	=	28.2	29.3
$X = 0.7832 \cdot R_x + 0.1972 \cdot R_z$	=	63.5	63.6
$Y = R_y$	=	62.5	62.2
$Z = 1.181 \cdot R_z$	=	33.3	34.6
$X + Y + Z$	=	159.3	160.4
$x = \dfrac{X}{X+Y+Z}$	=	0.3987	0.3964
$y = \dfrac{Y}{X+Y+Z}$	=	0.3923	0.3878
$Y = R_y$	=	62.5	62.2
$L^* = 116 \sqrt[3]{Y/Y_w} - 16$	=	83.2	83.0
$a^* = 500 (\sqrt[3]{X/X_w} - \sqrt[3]{Y/Y_w})$	=	6.3	7.1
$b^* = 200 (\sqrt[3]{Y/Y_w} - \sqrt[3]{Z/Z_w})$	=	39.1	37.1
$\Delta E^* = \sqrt{(\Delta L^*)^2 + (\Delta a^*)^2 + (\Delta b^*)^2}$	=	2.1	
X_w, Y_w, Z_w: Value for standard white $X_w = 97.28 / Y_w = 100 / Z_w = 116.14$			

Figure 10 Calculation example for green.

Safety and Quality

> 5 to 10 g of the test pigment (or pigment paste) is blended with 45 g of a glue solution A, and is further added to 100 g of dispersion paint (wallpaper paint).
>
> This mass is passed three times over a triple roller mill in order to achieve a uniform colorant (pigment) distribution.
>
> The paste obtained in this way is then applied onto a white cardboard C with low-absorption properties with a spatula B in a completely covering manner.
>
> After drying, the colorant is then compared with a standard (manufactured in the same way). Comparison is either visual or by using a color measuring device.
>
> A   Glue solution 10 g Optalin wallpaper glue dissolved in 1000 ml of water
>
> B   Spatula Frame type 360, Firma Erichsen GmbH&Co KG, Postfach 720, D 58675 Hemer/Germany
>
> C   Bristol cardboard, wood-free, white, coated, smooth surface, 369 g/m^2.

Figure 11   Test method for pigments.

8 Analysis

During the last 25 years, analytical chemistry has made significant progress. Limits of detection have been reached, which could not have been imagined years ago. The increased environmental consciousness of people has followed in the same way. With the currently available methods, everything can be detected. What do the ppm's[1] and ppb's of an element mean and how are they linked to the consumer?

By using food additives, the natural content of heavy metals should not be increased significantly. If a food colorant is added to food on a level of 50 g/100 kg (which results in a very intensive coloration) and this colorant has a permissible maximum concentration of 5 ppm arsenic, this results in an increase of 2.5 ppb (=0.0025 ppm) in food.

It should be noted that human food has always contained heavy toxic metals. A comparison of the cadmium level in cereal samples from 1835 and the period 1950 to 1979 has shown that the levels have always varied around the same content currently observed.[2] By respecting the purity requirements (see also section 8.1.1) for food colorants, food and drugs do not receive an additional dose of heavy metals.

8.1. Purity requirements

8.1.1. Colorants for food and drugs

Purity standards for food colorants have been established for all member countries of the European Community in the guidelines of 1962, which is still valid today. The revision of the purity standards on the level of the EU is still in the draft stage (as of December 1994).

In general purity standards, the maximum levels for heavy metals, aromatic amines, synthetic precursor products, colorant by-products, water-insoluble parts of water-soluble colorants and the ethyl-extractable parts are defined. Furthermore, the purity standards contain the requirement, that certain elements like cadmium, mercury, selenium, tellurium as well as polycyclic aromatic hydrocarbons and some very specific aromatics should not be found in food colorants. The notation "not contained" means "not detectable." As analytical methods have made quite some progress since 1962 this means not detectable by the methods of 1962. For mercury this means not detectable in 1962; today the maximum value is 1 ppm, and the detection limit is far below.

Specific purity standards are applicable for certain colorants and are restricted to special precursors of these colorants and their synthesis. The general and special purity standards for food products can be found in Table 17. It is the responsibility of the colorant manufacturer to comply with the legal purity standards. In the last few years it has become common practice, that the manufacturer issues a compliance certificate.

---

[1] ppm: Parts per million, e.g., 1 g/ton or 1 mg/kg; ppb: Parts per billion, e.g., 1 g/1000 tons or 1 mg/ton; 1 ppm = 1000 ppb

[2] Lorenz, Ocker, Brüggemann.Weigert and Sonneborn : Cadmiumgehalte in Getreideproben der Vergangenheit-Vergleich zur Gegenwart, Z.Lebensm.Unters.Forsch. (1986) 183: 402-405

Table 17 Purity standards for food colorants (source: Zusatzstoff-Verkehrs-Verordnung, December 20, 1977)

Apart from the described sodium compounds, the purity standards apply to the corresponding free acids, potassium, calcium and aluminum compounds. (1 mg/kg = 1 ppm)

1. General purity standards

Arsenic	Maximum 5 mg/kg
Lead	Maximum 20 mg/kg
Antimony, Copper, Chromium, Zinc, Barium sulfate	Individually maximum 100 mg/kg, in total maximum 200 mg/kg
Cadmium, Mercury, Selenium, Tellurium, Thallium, Uranium, Chromate and in diluted hydrochloric acid Soluble Barium compounds Poly-cyclic aromatic hydrocarbons with three or more condensed cores 2-Naphthyl amine, Benzidine, 4-Amino biphenyl (Xenylamine)	Not to be found
Other aromatic amines	Maximum 100 mg/kg
Other synthetic precursor products (as free aromatic amines)	Maximum 0.5%
By-products of colorants (isomer, homologues)	In total maximum 0.4%
Only for E 102 to E 110; E 122 to E 132 and E 142 and E 151	
- Water-insoluble parts	Maximum 0.2%
- Ethyl ether extractable parts	Maximum 0.2%

2. specific purity standards

E number C number		Purity standard
E 100		
E 101	Lumiflavin	Not detectable
E 102	Colorant by-product	Maximum 1%
E 104	May contain parts of mono-sulfon derivates, partially methylated	
E 110		
E 120	Uniform in chromatography	
E 122	Colorant by-product	Maximum 1%
E 123		
E 124		
E 127	Colorant by-product: Fluorescin; Inorganic iodide compounds	Maximum 3% Not detectable in UV light Maximum 0.3% as NaI

Table 17 continued

E number / C number		Purity standard
E 131	Colorant by-products:	Maximum 1%
	Water-insoluble:	Maximum 0.5%
	Chromium:	Maximum 20 mg/kg
E 132	Colorant by-products:	Maximum 1%
	Isatinsulfonic acid:	Maximum 1%
E 140		
E 141	Free, ionizable copper:	Maximum 200 mg/kg
	Solution in turpentine:	Clear
	Colorant by-products:	Maximum 1%
E 142		
E 150	pH value: minimum 1.8	
	Sulfurous acid (method Monier-Williams):	Maximum 0.1%
	Ammonia-Nitrogen (method Tillmanns-Mildner):	Maximum 0.5%
	Phosphate (as P_2O_5):	Maximum 0.5%
	4-Methyl imidazol:	Maximum 200 mg/kg
	based on product with a color intensity of 20,000 EBC units	
E 151	Colorant by-product:	Maximum 10%
	Synthesis intermediate product:	Maximum 1%
E 153	Cyclo-hexane extract (2 hours 10%)	
	- colorless	
	- practically non-fluorescent	
	- residue below 1 mg/kg	
	Alkali extract:	Colorless
	(20 minutes boiling in 1 N NaOH and filtration)	
E 160a	Uniform in chromatography	
E 160b	Crocetin not detectable	
E 160c to		
E 160f		
E 161 to		
E 161g		
E 162	Uniform in chromatography	
E 163		
E 170		
E 171	Hydrochloric acid extract:	Maximum 0.35%
	(boiling for 35 minutes on 0.5 N HCl, filtration, drying and ashing)	
	Antimony:	Maximum 100 mg/kg
	Soluble Barium compounds:	Maximum 5 mg/kg
E 172	Selenium:	Maximum 2 mg/kg
	Mercury:	Maximum 1 mg/kg
	(both in a 0.5 N HCl extract)	

(continued)

Table 17   continued

E number C number		Purity standard
E 173 to E 180		
C 2	Tetra and Hexa-methyl compound	Maximum 10%
C 3 to C 5		
C 7 to C 17		

8.1.2. Colorants for cosmetic products

Cosmetic colorants, which are also food colorants (and which had the same status earlier e.g., E 105, C.I. 13015) must meet the purity standards of food colorants.

For other cosmetic colorants there are special purity standards in the Kosmetik-Verordnung (cosmetic ordinance). In general they refer to organic precursor or by products that may be found in those colorants.

8.2. Identification of colorants

In the past, there have been numerous publications discussing the identification of food and cosmetic colorants on an individual basis. A comprehensive review "Anleitung zur Abtrennung und Identifizierung von Farbstoffen in gefärbten Lebensmitteln" (Procedures for the isolation and identification of food colorants in colored food) has been issued as communication XIV of the Farbstoff-Kommission of the Deutsche Forschungsgemeinschaft. This work has been complemented by communication XVII entitled "Identifizierung von Farbstoffen in Kosmetika" (Identification of colorants in cosmetics).

Identification of colorants by using chromatographic methods together with spectral photometry is relatively simple, as it is sufficient to identify the approved colorant (as other colorants are not approved and their use is considered a felony). Utilizing infrared spectroscopy (reference spectra are published in communication XVII) is not necessary. It is strongly discouraged to use spectral photometry as the single method for identification. In colorant blends, significant modifications can be observed because of the movement of absorption spectra and overlapping of absorption curves. For example a blend of 85% Yellow orange (E 110) and 15% Ponceau 4R (E 124) cannot practically be differentiated in the VIS spectrum from Orange II (C.I. 15510), but can be done efficiently by paper chromatography.

The identification of pigments is far more complicated than the identification of soluble colorants or aluminum lakes:

> Identification of inorganic pigments is done by the characteristic chemical reactions with specific reagents.
> Identification of organic pigments is done by disintegration of the colorant by using acid or dimethyl formamide followed by chromatography and/or VIS absorption spectroscopy.

8.2.1. Water-soluble colorants for food and cosmetics

There are two methods for the identification of water-soluble colorants, based on the current state of analytical chemistry:

Paper or thin layer chromatography
Spectral photometry

Relevant information can be found in the data sheets (see Section 9.2). There exist two other very simple methods:

> Dripping different reagents on a colored paper strip and observing of the resulting color reaction
> Observation of the solvent color of the colorant in concentrated sulfuric acid and the change in color when diluted with water (note: add acid into water and not vice-versa).

The necessary equipment for the chromatographic and droplet analysis is modest and can be procured with small amounts of money. Paper chromatography is a very old method, and it has been replaced in the modern laboratory by thin layer chromatography for good reason. Nevertheless it is well suited for the identification of water-soluble colorants, as the required analytical reagents are easily available and the developed chromatogram can be preserved after drying without further preparation.

8.2.1.1. Paper chromatography

a) **Material**

> Paper 2043b Mgl Schleicher & Schüll, Dassel
> Chromatography vessel (e.g., preservation glass), solvents (see data sheets in Chapter 9), tri-Sodium citrate-2-hydrate, ammonia 25%, distilled water, reagent glasses, micropipettes (manufactured by the extension of thin glass tubes in the flame of a Bunsen burner), measuring cylinder (100 mL), pair of scissors, and a ruler.

b) **Method**

Normally, the rising chromatography method is used. The general procedure has been described extensively in literature (see Section 10.5). The format of the chromatography paper does not play a role and depends on the dimension of the vessel. The maximum rising height is 30 cm, but even at rising heights of 15–20 cm a good separation is achieved. When the paper is prepared, consideration must be given to the aspect that the flow direction and orientation of the paper fiber are the same. Applying a small water droplet can check this; the droplet extends in the form of an ellipse, and the greatest diameter corresponds to the flow direction.

The starting line is marked with a pencil (about 2 cm above the bottom of the paper) as well as the end of the rising line (about 15–20 cm above the start line). Now a 1% solution of the colorant to be analyzed is prepared and is applied in small dots (diameter about 5 mm) on the starting line. This solution is then dried and the paper is then positioned in the vessel (hanging or standing), which contains the solvent. The vessel should have been filled at least 15 minutes prior to the analysis (filling level about 1–1.5 cm), so that the headspace is completely saturated. The lid of the vessel must closed tight.

Once the solvent has reached the upper pencil line, the chromatogram is removed and is dried. When solvents are used that contain pyridine, the procedure must be done under an extraction hood because of the toxicity involved. Colorants are very often characterized by their "Rf" value:

$$Rf = \frac{\text{Distance colorant} - \text{start point}}{\text{Distance solvent front} - \text{start point}} < 1$$

The reproducibility of the Rf value depends on many factors: age of the colorant solution, age of the solvent, solvent temperature, degree of headspace saturation, room temperature, and so forth. As it is very difficult to keep all parameters constant, it is common practice to use reference colorant solutions.

c) **Evaluation**

If the distances or Rf values of both color dots (sample and reference) are identical, and this is the case when a second solvent is used, then it can be assumed with a very high probability, that both colorants are identical.

An exception to this statement occurs for colorants such as Orange GGN (C.I. 15980, earlier E 111) and Yellow orange S (C.I. 15985, E 110), as the differences in their molecular structure are so small, that a chromatographic separation is not possible. To my knowledge, E 111 is no longer synthesized. There is a description of a method on how to distinguish those two colorants by reduction with Sn-II-chloride solution (in hydrochloric acid) (see communication XIV of the Farbstoff-Kommission of the Deutsche Forschungsgemeinschaft).

8.2.1.2. *Droplet reactions and solubility characteristics in concentrated sulfuric acid*

a) **Reagents**

10% acetic acid, 10% hydrochloric acid, 10% bicarbonate solution, 25% ammonia, 10% caustic, 98% sulfuric acid, 65% nitric acid

b) **Method**

0.5 g colorant is dissolved in 100 mL hot distilled water. A filter paper strip is immersed into this colorant solution and then dried in the open air. The above mentioned reagents are pipetted onto the colored and dried filter paper strip. The observed color changes are typical for the colorant, and can be used for identification purposes when a reference sample is available.

Colorant blends must first be separated with paper chromatography. For this purpose, the solution is applied in the form of a line (instead of a droplet) at the start line. The droplet reactions are done after drying the chromatogram in the areas of the separated line-like color zones.

The solution characteristics are determined in a reagent glass by using concentrated sulfuric acid. Then a droplet of the colored concentrated sulfuric acid is added to 10 mL water.

The reactions of the most common water-soluble food and cosmetic colorants are shown in Table 18. For summary purposes, only the clearly visible color changes are indicated for these droplet reactions.

8.2.1.3. *Spectral photometry*

In a spectral photometer the absorption spectra of heavily diluted colorant solutions are recorded in the visible range of 350-750 nm. The colorants are characterized by indicating the wavelength of the absorption maximum. This information is found in the data sheets (Section 9.2). In Table 19, synthetic water-soluble colorants are sorted based on the wavelength of the absorption maximum, which facilitates the identification.

Analysis

Table 18 Droplet reaction and solution colors in sulfuric acid

C.I. No.	Color of filter paper	Color modifications with							Solution	
		Acetic Acid 10%	Hydrochloric Acid 10%	Bicarbonate sol. 10%	Ammonia 25%	Caustic 10%	Sulfuric acid 65%	Nitric acid 65%	In conc. Sulfuric acid	Diluted with water
14720	Dark red		Brown				Blue black		Blue-violet	Red
14815	Yellow red			Yellow orange		Yellow	Red		Red	Orange
16185	Blue red				Light red	Brown	Violet		Blue-violet	Blue-red
16255	Red					Olive green	Violet		Red-violet	Light red
16290	Wine red		Yellow orange			Olive green	Violet		Blue-violet	Red
45170	Violet red		Yellow				Orange		Yellow	Red
45430	Pink red						Yellow orange		Red-brown	Yellow-red
10316	Light yellow		Discolored			Light red		Discolored	Brown	Yellow-green
13015	Light yellow		Red			Dark red	Orange	Red	Orange	
14270	Yellow orange	Reddish	Reddish		Yellow	Red brown ring			Yellow orange	Red
15510	Orange					Red brown ring	Dark red		Blue-red	Yellow orange
15980	Yellow orange					Discolored	Orange	Blue red	Red	Orange
15985	ellow orange						Orange		Red	Orange
19140	Light yellow								Yellow	Orange
45350	Yellow		Yellow green				Yellow		Yellow-green	Yellow
47005	Green yellow					Discolored			Orange	Green yellow Fluorescent Yellow-green
42051	Blue	Blue-green	Yellow					Yellow	Brown-olive	Yellow
42053	Blue green		Yellow	Blue-violet	Blue-violet	Blue-violet		Yellow orange	Brown	Green
42090	Blue		Yellow					Yellow orange	Brown-olive	Green
44090	Blue-greenish	Dark green	Yellow orange					Yellow orange	Brown	Green
61570	Turquoise			Blue	Blue	Blue	Olive	Discolored	Blue-green	Blue-green
73015	Grey-blue				Green with blue rim	Yellow with green rim	Dark blue	Discolored	Dark blue	Blue
28440	Dark blue		Yellow with Blue-green rim				Green	Green	Blue-green	Blue-violet
42640	Blue violet							Yellow	Brown	Green

8.2.2. Oil-soluble food and cosmetic colorants

8.2.2.1. Thin layer chromatography

a) **Material**

Kieselgel TLC foil or plates (e.g., Merck/Darmstadt, Schleicher & Schüll/Dassel, Woelm/Eschwege)
Cellulose TLC foil or plates (e.g., Merck/Darmstadt, Schleicher & Schüll/Dassel)

Tools and chemicals are described in Section 8.2.1.1 a.

Table 19 Absorption maximum of selected synthetic water-soluble food and cosmetic colorants (enumerated if several exist)

Wavelength	Color Index No. or description	Wavelength	Color Index No. or description
370	1.14700, 1.59040	504	1.18050
385	13015	505	15620
390	18820	507	45425
392	1.10316	510	16255, 24790
404	2.59040	516	14720
405	1.42090	520	16185, 16290
406	18965	525	1.75470
407	1.42045, 1.42080	527	45190
410	1.28440, 40215	528	45430
412	1.42051	530	17200, 1.18130, 45220
414	1.61570	532	2.18050
416	1.42100	543	42460
418	47005	546	42510
420	19120, 19140	554	45170
425	20170	560	50325
426	1.44025	562	2.18130
430	2.10316	566	45100
433	13065	567	2.75470
435	1.42170	575	2.28440
438	14270	577	1.61585
445	1.27775	580	60730, 1.42735
470	16230	582	2.27755
480	15980	584	42535
482	15510, 15985	606	2.42735
485	45350	610	2.61570, 73015
488	14815	612	44045
495	18736	613	20470
497	16035	618	1.74180
500	2.14700	624	2.61585

(continued)

Table 19 continued

Wavelength	Color Index No. or description	Wavelength	Color Index No. or description
627	2.42053	640	2.44025
632	2.42090, 44090	644	3.61570
633	2.42080	658	2.74180
635	2.42045	663	2.42170
638	2.42051, 2.42100	710	10020

Table 20 Absorption maximum of selected synthetic oil-soluble cosmetic colorants (enumerated in case of several maxima)

Wavelength nm	Color Index No.	Solvent
350	21230	1,1,1-Trichlor ethane or dimethyl formamide
352	1.26100	Dichloro methane
390	11920	1,1,1-Trichlor ethane
392	12010	1,1,1-Trichlor ethane
394	12700	1,1,1-Trichlor ethane
404	1.61565	1,1,1-Trichlor ethane or chloroform
494	12150	1,1,1-Trichlor ethane
515	2.26100	Dichloro methane
577	60725	Dimethyl formamide
580	1.61554	1,1,1-Trichlor ethane
592	1.61554	Methanol
604	2.61565	1,1,1-Trichlor ethane or chloroform
628	2.61554	1,1,1-Trichlor ethane
639	2.61554	Methanol
641	3.61565	1,1,1-Trichlor ethane or chloroform

8.2.3. Aluminum lakes

Aluminum lakes of water-soluble food colorants are dissolved in hydrochloric acid, filtered and identified in the same manner as water-soluble colorants (see 8.2.1). Absorption maximum of these solutions is identical with absorption maximum of the corresponding water-soluble colorants.

8.2.4. Pigments

The color of the pigment powder is an indication for the kind of pigment used.

- blue pigments	Indanthren blue RS (C.I.69880), Indanthren blue BC (C.I.69825), Indigo C.I.73000, Phtalocyanin pigments C.I.74100, C.I.74160, Ultramarine blue C.I.77007, Prussian blue C.I.77510
- brown pigments	Permanent brown FG (C.I.112480), in most cases blends of Iron oxide yellow (C.I.77492), Iron oxide red (C.I.77491) and Iron oxide black (C.I.77499), eventually merge together with Titanium dioxide (C.I.77891)
- yellow pigments	Organic Azopigments (brilliant yellow)(C.I.11680, 11710, 20040, 21100, 21108), Iron oxide yellow (C.I.77492) (mat yellow)
- green pigments	Chromium oxide (C.I.77288, 77289), Pigment green B (C.I.10016), Pigment Green 14C (C.I.77436), Phtalocyanin green (C.I.74260)
- orange and red pigments	Organic Azopigments C.I.11725, 12075, 21110, 21115, 12085, 12120, 12370, 12420, 12490, 15525, 15580, 15585, 15630, 15800, 15850, 15865, 15880), Alizarin (C.I.5800), Hostapermorange GR (C.I.71105), Iron-II-oxide (C.I.77489), Tetrachlor-thioindigo (C.I.73312), Indanthren brilliant pink RC (C.I.73360), Hostapermred EG (C.I.73905), C.I. Pigment Red 122 C.I.73915, Manganese phosphate (C.I.77745), Iron oxide red (C.I.77491), Aluminum silicate colored with iron oxide (C.I.77015)
- black pigments	Cola black (C.I.77266, 77267, 77268:1), Iron oxide black (C.I.77499)
- violet pigments	Ultramarine violet (C.I.77007), Sandorin violet BL (C.I.51319), C.I. Disperse violet 23C (C.I.60724), Indanthren violet RH (C.I.73385), Manganese violet (C.I.77742)
- white pigments	Normally Titanium dioxide (C.I.77891), possible are Aluminum oxide (C.I.77002, 77004), Barium sulfate (C.I.77120), chalk (C.I.77220), Gypsum (C.I.77231), Magnesium carbonate (C.I.77713), Zinc white (C.I.77497)
- shiny pigments	Metals such as aluminum (C.I.77000), silver (C.I.77820), copper (C.I.77400), gold (C.I.77480) as well as the other mother of pearl/titanium dioxide/mica blends, Guanin (C.I.75170), Bismuth oxichloride (C.I.77163)

8.2.4.1. Inorganic pigments

The identification of inorganic pigments is performed by standard methods of inorganic analysis.

The identification of Titanium dioxide (C.I.77891), Ultramarine (C.I.77007), Manganese violet (C.I.77742), Iron oxide (C.I.77491, 77492, 77499), Berlin blue (C.I.77510, 77520), Chromium in Chromium oxide, Chromium oxihydrate as well as Bismut and Aluminum has been described in detail in communication XVII, pages 40–47 of the Farbstoff-Kommission of the Deutsche Forschungsgemeinschaft.

8.2.4.2. Organic pigments (without lake)

In communication XVII of the Farbstoff-Kommission of the DFG, pages 47–49, there is a differentiation between lakes dissolved by acid, lakes dissolved by dimethyl formamide, hydrocarbons and phtalocyanines. Pigments soluble in dimethyl formamide can be identified by either spectrophotometry or by thin layer chromatography. Pigments identified by spectrophotometry are shown in Table 21 (sorted as a function of wavelength and absorption maximum in order to facilitate the location in the data sheets).

Table 21 Absorption maximum of selected organic cosmetic pigments (enumerated in case several maxima exist)

Wavelength nm	Color Index No.	Solvent
355	1.15865	Dimethyl formamide
357	1.11725	Dichloro methane
398	15880	Dimethyl formamide
409	11710	Chloroform
411	11680	Chloroform
417	1.15800	Dimethyl formamide
430	2.11725	Dichloro methane
	2.15880	Dimethyl formamide
450	2.15865	Dimethyl formamide
477	15585	Methanol
478	12075	Dichloro methane
480	15525	Dimethyl formamide
482	1.73905	Dimethyl formamide
485	12085	Chloroform
490	15630	Dimethyl formamide
500	2.15800	Dimethyl formamide
502	1.12730	Chloroform
504	3.15880	Dimethyl formamide
505	1.12490	Dichloro methane
513	2.73905	Dimethyl formamide
525	58000	Dimethyl formamide
527	2.12370	Chloroform
530	2.12490	Dichloro methane
535	73360	Dimethyl formamide
562	73385	Dimethyl formamide
568	3.15880	Dimethyl formamide
607	73000	Dimethyl formamide
625	69800	Dimethyl formamide

8.2.5. Isolation of the coloring agent in the finished product and its identification

The colorant intensity of the various colorants for food, drugs and cosmetics permits their application in sometimes extremely low concentrations. There it is possible, in very few cases, to identify the colorant directly and without isolation. This works mostly in clear and soluble products (e.g., foam bath, bathing salt, beverages), and only in cases where there is no overlapping of the absorption curves in spectrophotometric analysis.

When analyzing most of the approved food, drug or cosmetic colorants, it is necessary to enrich the colorant or to isolate them from the product in order to permit a clear identification.

8.2.5.1. Soluble coloring agents

The isolation of a soluble colorant will be successful, when the material to be analyzed is dissolved, and can be bound (after filtration) to an adsorbent. Specifically suited are:

> Polyamide powder which adsorbs all synthetics, water-soluble, acid[3] colorants, betanin, chlorophyll, anthocyan, carmine and water-soluble Annatto.
> Defatted sheep wool thread, which shows similar characteristics as polyamide powder.
> Carboxylmethyl cellulose, which adsorbs all synthetic basic[4] colorants.
> Bentonite which is suitable for the adsorption of carotenoids and Riboflavin and Talcum, which adsorbs Chlorophyll.

a) **Working principle for the isolation of colorants from a water-soluble product**

As a function of color intensity, 0.5–5 g finished product are blended with 10 times the amount of distilled water, the blend is heated, filtered and—if it does not react in an acidic manner—acidified with acetic acid. 0.5–1 g polyamide powder are then added to the solution and mixed thoroughly. After adsorption of the colorant to the polyamide powder, the suspension is poured into the prepared chromatography column; the column is washed multiple times with hot distilled water and thereafter with methanol in order to remove various different byproducts from the test material. Finally the adsorbed colorant is extracted with 5% methanolic ammonia solution. The extract is acidified with acetic acid, concentrated (e.g., by sublimation) and then analyzed with a spectrophotometer or by thin layer chromatography.

b) **Other information**

Communication XIV of the Farbstoff-Kommission of the DFG describes in detail:

> Separation of colorants from water-soluble food and food that can be blended with water, e.g., jams, marmalades, sweets, carbonated beverage powder, liqueurs, gelatin and pectin-containing food products, gelatin capsules, candied and preserved food;

---

[3] e.g., all sulfonic acid groups containing water-soluble colorants such as Tartrazine E 102.
[4] e.g., Fuchsin and methyl violet.

- Separation of colorants from protein-containing food products, e.g., meat, sausages and patés, raw sausage, fish products, dairy products, toffees, marchpane or similar products, egg liqueur, mustard;
- Separation of colorants from starch-based products, e.g., pudding powder, flour, cookies, pastry and pasta products, cereals;
- Separation of colorants from different food products, e.g., color traces in wine and fruit juice, fats and oils, chocolate, chewing gum, coatings made of paraffin, wax or resin, surface coloring of smoked products, truffle imitations in sausage, surface coating of sausages and colored eggs.

In communication XVII of the Farbstoff-Kommission of the DFG, the isolation and identification of colorants from cosmetic products is described for:

- hair shampoo, hair washing solutions and perm solutions
- foam bath, shower gel and cream bath products, bathing salt, bathing tablets, bathing solution with herbs, bathing oils
- mouth wash water, toothpaste, cleaning tablets, adhesion cream for artificial teeth, colorants for tooth coating residues
- lipstick and crème rouge, skin cream
- soap
- nail polish
- eye makeup

8.2.5.2. Lakes and pigments

In contrast to the water-soluble colorants, lakes and pigments cannot be isolated by adsorption from the colored finished product. Fat products and other components of the pigment must be separated from the product, e.g., even soluble colorants, before the pigment is isolated from a residue.

In communication XVII of the Farbstoff-Kommission of the DFG the following general method is described:

For the proof and identification of colorants, a separation of lipophilic substances and water-soluble colorants is necessary. Thereafter inorganic pigments and pigments existing as organic colorants can be identified.

Method
5 to 25 g material is extracted with acetic acid ethyl ester and Dichloro methane to remove lipophilic substances and with methanol to remove soluble organic colorants, filtrate the insoluble pigments (eventually by centrifugation), wash the filter residue with methanol and dry in a drying cabinet. Split this residue into several equal parts (by disintegration of this residue) for the following reactions; the color in itself indicates the type of pigment."

For the following identification reactions see 8.2.4.

9 Data Sheets of Colorants for Food, Drugs and Cosmetics

By extending the first edition, colorants of the European Union (EU) as well as products which are approved outside the EU for various applications, (i.e., the United States of America and other countries) are covered in this edition.

The data sheets of the colorants are sorted according to the increasing Color Index numbers. Colorants without a Color Index number can be found at the end of the chapter, sorted alphabetically by name.

9.1. Explanations of the data sheets

9.1.1. Names

Listed are:

- a known trivial name of the colorant
- Color Index generic name (C.I.) of the colorant
- if available, the name according to the Code of Federal Regulations 21 (CFR21) of the U.S. or the CTFA adopted name
- if available, the Japanese name
- CAS number, EINECS number
  The CAS number (CAS = Chemical Abstract System) is a randomly progressing enumeration of the globally used Chemical Abstract System which is used by the search machine of the Chemical Abstract System and yields all literature information about the described chemicals. For various colorants there exist multiple CAS numbers. Here we use only the one which is mentioned most often in the literature.
  EINECS (European inventory of existing commercial chemical substances) is a multi-volume publication of the European Commission. The CAS number of a chemical corresponds with the EINECS number as long as a manufacturer has registered the product with EINECS.
- In differentiation from the first edition, the names and numbers of the colorants according to DFG (e.g., L-Grün 1, C-Grün) or EU directive 1976 (e.g., Grün-11 II, 2) are no longer mentioned, as it was never implemented with colorant manufacturers as well as their users, and on the other hand, it has no more importance in the EU with the implementation of cosmetic application groups.
- INCI (International Cosmetic Ingredient Dictionary) names: The INCI name of a cosmetic colorant is normally identical with the Color Index genereic name or the CTFA name (e.g., for tartrazine C.I.19140: C.I. Acid Yellow 23 or FD&C Yellow # 5 for the colorant with an FDA certificate).

9.1.2. Chemical name

At a variance to the IUPAC nomenclature and the ring-books of the Deutsche Forschungsgemeinschaft, the chemical name for the colorants is given mostly in the simplified, old way. For the Azo-colorants and -pigments, the name corresponds with the indications of the Color Index. Diazo and coupling compounds are also indicated. The arrow symbolizes the Azo-bridge.

Colorants indicated with (X) are approved in the EU in the described form as well as the Barium, Strontium or Zirconium compounds.

9.1.3. Color and solubility

As a principle, for soluble colorants the color of a diluted solution is indicated; for pigments and paint lacquer the appearance of the powder is indicated.

9.1.4. Chromatography

The Rf-value is not mentioned due to the difficult reproducibility.

9.1.5. Spectral photometry

In some cases, data differ between the Farbstoff-Kommission of the DFG and their own assays. In these cases, both data are mentioned (with indication of the source).

9.1.6. Major applications

Information on major applications is based on information from various colorant manufacturers, the DFG Farbstoff-Kommission and own experiences.

9.1.7. Toxicological and dermatological information

The following acronyms are used :

- LD50   Unless otherwise indicated the acute oral toxicity (LD50 p.o) has been tested.
  i.p.: intraperitonal, i.e., injection into the...
- ADI   Acceptable Daily Intake in mg/kg body weight. The ADI was defined in 1975 by the SCF as 1% of the dosage, which has no adverse effect during a life-long intake during animal trials.
- SCF   Scientific Committee for Food, an organization of the European Union.
- WHO   World Health Organization, an organization of the United Nations.

A summary of the biological-toxicological research can be found in "Kosmetische Färbemittel/Farbstoff-Kommission der Deutschen Forschungsgemeinschaft, 3. völlig überarbeitet Auflage, Weinheim, VCH 1991."

9.1.8. Certification status

The selection of the countries has been done in such a way, from where reliable information was available (see 10.6). In the expanded first edition, numerous countries have been incorporated. For the countries mentioned below, some peculiarities must be mentioned. General statements such as:

"EU-approved colorants are accepted for cosmetics" or
"EU- or US-approved colorants are accepted for cosmetics" etc.

are not repeated in the data sheets. For research on a specific country, it is strongly recommended to check first, if there is any mention in the list below.

European Union	Food :

Until December 31, 1995 the current national regulations are valid. They are no longer considered in the edition of this book. All information is now based on the EU Colorant Guideline 94/36/EU, dated June 30, 1994.

Drugs:
Food colorants mentioned in the above EU guideline are not approved for drugs in all countries for the time being. Detailed information can be found in the data sheets.

Cosmetics :
Cosmetic application groups 1–4 are defined as follows:

Group 1/
These colorants can be used for all cosmetic preparations.

Group 2/
These colorants cannot be used for cosmetic preparations, which are in contact with the mucous membranes of the eye, especially those for makeup removal products.

Group 3/
These colorants cannot be used for cosmetic preparations, and definitely should not come in contact with the mucous membrane.

Group 4/
These colorants can only be used for cosmetic preparations, even when in contact with the skin for only a short time.

Australia	EU- or US-approved cosmetic colorants are accepted.
Chile	·US-approved cosmetic colorants are accepted.
China (PRC)	US-approved cosmetic colorants are accepted.

Costa Rica	All synthetic food colorants are not approved (Permanent Secretary of the General Treaty of Central American Economic Integration, 1983).
Ecuador	US-approved cosmetic colorants are accepted.
El Salvador	All synthetic food colorants are not approved (Permanent Secretary of the General Treaty of Central American Economic Integration, 1983)
Finland	EU-approved cosmetic colorants are accepted.
Guatemala	All synthetic food colorants are not approved (Permanent Secretary of the General Treaty of Central American Economic Integration, 1983).
Honduras	All synthetic food colorants are not approved (Permanent Secretary of the General Treaty of Central American Economic Integration, 1983).
Hong Kong	EU-, Japan- and US-approved cosmetic colorants are accepted.
Iraq	There is no national positive list for food colorants. Colorants which are approved in their country of origin are accepted (1985)
Jamaica	EU- or US-approved cosmetic colorants are accepted.
Japan	"Quasi-drugs" are defined as follows: • Products for a prophylactic treatment of nausea and non-well being, bad breath or body smell • Products for the prophylactic treatment of heat pricks, skin rash and similar symptoms • Products for the prophylactic treatment against hair loss, for the growth of hair and for hair removal • Hair dyes • Perm products • Products which combine a prophylactic effect with symptoms of pimples, skin rashes, itchy skin, rashes, frost bite and disinfection of the skin and other oral areas • Bathing products (apart from cosmetic bathing products)
Canada	US-approved cosmetic colorants are accepted.
Colombia	US-approved cosmetic colorants are accepted.
Malaysia	EU- or US-approved cosmetic colorants are accepted.
Mexico	US-approved cosmetic colorants are accepted, EU-approved cosmetic colorants are accepted too if registered accordingly.
New Zealand	EU-approved cosmetic colorants are accepted.

Nicaragua	All synthetic food colorants are not approved (Permanent Secretary of the General Treaty of Central American Economic Integration, 1983).
Norway	All synthetic food colorants are not approved. EU-approved cosmetic colorants are accepted.
Austria	EU-approved cosmetic colorants are accepted.
Pakistan	Food colorants approved in Europe are accepted (1988).
Panama	US-approved cosmetic colorants are accepted.
Peru	US-approved cosmetic colorants are accepted.
Romania	No information available regarding a positive list for cosmetic colorants.
Saudi Arabia	EU-approved cosmetic colorants are accepted.
Sweden	EU-approved cosmetic colorants are accepted.
Switzerland	EU-approved cosmetic colorants are accepted.
Singapore	No information available regarding a positive list for cosmetic colorants.
South Africa	The application groups for cosmetic colorants are identical in their definition with those of the EU.
Trinidad & Tobago	US-approved cosmetic colorants are accepted.
Turkey	The application groups for cosmetic colorants are identical in their definition with those of the EU.
Hungary	The application groups for cosmetic colorants are identical in their definition with those of the EU. Note: In the majority of cases, colorants are put into application groups with lower dosages.
USA	Soap is not considered a cosmetic preparation.

NOTE: Information received after March 31, 1995 was not considered.

C.I.10006

Name	EU-Nr.	C.I.Nr.	Class	Chemical name / formula
Pigmentgrün B C.I. Pigment Green 8		10006	Nitroso-naphtol	1-Hydroxyimino-2-(1H)-naphathalinon, Iron-III-complex

Color	Green pigment
Solubility	Low solubility in water and methanol, available commercially as water-dispersible pigment
Chromatography DC Carrier	Source : Communication XVII DFG Farbstoff-Kommission Kieselgel Acetic acid ester 11 ml + Pyridine 5 ml + Water 4 ml
Spectralphotometry Solvent Absorption maximum	Source : own assay of the water-dispersible form Water 406, 666 nm, minimum 556 nm
Main applications Cosmetics	This colorant is available commercially as a pigment as well as in the form of water-dispersible pigment - toilet soap (pigment and water-dispersible form) - liquid soap, shampoo, shower gel (only in water-dispersible form)

Toxicological and dermatological data		Source
LD50 tested on rats	> 10000 mg/kg	Kosmet. Färbemittel 3. ed., 1991
Skin compatibility tested on rabbits	non-irritant	
Mucous membrane compatibility tested on a rabbit eye	non-irritant	

Certification status

European Union	Approved for the coloration of cosmetics of group 4 (only short residence time on skin)
Australia	EU- or US-approved cosmetic colorants are accepted
Bulgaria	Not approved for cosmetics
Japan	Not approved for food, drugs and cosmetics
Malta	Not approved for cosmetics
Poland	Not approved for cosmetics
South Africa	Approved for the coloration of cosmetics of group 4 (only short residence time on skin)

Turkey	Approved for the coloration of cosmetics of group 4 (only short residence time on skin)
Hungary	Approved for the coloration of cosmetics of group 4 (only short residence time on skin)
USA	Not approved for food, drugs and cosmetics

For acceptance of this colorant in other countries, based on above mentioned approvals, see also 9.1.8.

C.I.10020

Name	EU-No.	C.I. No.	Class	Chemical name/ formula
Grün PLX C.I. Acid Green 1 Green #401 (Japan) CAS # 19381-50-1 EINECS # 243-010-2	C 7	10020	Nitroso-naphtol	5,6-Dihydro-5-hydroxy-imino-6-oxo-naphthalin sulfonic acid, sodium salt Iron-III-complex

Color	Green solution in water
Solubility	Soluble in water (at 25 °C about 25 g/l)
Chromatography DC Carrier	Source : Communication XVII DFG Farbstoff-Kommission Kieselgel Tert. butanol 40 ml + Methyl ethyl ketone 25 ml + Water 4 ml
Spectral photometry Solvent Absorption maximum	Source : Ringbuch Kosmetische Färbemittel 1984 Water 710 nm (own assay 716 nm)
Main applications Cosmetics	- alcohol-based perfumes, facial solutions - toilet soap - liquid soap, shampoo, shower gel , foam bath

Toxicological and dermatological data		Source
LD50 tested on rats	> 10000 mg/kg	Kosmet. Färbemittel 3. ed., 1991
Skin compatibility tested on rabbits	non-irritant	
Mucous membrane compatibility tested on a rabbit eye	non-irritant	

Certification status

European Union	Approved for the coloration of cosmetics of group 3 (not on mucous membranes)
	According to Colorant guideline 94/36/EU dd. 30.6.96 not approved anymore for food surface stamps and for the coloration of egg shells
Hungary	Approved for the coloration of cosmetics of group 3 (not on mucous membranes)
Israel	Approved for drugs and cosmetics
Japan	Approved for drugs, "quasi-drugs" and cosmetics for external applications, but not on mucous membranes
Korea (South)	Approved for cosmetics
Malta	Not approved for cosmetics
Poland	Approved for cosmetics
South Africa	Approved for the coloration of cosmetics of group 3 (not on mucous membranes)
Taiwan	Approved for facial toning masks, not for cosmetics
Thailand	Approved for cosmetics, but not for application to eyes and mucous membranes
Turkey	
USA	Not approved for food, drugs and cosmetics

Acceptance of this colorant in other countries, based on above mentioned approvals, see also 9.1.8.

C.I.10316

Name	EU-No.	C.I. No.	Class	Chemical name/ formula
Naphtholgelb S C.I. Acid Yellow 1 Ext.D&C Yellow # 7 (CTFA adopted name) Yellow # 403 (Japan) CAS # 846-70-8 EINECS # 212-690-2		10316	Nitro	8-Hydroxy-5,7-dinitro-2-naphthalin sulfonic acid, sodium salt (X)
Color	Yellow solution in water			
Solubility	Soluble in water			
Chromatography DC Carrier	Source : own assay Schleicher & Schüll 2043b Mgl Acetic acid ester 11 ml + Pyridine 5 ml + Water 4 ml			

Data Sheets

Spectral photometry
Solvent
Absorption maximum

Source : own assay
Water
392, 430 nm; minimum at 406 nm

Main applications
Cosmetics
- toilet soap
- liquid soap, shampoo, shower gel (only in water-dispersible form)

Toxicological and dermatological data		Source
LD50 tested on rats	7200 mg/kg	Kosmet. Färbemittel 3. ed., 1991
Skin compatibility tested on rabbits	non-irritant	
Mucous membrane compatibility tested on a rabbit eye	non-irritant	

Certification status

European Union	Approved for the coloration of cosmetics of group 2 (not on eyes)
Argentina	Approved for cosmetics for external applications, but not on eyes and lips
Brazil	Approved for cosmetics for external applications, but not on eyes and lips
Bulgaria	Not approved for cosmetics
Dominican Republic	Approved for food
Hungary	Approved for the coloration of cosmetics of group 2 (not on eyes)
Japan	Approved for drugs, "quasi-drugs" and cosmetics for external applications, but not on mucous membranes
Korea (South)	Approved for cosmetics
Peru	Approved for food
Philippines Poland	Approved for cosmetics for external applications, but not on eyes and lips
South Africa	Approved for the coloration of cosmetics of group 2 (not on eyes)
Taiwan	Approved for facial toning masks (sodium and potassium salt, aluminum-lake), not for cosmetics
Thailand	Approved for cosmetics for external applications, but not on eyes and lips
Turkey	Approved for the coloration of cosmetics of group 2 (not on eyes)
USA	Not approved for food
	Approved for drugs and cosmetics for external applications, but not on eyes and lips
	Utilization requires FDA certificate

Acceptance of this colorant in other countries, based on above mentioned approvals, see also 9.1.8.

C.I.10380

Name	EU-Nr.	C.I.Nr.	Class	Chemical name / formula
Oil yellow AB C.I. Solvent Yellow 6 Yellow # 405 (Japan) CAS # 131-79-5 EINECS # unknown		10380	Monoazo	Aniline→ 2-Naphthylamine
Color	Yellow-orange solution in ethanol			
Solubility	Soluble in ethanol, insoluble in water			
Chromatography	Data unknown			
Spectral photometry	Data unknown			
Main applications	Data unknown			

Toxicological and dermatological data		Source
LD50 tested on rates	< 1.0 g/kg	Communication 6 DFB, 2nd ed. 1957, p. 4

Certification status

European Union	Not approved for food, drugs and cosmetics
Japan	Approved for drugs, "quasi-drugs" and cosmetics for external applications, but not on mucous membranes
Taiwan	Approved for facial toning masks, not for cosmetics
USA	Not approved for food, drugs and cosmetics

Acceptance of this colorant in other countries, based on abovementioned approvals, see also 9.1.8.

C.I.11390

Name	EU-Nr.	C.I.Nr.	Class	Chemical name / formula
C.I. Solvent Yellow 6 Yellow # 405 (Japan) CAS # 131-79-5 EINECS # unknown		11390	Monoazo	o-Toluidin→ 2-Naphthylamine

Color	yellow-red solution in ethanol
Solubility	soluble in ethanol, insoluble in water
Chromatography DC Carrier	data unknown
Spectral photometry Solvent Absorption maximum	data unknown
Main applications	data unknown

Toxicological and dermatological data	**Source**
data unknown	

Certification status

European Union	Not approved for food, drugs and cosmetics
Japan	Approved for drugs, "quasi-drugs" and cosmetics for external applications, but not on mucous membranes
Taiwan	Approved for facial toning masks, not for cosmetics
USA	Not approved for food, drugs and cosmetics

Acceptance of this colorant in other countries, based on above mentioned approvals, see also 9.1.8.

C.I.11680

Name	EU-No.	C.I. No.	Class	Chemical name/ formula
Hansagelb G C.I. Pigment Yellow 1 Yellow # 401 (Japan) CAS # 2512-29-0 EINECS # 219-730-8		11680	Monoazo	2-Nitro-p-toluidine→ Acetoacetanilide
Color	Yellow pigment, available commercially in water-dispersible form			
Solubility	Soluble in chloroform, insoluble in water			

Chromatography DC Carrier	Source : Communication XVII DFG Farbstoff-Kommission Kieselgel benzol 90 ml + Acetone 10 ml
Spectral photometry Solvent Absorption maximum	Source : Ringbook Kosmetische Färbemittel 1984 Chloroform 411 nm
Main applications Cosmetics	- toilet soap

Toxicological and dermatological data		Source
LD50 tested on rats	> 8000 mg/kg	Kosmet. Färbemittel 3. ed., 1991
Skin compatibility tested on rabbits	non-irritant	
Mucous membrane compatibility tested on a rabbit eye	weak, reversible reddening	

Certification status	
European Union	Approved for the coloration of cosmetics of group 3 (not on mucous membranes)
Argentina	Approved for cosmetics, except for application to eyes and lips
Hungary	Approved for the coloration of cosmetics of group 3 (not on mucous membranes)
Japan	Approved for drugs, "quasi-drugs" and cosmetics for external applications, but not on mucous membranes
Korea (South)	Approved for cosmetics
Malta	Not approved for cosmetics
Poland	Approved for cosmetics
South Africa	Approved for the coloration of cosmetics of group 3 (not on mucous membranes)
Turkey	Approved for the coloration of cosmetics of group 3 (not on mucous membranes)
USA	Not approved for food, drugs and cosmetics

Acceptance of this colorant in other countries, based on above mentioned approvals, see also 9.1.8.

C.I.11710

Name	EU-No.	C.I. No.	Class	Chemical name/ formula
Hansagelb 10G C.I. Pigment Yellow 3		11710	Monoazo	4-chlor-2-nitro-anilin →

Data Sheets

CAS # 6486-23-3
EINECS # 229-355-1

o-chlor-aceto-acetanilide

Color	Yellow pigment
Solubility	Soluble in chloroform, insoluble in water and ethanol
Chromatography DC Carrier	Source : Communication XVII DFG Farbstoff-Kommission Kieselgel Benzol 90 ml + Acetone 10 ml
Spectral photometry Solvent Absorption maximum	Source : Ringbook Kosmetische Färbemittel 1984 Chloroform 409 nm
Main applications Cosmetics	- toilet soap

Toxicological and dermatological data

		Source
LD50 tested on rats	> 8000 mg/kg	Kosmet. Färbemittel 3. ed., 1991
Skin compatibility tested on rabbits	non-irritant	
Mucous membrane compatibility tested on a rabbit eye	non-irritant	

Certification status

European Union	Approved for the coloration of cosmetics of group 3 (not on mucous membranes)
Bulgaria	Not approved for cosmetics
Hungary	Approved for the coloration of cosmetics of group 3 (not on mucous membranes)
Japan	Not approved for food, drugs and cosmetics
Malta	Not approved for cosmetics
South Africa	Approved for the coloration of cosmetics of group 3 (not on mucous membranes)
Turkey	Approved for the coloration of cosmetics of group 3 (not on mucous membranes)
USA	Not approved for food, drugs and cosmetics

Acceptance of this colorant in other countries, based on above mentioned approvals, see also 9.1.8.

C.I.11725

Name	EU-No.	C.I. No.	Class	Chemical name/formula
Hansagelb 3R C.I. Pigment Orange 1 Orange # 401 (Japan) CAS # 6371-96-6 EINECS # unknown		11725	Monoazo	2-Nitro-p-anisidine → o-Acetoacettoluidid

Color	Orange pigment
Solubility	Soluble in chloroform, insoluble in water and ethanol
Chromatography DC Carrier	Source : Communication XVII DFG Farbstoff-Kommission Kieselgel Benzol 90 ml + Acetone 10 ml
Spectral photometry Solvent Absorption maximum	Source : Ringbook Kosmetische Färbemittel 1984 Dichloromethane 357, 430 nm
Main applications Cosmetics	- toilet soap

Toxicological and dermatological data		Source
LD50 tested on rats	> 10000 mg/kg	Kosmet. Färbemittel 3. ed., 1991
Skin compatibility tested on rabbits	non-irritant	
Mucous membrane compatibility tested on a rabbit eye	non-irritant	

Certification status	
European Union	Approved for the coloration of cosmetics of group 4 (only for a short residence time on skin)
Bulgaria	Not approved for cosmetics
Hungary	Approved for the coloration of cosmetics of group 3 (not on mucous membranes)
Japan	Approved for drugs, "quasi-drugs" and cosmetics for external applications, but not on mucous membranes
South Africa	Approved for the coloration of cosmetics of group 4 (only for a short residence time on skin)
Turkey	Approved for the coloration of cosmetics of group 4 (only for a short residence time on skin)
USA	Not approved for food, drugs and cosmetics

Acceptance of this colorant in other countries, based on above mentioned approvals, see also 9.1.8.

C.I.11920

Name	EU-No.	C.I. No.	Class	Chemical name/ formula
Sudanorange G C.I. Solvent Orange 3 C.I. Food Orange 3 CAS # 201-85-6 EINECS # unknown		11920	Monoazo	Aniline → Resorcin
Color	Orange solution in chloroform			
Solubility	Soluble in ethanol, ether, halogenated hydrocarbons, vegetable fats and oils, low solubility in paraffin and water			
Chromatography DC Carrier	Source : own assay Kieselgel Benzol			
Spectral photometry Solvent Absorption maximum	Source : own assay 1,1,1,-Trichloroethane 390 nm			
Main applications Cosmetics	- bathing oils, creamy bath shampoos - sun lotion and after-sun products - body- and massage oils - transparent soaps			

Toxicological and dermatological data		Source
LD50 tested on rats	> 5000 mg/kg	Kosmet. Färbemittel 3. ed., 1991
Skin compatibility tested on rabbits	non-irritant	
Mucous membrane compatibility tested on a rabbit eye	non-irritant	

Certification status

European Union	Approved for the coloration of cosmetics of group 1 (all cosmetic products)
Hungary	Approved for the coloration of cosmetics of group 1 (all cosmetic products)
Japan	Not approved for food, drugs and cosmetics
Thailand	Approved for cosmetics
Turkey	Approved for the coloration of cosmetics of group 1 (all cosmetic products)
USA	Not approved for food, drugs and cosmetics

Acceptance of this colorant in other countries, based on above mentioned approvals, see also 9.1.8.

C.I.12010

Name	EU-No.	C.I. No.	Class	Chemical name/ formula
Ceresbraun B C.I. Solvent Red 3 CAS # 6435-42-8 EINECS # 229-439-8		12010	Monoazo	p-Phenetidine → 1-Naphthol

Color	Brown solution in 1,1,1-Trichlorethane
Solubility	Soluble in ethanol, halogenated hydrocarbons, and oils, insoluble in water
Chromatography DC Carrier	Source : own assay Kieselgel Benzol
Spectral photometry Solvent Absorption maximum	Source : Ringbook Kosmetische Färbemittel 1984 and own assay 1,1,1,-Trichloroethane 392 nm
Main applications Cosmetics	- bathing oils, creamy bath shampoos - sun lotion and after-sun products - body- and massage oils - transparent soaps

Toxicological and dermatological data		Source
LD50 tested on rats	11300 mg/kg	Kosmet. Färbemittel 3. ed., 1991
Skin compatibility tested on rabbits	non-irritant	
Mucous membrane compatibility tested on a rabbit eye	light reversible reddening	

Certification status	
European Union	Approved for the coloration of cosmetics of group 3 (not on mucous membranes)
Hungary	Approved for the coloration of cosmetics of group 4 (only for a short residence time on skin)
Japan	Not approved for food, drugs and cosmetics
Poland	Approved for cosmetics
Turkey	Approved for the coloration of cosmetics of group 3 (not on mucous membranes)
USA	Not approved for food, drugs and cosmetics

Acceptance of this colorant in other countries, based on above mentioned approvals, see also 9.1.8.

Data Sheets

C.I.12075

Name	EU-No.	C.I. No.	Class	Chemical name/formula
Permanentrot GG C.I. Pigment Orange 5 Orange # 203 (Japan) CAS # 3468-63-1 EINECS # unknown		12075	Monoazo	2,4-Dinitroanilin → 2-Naphthol, (X)

Color	Orange pigment
Solubility	Soluble in halogenated hydrocarbons, insoluble in water
Chromatography DC Carrier	Source : Communication XVII DFG Farbstoff-Kommission Kieselgel Benzol 90 ml + Acetone 10 ml
Spectral photometry Solvent Absorption maximum	Source : Communication XVII DFG Farbstoff-Kommission Dichloromethane 478 nm
Main applications Cosmetics	- lipstick - toilet soap

Toxicological and dermatological data		Source
LD50 tested on rats	>10000 mg/kg	Safety data sheet Sicomet Orange P12075 BASF

Certification status

European Union	Not approved for cosmetics
Argentina	Approval status pending
Israel	Not approved for cosmetics
Japan	Approved for drugs, "quasi-drugs" and cosmetics for external application
Korea (South)	Approved for cosmetics
Taiwan	Approved for cosmetics
USA	Not approved for cosmetics

Acceptance of this colorant in other countries, based on above mentioned approvals, see also 9.1.8.

C.I.12085

Name	EU-No.	C.I. No.	Class	Chemical name/formula
Permanentrot R C.I. Pigment Red 4 D&C Red # 36 (CTFA adopted name) Red # 228 (Japan) CAS # 2814-77-9 EINECS # 220-562-2		12085	Monoazo	2-Chlor-4-nitro-aniline → 2-Naphthol

Color	Red pigment
Solubility	Soluble in chloroform, less soluble in ethanol, acetone and benzol, insoluble in water
Chromatography DC Carrier	Source : Communication XVII DFG Farbstoff-Kommission Kieselgel Benzol
Spectral photometry Solvent Absorption maximum	Source : Communication XVII DFG Farbstoff-Kommission Chloroform 485 nm
Main applications Cosmetics	- lipstick - Make-up - toilet soap (brown discoloration during longer storage)

Toxicological and dermatological data		Source
LD50 tested on rats	> 10000 mg/kg	Kosmet. Färbemittel 3. ed., 1991
Skin compatibility tested on rabbits	non-irritant	
Mucous membrane compatibility tested on a rabbit eye	light reversible reddening	

Certification status	
European Union	Approved for the coloration of cosmetics of group 1 (all cosmetic products, max. level not more 3% of total mass)
Argentina	Approved for cosmetics, but not for application in the eye area Maximum dosage level in products for the lip area 3%, in tooth care products max. 0.1 %
Brazil	Approved for cosmetics, but not for application in the eye area
Hungary	Approved for the coloration of cosmetics of group 1 (all cosmetic products, max. level not more 3% of total mass)

Japan	Approved for drugs, "quasi-drugs" and cosmetics for external applications, but not on mucous membranes
Korea (South)	Approved for cosmetics
Philippines	Approved for cosmetics, but not for application in the eye area
Poland	Approved for cosmetics
South Africa	Approved for the coloration of cosmetics of group 1 (all cosmetic products, max. level not more 3% of total mass)
Taiwan	Approved for cosmetics
Thailand	Approved for cosmetics
Turkey	Approved for the coloration of cosmetics of group 4 (only for a short residence time on skin)
USA	Not approved for food Approved for drugs with many restrictions (see CFR21, §74.1336) Approved for cosmetics, but for application in the eye area Maximum dosage in products for the lip area 3% Utilization requires FDA certificate
Venezuela	Approved for cosmetics, but for application in the eye area

Acceptance of this colorant in other countries, based on above mentioned approvals, see also 9.1.8.

C.I.12100

Name	EU-No.	C.I. No.	Class	Chemical name/formula
C.I. Solvent Orange 2 Orange # 403 (Japan) CAS # 2646-17-5 EINECS # unknown		12100		o-Toluidine → 2-Naphthol
Color	Orange-red solution in ethanol			
Solubility	Low solubility in ethanol, acetone and benzol			
Chromatography	Source : no data available			
Spectral photometry	Source : no data available			
Main applications	No information available			
Toxicological and dermatological data				Source
No information available				

Certification status

European Union	Not approved for food, drugs and cosmetics
Japan	Approved for drugs, "quasi-drugs" and cosmetics for external applications, but not on mucous membranes
Taiwan	Approved for facial toning masks, but not for cosmetics
USA	Not approved for food, drugs and cosmetics

Acceptance of this colorant in other countries, based on above mentioned approvals, see also 9.1.8.

C.I.12120

Name	EU-No.	C.I. No.	Class	Chemical name/formula
Hansarot B C.I. Pigment Red 3 Red # 221 (Japan) CAS # 2425-85-6 EINECS # unknown		12120	Monoazo	2-Nitro-p-toluidine → 2-Naphthol

Color	Red pigment
Solubility	Low solubility in ethanol, acetone, benzol
Chromatography	No information available
Spectral photometry	No information available
Main applications	No information available

Toxicological and dermatological data		Source
LD50 tested on rats	> 10000 mg/kg	Kosmet. Färbemittel 3. ed., 1991
Skin compatibility tested on rabbits	non-irritant	
Mucous membrane compatibility tested on a rabbit eye	non-irritant	

Certification status

European Union	Approved for the coloration of cosmetics of group 4 (only short residence time on skin)
Argentina	Approved for cosmetics, but not for application in the eye and lip area

Data Sheets

Hungary	Approved for the coloration of cosmetics of group 4 (only short residence time on skin)
Japan	Approved for drugs, "quasi-drugs" and cosmetics for external applications, but not on mucous membranes
Korea (South)	Approved for cosmetics, but not for application in the eye and lip area
South Africa	Approved for the coloration of cosmetics of group 4 (only short residence time on skin)
Taiwan	Approved for cosmetics
Thailand	Approved for cosmetics
Turkey	Approved for the coloration of cosmetics of group 4 (only short residence time on skin)
USA	Not approved for food, drugs and cosmetics

Acceptance of this colorant in other countries, based on above mentioned approvals, see also 9.1.8.

C.I.12140

Name	EU-No.	C.I. No.	Class	Chemical name/formula
Sudanorange RR C.I. Solvent Orange 7 Red # 505 (Japan) CAS # 3118-97-6 EINECS # unknown		12140	Monoazo	2,4-Xylidine → 2-Naphthol
Color	Red-orange solution in ethanol			
Solubility	Less soluble in ethanol, acetone, benzol			
Chromatography	No information available			
Spectral photometry	No information available			
Main applications	No information available			

Toxicological and dermatological data		Source
LD50 tested on rats	No information available	Communication 6 DFG 2. ed., 1957, p. 13

Certification status	
European Union	Not approved for food, drugs and cosmetics

Japan	Approved for drugs, "quasi-drugs" and cosmetics for external applications, but not on mucous membranes
Taiwan	Approved for facial toning masks, but not for cosmetics
USA	Not approved for food, drugs and cosmetics

Acceptance of this colorant in other countries, based on above mentioned approvals, see also 9.1.8.

C.I.12150

Name	EU-No.	C.I. No.	Class	Chemical name/formula
Sudanrot G C.I. Solvent Red 1 CAS # 1229-55-6 EINECS # 214-968-9	C 10	12150	Monoazo	o-Anisidine → 2-Naphthol
Color	Red solution in 1,1,1-Trichloroethane			
Solubility	Soluble in halogenated hydrocarbons and oils, insoluble in water			
Chromatography DC Solvent	Kieselgel Benzol			
Spectral photometry Solvent Absorption maximum	1,1,1-Trichloroethane 494 nm			
Main applications Cosmetics	- lipsticks - bathing oils, creamy bathing solutions - sun-lotion and after-sun products - body and massage-oils			

Toxicological and dermatological data		Source
LD50 tested on rats	> 5000 mg/kg	Safety data sheet Sicomet Rot F12150 BASF (3.12.1985)
Skin compatibility tested on rabbits	slightly irritating	
Mucous membrane compatibility tested on a rabbit eye	non-irritant	

Data Sheets

Certification status

European Union	Approved for the coloration of cosmetics of group 1 (all cosmetic products)
Bulgaria	Approved for cosmetics, but not for application in the eye and lip area
Hungary	Approved for the coloration of cosmetics of group 4 (only short residence time on skin)
Japan	Not approved for food, drugs and cosmetics
South Africa	Approved for the coloration of cosmetics of group 1 (all cosmetic products)
Thailand	Approved for cosmetics
Turkey	Approved for the coloration of cosmetics of group 1 (all cosmetic products)
USA	Not approved for food, drugs and cosmetics

Acceptance of this colorant in other countries, based on above mentioned approvals, see also 9.1.8.

C.I.12156

Name	EU-No.	C.I. No.	Class	Chemical name/ formula
C.I. Solvent Red 80 Citrus Red #2 (CFR21) CAS # 6358-53-8 EINECS # unknown		12156	Monoazo	2,5-Dimethoxy-aniline → 2-Naphthol

Color	Red solution in chloroform
Solubility	Soluble in chloroform, partially soluble in ethanol and oils, insoluble in water
Chromatography	No information available
Spectral photometry Solvent Absorption maximum	Source : Marmion, Handbook of U.S. Colorants Chloroform 515 nm
Main applications	Coloring of orange peels

Toxicological and dermatological data	Source
No information available	

Certification status

European Union	Not approved for food, drugs and cosmetics
Japan	Not approved for food, drugs and cosmetics
USA	Approved for the coloration of orange peels (maximum dosage 2 ppm based on the entire fruit
	Utilization requires FDA certificate

Acceptance of this colorant in other countries, based on above mentioned approvals, see also 9.1.8.

C.I.12245

Name	EU-No.	C.I. No.	Class	Chemical name/ formula
Arianor Madder Red C.I. Basic Red 76 C-ext. Rot 64 CAS # 68391-30-0 EINECS # unknown		12245		o-Anisidine → (7-Hydroxy-2-naphthyl)-trimethyl-ammonium-chloride
Color	Red solution in water			
Solubility	Soluble in water and ethanol			
Chromatography DC Carrier	Source : own assay Schleicher & Schüll 2043b Mgl 2 g tri-sodiumcitrate-2-hydrate in 100 ml ammonia 5%			
Spectral photometry Solvent Absorption maximum	Source : own assay Water 496 nm			
Main applications	hair coloration			

Toxicological and dermatological data		Source
LD50 tested on rats	16 g/kg	Ringbook Kosmetische Färbemittel 1984
Skin compatibility tested on rabbits	no observation	
Mucous membrane compatibility tested on a rabbit eye	no observation	

Data Sheets

Certification status

European Union	Not approved for food, drugs and cosmetics. Approved for hair dying preparations
Japan	Not approved for food, drugs and cosmetics. Approval status for hair dying is not known
USA	Not approved for food, drugs and cosmetics. Approval status for hair dying is not known

Acceptance of this colorant in other countries, based on above mentioned approvals, see also 9.1.8.

C.I.12250

Name	EU-No.	C.I. No.	Class	Chemical name/formula
Arianor Mahogany C.I. Basic Brown 16 C-ext. Braun 5 CAS # 26381-41-9 EINECS # unknown		12250		p-Amino-acetanilide → (7-Hydroxy-2-naphthyl)-trimethyl-ammonium-chloride and splitting of the acetyl group

Color	Brown solution in water
Solubility	Soluble in water and ethanol
Chromatography DC Carrier	Source : own assay Schleicher & Schüll 2043b Mgl 2 g tri-sodiumcitrate-2-hydrate in 100 ml ammonia 5%
Spectral photometry Solvent Absorption maximum	Source : own assay Water 478 nm
Main applications	Hair coloration

Toxicological and dermatological data		Source
LD50 tested on rats	2-4 g/kg	Ringbook Kosmetische Färbemittel 1984
Skin compatibility tested on rabbits	no observation	
Mucous membrane compatibility tested on a rabbit eye	no observation	

Certification status

European Union	Not approved for food, drugs and cosmetics. Approved for hair dying preparations
Japan	Not approved for food, drugs and cosmetics. Approval status for hair dying is not known
USA	Not approved for food, drugs and cosmetics. Approval status for hair dying is not known

Acceptance of this colorant in other countries, based on above mentioned approvals, see also 9.1.8.

C.I.12251

Name	EU-No.	C.I. No.	Class	Chemical name/ formula
Arianor Sienna Brown C.I. Basic Brown 17 C-ext. Braun 6 CAS # 30075-29-7 EINECS # unknown		12251		4-Amino-3-nitro-acetanilide → (7-Hydroxy-2-naphthyl)-trimethyl-ammonium-chloride and splitting of the acetyl group
Color	Brown solution in water			
Solubility	Soluble in water and ethanol			
Chromatography DC Carrier	Source : own assay Schleicher & Schüll 2043b Mgl 2 g tri-sodiumcitrate-2-hydrate in 100 ml ammonia 5%			
Spectral photometry Solvent Absorption maximum	Source : own assay Water 450 nm			
Main applications	Hair coloration			

Toxicological and dermatological data		Source
LD50 tested on rats	8-16 g/kg	Ringbook Kosmetische Färbemittel 1984
Skin compatibility tested on rabbits	no observation	
Mucous membrane compatibility tested on a rabbit eye	no observation	

Certification status

European Union	Not approved for food, drugs and cosmetics. Approved for hair dying preparations
Japan	Not approved for food, drugs and cosmetics. Approval status for hair dying is not known
USA	Not approved for food, drugs and cosmetics. Approval status for hair dying is not known

Acceptance of this colorant in other countries, based on above mentioned approvals, see also 9.1.8.

C.I.12315

Name	EU-No.	C.I. No.	Class	Chemical name/ formula
C.I. Pigment Red 22 Red # 404 (Japan) CAS # 6448-95-9 EINECS # unknown		12315	Monoazo	5-Nitro-o-toluidine → 3-Hydroxy-2-naphthanilide

Color	Red pigment
Solubility	Insoluble in water
Chromatography	No information available
Spectral photometry	No information available
Main applications	No information available

Toxicological and dermatological data		Source
No information available		

Certification status

European Union	Not approved for food, drugs and cosmetics
Japan	Approved for drugs, "quasi-drugs" and cosmetics for external applications, but not on mucous membranes
Korea (South)	Approved for cosmetics
Taiwan	Approved for facial toning masks, but not for cosmetics
USA	Not approved for food, drugs and cosmetics

Acceptance of this colorant in other countries, based on above mentioned approvals, see also 9.1.8.

C.I.12370

Name	EU-No.	C.I. No.	Class	Chemical name/ formula
Permanentrot FGR C.I. Pigment Red 112 CAS # 6536-46-29 EINECS # unknown		12370	Monoazo	2,4,5-Trichloroaniline → 3-Hydroxy-2-naphtho-o-toluidine
Color	Red solution in chloroform			
Solubility	Soluble in chloroform and Dimethyl formamid, insoluble in water and ethanol			
Chromatography DC Carrier	Source : Communication XVII DFG Farbstoff-Kommission Kieselgel Benzol 90 ml + Acetone 10 ml			
Spectral photometry Solvent Absorption maximum	Source : Ringbook Kosmetische Färbemittel 1984 Chloroform 502, 527 nm			
Main applications	No information available			

Toxicological and dermatological data		Source
LD50 tested on rats	10000 mg/kg	Kosmetische Färbemittel 3. ed., 1991
Skin compatibility tested on rabbits	non-irritant	
Mucous membrane compatibility tested on a rabbit eye	non-irritant	

Certification status

European Union	Approved for the coloration of cosmetics of group 4 (only for short residence time on skin)
Bulgaria	Not approved for cosmetics
Hungary	Approved for the coloration of cosmetics of group 4 (only for short residence time on skin)
Japan	Not approved for food, drugs and cosmetics
Poland	Not approved for cosmetics
South Africa	Approved for the coloration of cosmetics of group 4 (only for short residence time on skin)
Turkey	Approved for the coloration of cosmetics of group 4 (only for short residence time on skin)
USA	Not approved for food, drugs and cosmetics. Approval status for hair dying is not known

For acceptance of this colorant in other countries, based on above mentioned approvals, see also 9.1.8.

C.I.12420

Name	EU-No.	C.I. No.	Class	Chemical name/ formula
Permanentrout F4RH C.I. Pigment Red 7 CAS # 6471-51-89 EINECS # unknown		12420	Monoazo	4-Chlor-o-toluidine → 4'-Chlor-3-hydroxy-2-naphtho-o-toluidine

Color	Red pigment
Solubility	Insoluble in water
Chromatography	No information available
Spectral photometry	No information available
Main applications	No information available

Toxicological and dermatological data		Source
LD50 tested on rats	> 5000 mg/kg	Kosmetische Färbemittel 3. ed., 1991
Skin compatibility tested on rabbits	non-irritant	
Mucous membrane compatibility tested on a rabbit eye	non-irritant	

Certification status

European Union	Approved for the coloration of cosmetics of group 4 (only for short residence time on skin)
Bulgaria	Not approved for cosmetics
Hungary	Approved for the coloration of cosmetics of group 4 (only for short residence time on skin)
Japan	Not approved for food, drugs and cosmetics
Malta	Not approved for cosmetics
Poland	Not approved for cosmetics
South Africa	Approved for the coloration of cosmetics of group 4 (only for short residence time on skin)
Turkey	Approved for the coloration of cosmetics of group 4 (only for short residence time on skin)
USA	Not approved for food, drugs and cosmetics

For acceptance of this colorant in other countries, based on above mentioned approvals, see also 9.1.8.

C.I.12480

Name	EU-Nr.	C.I.Nr.	Class	Chemical name / formula
Permanentbraun FG C.I. Pigment Brown 1 CAS # 6410-40-8 EINECS # unknown		12480	Monoazo	2,5-Dichloroaniline → 3-Hydroxy-2', 5'-dimethoxy-2-naphthanilide
Color	brown pigment			
Solubility	insoluble in water			
Chromatography	no information available			
Spectral photometry	no information available			
Main applications	no information available			

Toxicological and dermatological data		Source
LD50 tested on rats	> 15000 mg/kg	Kosmetische Färbemittel 3. ed., 1991
Skin compatibility tested on rabbits	non-irritant	
Mucous membrane compatibility tested on a rabbit eye	non-irritant	

Certification status

European Union	Approved for the coloration of cosmetics of group 4 (only for short residence time on skin)
Bulgaria	Not approved for cosmetics
Hungary	Approved for the coloration of cosmetics of group 4 (only for short residence time on skin)
Japan	Not approved for food, drugs and cosmetics
Malta	Not approved for cosmetics
Poland	Not approved for cosmetics
South Africa	Approved for the coloration of cosmetics of group 4 (only for short residence time on skin)
Turkey	Approved for the coloration of cosmetics of group 4 (only for short residence time on skin)
USA	Not approved for food, drugs and cosmetics

For acceptance of this colorant in other countries, based on above mentioned approvals, see also 9.1.8.

C.I.12490

Name	EU-No.	C.I. No.	Class	Chemical name/ formula
Permanentcarmin FB C.I. Pigment Red 5 CAS # 6410-41-9 EINECS # 229-107-2		12490	Monoazo	N1,N1-Diethyl-4-methoxy-methanil-amide → 5'-Chlor-3-hydroxy-2',4'-dimethoxy-2-naphthanilide

Color	Red pigment, also available commercially in water-dispersible form
Solubility	Soluble in Dichloromethane, insoluble in water and ethanol
Chromatography DC Carrier	Source : Communication XVII DFG Farbstoff-Kommission Kieselgel Chloroform 90 ml + Ethanol 10 ml + Formic acid 98% 6 ml
Spectral photometry Solvent Absorption maximum	Source : own assay of the water-dispersible form Water 522, 564 nm
Solvent Absorption maximum	Dichloromethane (Source Communication XVII DFG Farbstoff-Kommission, assay of the pigment) 505, 530 nm
Main applications Cosmetics	- Make-up, lipstick (pigment) - toilet soap (pigment and water-dispersible form)

Toxicological and dermatological data		Source
LD50 tested on rats	> 10000 mg/kg	Kosmet. Färbemittel 3. ed., 1991
Skin compatibility tested on rabbits Mucous membrane compatibility tested on a rabbit eye	non-irritant light reversible reddening	

Certification status	
European Union	Approved for the coloration of cosmetics of group 1 (all cosmetic products)
Argentina	Approved only for soaps
Hungary	Approved for the coloration of cosmetics of group 1 (all cosmetic products)

Japan	Not approved for food, drugs and cosmetics
Poland	Approved for cosmetics
South Africa	Approved for the coloration of cosmetics of group 1 (all cosmetic products)
Thailand	Approved for cosmetics
Turkey	Approved for the coloration of cosmetics of group 1 (all cosmetic products)
USA	Not approved for food, drugs and cosmetics

For acceptance of this colorant in other countries, based on above mentioned approvals, see also 9.1.8.

C.I.12700

Name	EU-No.	C.I. No.	Class	Chemical name/formula
Sudangelb G C.I. Solvent Yellow 16 CAS # 4314-14-1 EINECS # 224-330-1		12700	Monoazo	Aniline → 3-Methyl-1-phenyl-5-pyrazalone

Color	Yellow solution in ethanol
Solubility	Soluble in ethanol and halogenated hydrocarbons
Chromatography DC Carrier	Source : own assay Kieselgel Benzol
Spectral photometry Solvent Absorption maximum	Source : own assay 1,1,1-Trichloroethane 522, 564 nm
Main applications	No information available

Toxicological and dermatological data		Source
LD50 tested on rats	> 15000 mg/kg	Kosmetische Färbemittel 3. ed., 1991
Skin compatibility tested on rabbits	non-irritant	
Mucous membrane compatibility tested on a rabbit eye	non-irritant	

Certification status	
European Union	Approved for the coloration of cosmetics of group 4 (only short residence time on skin)

Bulgaria	Not approved for cosmetics
Hungary	Approved for the coloration of cosmetics of group 4 (only short residence time on skin)
Japan	Not approved for food, drugs and cosmetics
Poland	Not approved for cosmetics
South Africa	Approved for the coloration of cosmetics of group 4 (only short residence time on skin)
Turkey	Approved for the coloration of cosmetics of group 4 (only short residence on skin)
USA	Not approved for food, drugs and cosmetics

For acceptance of this colorant in other countries, based on above mentioned approvals, see also 9.1.8.

C.I.12719

Name	EU-No.	C.I. No.	Class	Chemical name/ formula
Arianor Straw Yellow C.I. Basic Yellow 76 C-ext. Gelb 25 CAS # 68391-31-1 EINECS # unknown		12719	Monoazo	(m-Aminophenyl)-trimethyl-m-ammoniumchloride → 3-Methyl-1-phenyl-5-pyrazalone
Color	Yellow solution in water			
Solubility	Soluble in water and ethanol			
Chromatography DC Carrier	Source : own assay Schleicher & Schüll 2043 b Mgl 2 g Tri-sodium-citrate-2-hydrate in 100 ml ammonia 5 %			
Spectral photometry Solvent Absorption maximum	Source : own assay Water 384 nm			
Main applications	Hair dying			

Toxicological and dermatological data		Source
LD50 tested on rats	1-2 g/kg	Ringbook Kosmetische Färbemittel 3. ed., 1991
Skin compatibility tested on rabbits	no observation	
Mucous membrane compatibility tested on a rabbit eye	no observation	

Certification status

European Union	Not approved for food, drugs and cosmetics
	Approved for hair dying preparations
Japan	Not approved for food, drugs and cosmetics
	Approval status for hair dying not known
USA	Not approved for food, drugs and cosmetics
	Approval status for hair dying not known

For acceptance of this colorant in other countries, based on above mentioned approvals, see also 9.1.8.

C.I.13015

Name	EU-No.	C.I. No.	Class	Chemical name/ formula
Echtgelb C.I. Food Yellow 2 C.I. Acid Yellow 9 CAS # 2706-28-71 EINECS # 220-293-0	previously E 105	13015	Monoazo	p-Amino-azobenzol-2,4'-disulfonic acid, sodium salt
Color	Yellow solution in water			
Solubility	Soluble in water (at 20 °C about 40 g/l), low solubility in ethanol			
Chromatography DC Carrier	Source : own assay Schleicher & Schüll 2043 b Mgl Acetic acid ester 11 ml + Pyridine 5 ml + Water 4 ml			
Spectral photometry Solvent Absorption maximum	Source : Ringbook Kosmetische Färbemittel 1984 and own assay Water 385 nm			
Main applications Cosmetics	- shampoo, foam bath, shower gel - liquid soap, toilet soap			

Toxicological and dermatological data		Source
LD50 tested on rats	> 10000 mg/kg	Kosmetische Färbemittel 3. ed., 1991
Skin compatibility tested on rabbits	non-irritant	
Mucous membrane compatibility tested on a rabbit eye	non-irritant	Safety data sheet Spezialgelb S Bayer 1986

Certification status

European Union	Approved for the coloration of cosmetics of group 1 (all cosmetic products)
Brazil	Not approved for food
Egypt	Approved for drugs
Hungary	Approved for the coloration of cosmetics of group 1 (all cosmetic products)
Japan	Not approved for food, drugs and cosmetics
Poland	Approved for cosmetics
South Africa	Approved for the coloration of cosmetics of group 1 (all cosmetic products)
Taiwan	Approved for cosmetics
Thailand	Approved for cosmetics
Turkey	Approved for the coloration of cosmetics of group 1 (all cosmetic products)
USA	Not approved for food, drugs and cosmetics

For acceptance of this colorant in other countries, based on above mentioned approvals, see also 9.1.8.

C.I. 13058

Name	EU-No.	C.I. No.	Class	Chemical name/ formula
C.I. Pigment Red 100 D&C Red # 39 (CTFA adopted name) CAS # unknown EINECS # unknown		13058	Monoazo	Anthranil acid → 2,2'-(Phenyl-imino) diethanol

Color	Red pigment
Solubility	Low solubility in water, ethanol, ether and acetone
Chromatography	No information available
Spectral photometry	No information available
Main applications	Disinfection agents

Toxicological and dermatological data	Source
No information available	

Certification status

European Union	Not approved for food, drugs and cosmetics
Japan	Not approved for food, drugs and cosmetics
Taiwan	Approved for cosmetics
USA	Approved only for drugs with external application ("quaternary ammonium type germicidal solutions"), maximum dosage 0.1% based on finished product (drug)
	Utilization requires FDA certificate

Acceptance of this colorant in other countries, based on above mentioned approvals, see also 9.1.8.

C.I.13065

Name	EU-No.	C.I. No.	Class	Chemical name/ formula
Metanilgelb C.I. Acid Yellow 36 Yellow # 406 (Japan) CAS # 587-98-4 EINECS # 209-608-2		13065	Monoazo	Metanil acid → Diphenylamine, sodium salt
Color	Yellow solution in water			
Solubility	Soluble in water (at 20 °C about 10 g/l),			
Chromatography DC Carrier	Source : own assay Schleicher & Schüll 2043 b Mgl 2 g tri-Sodiumcitrate-2-hydrate in 100 ml ammonia 5%			
Spectral photometry Solvent Absorption maximum	Source : Ringbook Kosmetische Färbemittel 1984 and own assay Water 433 nm			
Main applications Cosmetic	- shampoo, foam bath, shower gel - liquid soap, toilet soap			

Toxicological and dermatological data		Source
LD50 tested on rats	ca. 3600 mg/kg	Safety data sheet Basaacid Gelb 230
Skin compatibility tested on rabbits	non-irritant	Bayer 1981
Mucous membrane compatibility tested on a rabbit eye	slight irritant	

Certification status

European Union	Not approved for cosmetics
Argentina	Approved only for soap
Israel	Not approved for cosmetics
Japan	Approved for drugs, "quasi-drugs" and cosmetics for external applications, also in the form of aluminum-lakes, but not on mucous membranes
Korea (South)	Approved for cosmetics
Philippines	Approved for cosmetics
Poland	Approved for cosmetics, but not for application in the eye area and on mucous membranes
Taiwan	Approved for facial toning masks, also in the form of aluminum-lakes, but not for cosmetics
Thailand	Approved for cosmetics, but not for application in the eye area and on mucous membranes
USA	Not approved for food, drugs and cosmetics

For acceptance of this colorant in other countries, based on above mentioned approvals, see also 9.1.8.

C.I.14270

Name	EU-No.	C.I. No.	Class	Chemical name/ formula
Chryosin S C.I. Food Yellow 8 CAS # 547-57-92 EINECS # unknown	previously E 103	14270	Monoazo	Sulfanil acid → Resorcin, sodium salt
Color	Yellow solution in water and ethanol			
Solubility	Soluble in water and methanol, insoluble in chloroform.			
Chromatography DC Carrier	Source : communication XVII DFG Farbstoff-Kommission Kieselgel Acetic acid ester 11 ml + Ammonia 25% 10 ml + Methanol 20 ml			
Spectral photometry Solvent Absorption maximum Solvent Absorption maximum	Source : Ringbook Kosmetische Färbemittel 1984 Water 438 nm Source: Communication XVII DFG Farbstoff-Kommission 425 nm			
Main applications	Unknown			

Toxicological and dermatological data		Source
LD50 tested on rats	> 1000 mg/kg	Ringbook Kosmetische Färbemittel 1984
Skin compatibility tested on guinea pigs	non-irritant	

Certification status

European Union	Approved for the coloration of cosmetics of group 1 (all cosmetic preparations)
Hungary	Approved for the coloration of cosmetics of group 1 (all cosmetic preparations)
Japan	Not approved for food, drugs and cosmetics
South Africa	Approved for the coloration of cosmetics of group 1 (all cosmetic preparations)
Thailand	Approved for cosmetics
Turkey	Approved for the coloration of cosmetics of group 1 (all cosmetic preparations)
USA	Not approved for food, drugs and cosmetics

For acceptance of this colorant in other countries, based on above mentioned approvals, see also 9.1.8.

C.I.14600

Name	EU-No.	C.I. No.	Class	Chemical name/formula
Orange 1 C.I. Acid Orange 20 Orange # 20 (Japan) CAS # 523-44-4 EINECS # unknown		14600	Monoazo	Sulfanil acid → 1-Naphthol, sodium salt
Color	Brown-orange solution in water			
Solubility	Soluble in water, low solubility in ethanol and acetone, insoluble in most of the organic solvents			
Chromatography	No information available			
Spectral photometry	No information available			
Main applications	No information available			

Toxicological and dermatological data		Source
LD50 tested on rats (i.p.)	1000 mg/kg	Communication 6/DFG 2. ed., 1957, p.25

Certification status

European Union	Not approved for food, drugs and cosmetics
Japan	Approved for drugs, "quasi-drugs" and cosmetics for external applications, also in the form of Barium- and Aluminum-lakes, but not mucous membranes
Taiwan	Approved for facial toning masks, also in the form of Barium- and Aluminum-lakes, but not for cosmetics
USA	Not approved for food, drugs and cosmetics

For acceptance of this colorant in other countries, based on above mentioned approvals, see also 9.1.8.

C.I.14700

Name	EU-No.	C.I. No.	Class	Chemical name/formula
Ponceau SX C.I. Food Red 1 FD&C Red #3 (CTFA adopted name) Red # 504 (Japan) CAS # 4548-53-2 EINECS # unknown		14700	Monoazo	5-Amino-2,4-xylol-sulfoacid → Neville Winther's acid, sodium salt
Color	Yellow-red solution in water			
Solubility	Soluble in water and methanol			
Chromatography DC Carrier	Source : communication XVII DFG Farbstoff-Kommission Kieselgel Acetic acid ester 11 ml + Pyridine 5 ml + Water 4 ml			
Spectral photometry Solvent Absorption maximum	Source : Communication XVII DFG Farbstoff-Kommission Water 370, 500 nm			
Main applications Cosmetics	- toilet soap - alcohol-based perfumes			

Toxicological and dermatological data		Source
LD50 tested on rats	> 21000 mg/kg	Kosmetische Färbemittel 3. ed., 1991
Skin compatibility tested on rabbits	non-irritant	
Mucous membrane compatibility tested on a rabbit eye	non-irritant	

Certification status

European Union	Approved for the coloration of cosmetics of group 1 (all cosmetic preparations)
Argentina	Approved for cosmetics, but not for application in the eye area
Brazil	Approved for cosmetics, but not for application in the eye and lip area
Bulgaria	Not approved for cosmetics
Hungary	Approved for the coloration of cosmetics of group 1 (all cosmetic preparations)
Japan	Approved for drugs, "quasi-drugs" and cosmetics, also in the form of Aluminum-lakes, but not on mucous membranes
Korea (South)	Approved for cosmetics
Philippines	Approved for cosmetics, but not for applications in the eye and lip area
Poland	Not approved for cosmetics
South Africa	Approved for the coloration of cosmetics of group 1 (all cosmetic preparations)
Taiwan	Approved for cosmetics
Turkey	Approved for the coloration of cosmetics of group 1 (all cosmetic preparations)
USA	Not approved for food, drugs and cosmetics
Venezuela	Approved for cosmetics, but not for application in the eye and lip area

For acceptance of this colorant in other countries, based on above mentioned approvals, see also 9.1.8.

C.I.14720

Name	EU-No.	C.I. No.	Class	Chemical name/ formula
Azorubin Carmoisin C.I. Food Red 3 C.I. Acid Red 14 CAS # 3567-69-9 EINECS # 222-657-4	E 122	14720	Monoazo	Naphthoic acid → Neville Winther's acid, sodium salt

Data Sheets

Azorubin-lake   E 122   14720   Monoazo -, Aluminum-lake
CAS # unknown
EINECS # unknown

Color	Sodium salt red solution in water, Aluminum-lake red powder
Solubility	Sodium salt soluble in water (at 20 °C about 70 g/l) and methanol, insoluble in Dichloro methane. Aluminum-lakes insoluble in water, soluble in diluted hydrochloric acid.
Chromatography DC Carrier	Source : own assay Schleicher & Schüll 2043 b Mgl Acetic acid ester 11 ml + Pyridine 5 ml + Water 4 ml
Spectral photometry Solvent Absorption maximum	Source : own assay Water 516 nm

Main applications
Food   - beverages, candies, dessert products, fruit preserves, artificial ice-cream
Drugs   - widely utilized, Aluminum-lakes used for the coloration of capsules

Toxicological and dermatological data		Source
LD50 tested on rats	> 10000 mg/kg	Kosmetische Färbemittel 3. ed., 1991
Sensitivity tested on guinea pigs	not sensitive	
ADI-value (EEC-Color Group 1983)	0 -4.0 mg/kg	

Certification status

European Union	Approved for the coloration of certain food (see 2.4.1), drugs and cosmetics of group 1 (all cosmetic preparations).
Australia	Approved for certain food products.
Chile	Approved for food.
Cyprus	Approved for certain food products.
Egypt	Approved for food.
Hungary	Approved for certain food products. Approved for the coloration of cosmetics of group 1 (all cosmetic preparations).
India	Approved for food.
Iran	Approved for food.
Israel	Approved for food.
Japan	Not approved for food, drugs and cosmetics.
Kenya	Approved for food.
Korea (South)	Approved for food.
Malaysia	Approved for certain food products.
New Zealand	Approved for certain food products.
Poland	Approved for cosmetics.

Saudi Arabia	Approved for food.
Singapore	Approved for food.
South Africa	Approved for certain food products. Approved for the coloration of cosmetics of group 1 (all cosmetic preparations).
Switzerland	Approved for certain food products and drugs.
Syria	Approved for food.
Taiwan	Approved for cosmetics.
Thailand	Approved for food and cosmetics.
Turkey	Approved for the coloration of cosmetics of group 1 (all cosmetic preparations).
Tunisia	Approved for certain food products.
United Arab Emirates	Approved for food.
USA	Not approved for food, drugs and cosmetics.

For acceptance of this colorant in other countries, based on above mentioned approvals, see also 9.1.8.

C.I. 14815

Name	EU-No.	C.I. No.	Class	Chemical name/formula
Scharlach GN C.I. Acid Dye CAS # 3257-28-1 EINECS # unknown	Previously E 125	14815	Monoazo	2-Amino-3,5-xylol-sulfoacid $\rightarrow$ 1-Naphthol-5-sulfo acid, sodium salt
Color	Red solution in water			
Solubility	Soluble in water and methanol, insoluble in chloroform			
Chromatography DC Carrier	Source : own assay Schleicher & Schüll 2043 b Mgl Acetic acid ester 11 ml + Pyridine 5 ml + Water 4 ml			
Spectral photometry Solvent Absorption maximum	Source : Ringbook Kosmetische Färbemittel and own assay Water 488 nm, minimum at 400 nm			
Main applications Cosmetics	- shampoo, foam bath, shower gel - liquid soap			

Toxicological and dermatological data		Source
LD50 tested on rats	> 2000 mg/kg	Kosmetische Färbemittel 3. ed., 1991
Sensitivity tested on guinea pigs	not sensitive	

Certification status

European Union	Approved for the coloration of cosmetics of group 1 (all cosmetic preparations).
Brazil	Not approved for food.
Hungary	Approved for the coloration of cosmetics of group 1 (all cosmetic preparations).
Iran	Approved for food.
Japan	Not approved for food, drugs and cosmetics.
Poland	Approved for cosmetics.
South Africa	Approved for the coloration of cosmetics of group 1 (all cosmetic preparations).
Thailand	Approved for cosmetics.
Turkey	Approved for the coloration of cosmetics of group 1 (all cosmetic preparations).
USA	Not approved for food, drugs and cosmetics.

For acceptance of this colorant in other countries, based on above mentioned approvals, see also 9.1.8.

C.I.15510

Name	EU-No.	C.I. No.	Class	Chemical name/ formula
Orange II C.I. Acid Orange 7 D&C Orange # 4 (CTFA adopted name) Orange # 205 (Japan) CAS # 633-96-5 EINECS # 211-199-0		15510	Monoazo	Sulfanil acid → 2-Naphthol, sodium salt
Color	Orange solution in water			
Solubility	Soluble in water (at 20 °C about 50 g/l) and ethanol, low solubility in chloroform			
Chromatography DC Carrier	Source : own assay Schleicher & Schüll 2043 b Mgl Acetic acid ester 11 ml + Pyridine 5 ml + Water 4 ml			

Spectral photometry
Solvent water
Absorption maximum 482 nm

Source : own assay

Main applications
Cosmetics
- shampoo, foam bath, shower gel
- liquid soap

Toxicological and dermatological data		Source
LD50 tested on rats	> 10000 mg/kg	Kosmetische Färbemittel 3. ed., 1991
Skin compatibility tested on rabbits	non-irritant	
Mucous membrane compatibility tested on a rabbit eye	non-irritant	

Certification status

European Union	Approved for the coloration of cosmetics of group 2 (not on eyes).
Argentina	Approved for cosmetics, but not for application in the eye area or on mucous membranes.
Brazil	Approved for cosmetics, but not for application in the eye area or on mucous membranes.
Hungary	Approved for the coloration of cosmetics of group 2 (not on eyes).
Israel	Approved for drugs and cosmetics.
Japan	Approved for drugs, "quasi-drugs" and cosmetics for external application, also in the form of Aluminum-, Barium- and Zirconium-compound.
Korea (South)	Approved for cosmetics.
Poland	Approved for cosmetics, but not for application in the eye area and on mucous membranes.
South Africa	Approved for the coloration of cosmetics of group 2 (not on eyes).
Taiwan	Approved for cosmetics, also in the form of Aluminum-, Barium- and Zirconium-compound.
Turkey	Approved for the coloration of cosmetics of group 2 (not on eyes).
USA	Approved for external applications of drugs and cosmetics, but not for application in the eye area and on mucous membranes.
Venezuela	Approved for cosmetics, but not for application in the eye and lip area.

For acceptance of this colorant in other countries, based on above mentioned approvals, see also 9.1.8.

Data Sheets

C.I. 15525

Name	EU-No.	C.I. No.	Class	Chemical name/ formula
Permanentrot-toner NCR C.I. Pigment Red 68 CAS # 5850-80-6 EINECS # unknown		15525	Monoazo	5-Amino-2-chlor-4-sulfo-benzoic acid → 2-Naphthol, calcium salt

Color	Red pigment
Solubility	Soluble in Dimethyl formamide, insoluble in water and ethanol
Chromatography DC Carrier	Source : Communication XVII DFG Farbstoff-Kommission Kieselgel Acetic acid ester 11 ml + Pyridine 5 ml + Water 4 ml
Spectral photometry Solvent Absorption maximum	Source : Communication XVII DFG Farbstoff-Kommission Dimethylformamide 480 nm
Main applications Cosmetics	- lipstick, make-up

Toxicological and dermatological data		Source
LD50 tested on rats	> 15000 mg/kg	Kosmetische Färbemittel 3. ed., 1991
Skin compatibility tested on rabbits	non-irritant	
Mucous membrane compatibility tested on a rabbit eye	non-irritant	

Certification status	
European Union	Approved for the coloration of cosmetics of group 1 (all cosmetic products).
Bulgaria	Not approved for cosmetics.
Hungary	Approved for the coloration of cosmetics of group 1 (all cosmetic products).
Japan	Not approved for food, drugs and cosmetics.
Poland	Not approved for cosmetics.
South Africa	Approved for the coloration of cosmetics of group 1 (all cosmetic products).
Thailand	Approved for cosmetics, but not for application in the eye area.
Turkey	Approved for the coloration of cosmetics of group 1 (all cosmetic products).
USA	Not approved for food, drugs and cosmetics.

For acceptance of this colorant in other countries, based on above mentioned approvals, see also 9.1.8.

C.I.15580

Name	EU-No.	C.I. No.	Class	Chemical name/formula
Pheliorot RMT C.I. Pigment Red 51 CAS # 5850-87-3 EINECS # unknown		15580	Monoazo	4-Amino-o-toluol-sulfo acid → 2-Naphthol, barium salt
Color	Red pigment			
Solubility	Soluble in Dimethylformamide, insoluble in water			
Chromatography	No information available			
Spectral photometry Solvent Absorption maximum	Source : own assay Dimethylformamide 486 nm			
Main applications	No information available			
Toxicological and dermatological data			Source	
No information available				
Certification status				

European Union	Approved for the coloration of cosmetics of group 1 (all cosmetic products).
Bulgaria	Approved for cosmetics, but not for application in the eye area.
Hungary	Approved for the coloration of cosmetics of group 1 (all cosmetic products).
Japan	Not approved for food, drugs and cosmetics.
Poland	Approved for cosmetics, but not for application in the eye area.
Turkey	Approved for the coloration of cosmetics of group 1 (all cosmetic products).
USA	Not approved for food, drugs and cosmetics.

For acceptance of this colorant in other countries, based on above mentioned approvals, see also 9.1.8.

C.I.15585

Name	EU-No.	C.I. No.	Class	Chemical name/formula
Lackrot C C.I. Pigment Red 53 Red # 203 (Japan) CAS # 2092-56-0 EINECS # unknown		15585	Monoazo	2-Amino-5-chlor-p-toluol-sulfo acid → 2-Naphthol, Sodium salt

Data Sheets

C.I. Pigment Red 53:1 Red # 204 (Japan) CAS # 5160-02-1 EINECS # unknown	15585:1	Monoazo	-, Barium salt
C.I. Pigment Red 53:2 CAS # 67990-35-6 EINECS # unknown	15585:2	Monoazo	-, Calcium salt

Color	Red pigment
Solubility	Sodium salt low solubility in water and ethanol, Barium- and Calcium salts insoluble in water
Chromatography DC Carrier	of the Barium salt Source : Communication XVII DFG Farbstoff-Kommission Kieselgel Acetic acid ester 11 ml + Pyridine 5 ml + Water 4 ml
Spectral photometry Solvent Absorption maximum	of the Barium salt Source : Communication XVII DFG Farbstoff-Kommission Methanol 477 nm
Main applications Cosmetics	- lipstick, make-up - toilet soap

Toxicological and dermatological data	**Source**
No information available	

Certification status

1) C.I.15585 (Sodium salt)

European Union	Not approved for cosmetics.
Argentina	Approved for cosmetics, maximum dosage in products for the lip area 3%, for tooth care products 0.1%.
Japan	Approved for drugs, "quasi-drugs" and cosmetics for external applications.
Korea (South)	Approved for cosmetics.
Taiwan	Approved for cosmetics.
Thailand	Approved for cosmetics, maximum dosage in oral products 6%.
USA	Not approved for food, drugs and cosmetics.

For acceptance of this colorant in other countries, based on above mentioned approvals, see also 9.1.8.

2) C.I.15585:1 (Barium salt)

European Union	Not approved for cosmetics.
Argentina	Approved for cosmetics, maximum dosage in products for the lip area 3%, for tooth care products 0.1%.
Brazil	Approved for cosmetics, but not for application in the eye area.
Japan	Approved for drugs, "quasi-drugs" and cosmetics for external applications.
Korea (South)	Approved for cosmetics.
Philippines	Approved for cosmetics, but not for application in the eye area.
Poland	Approved for cosmetics.
South Africa	Not approved for cosmetics.
Taiwan	Approved for cosmetics.
Thailand	Approved for cosmetics.
USA	Not approved for drugs and cosmetics.

For acceptance of this colorant in other countries, based on above mentioned approvals, see also 9.1.8.

3) C.I.15585:2 (Calcium salt)

European Union	Not approved for cosmetics.
Japan	Approved for drugs, "quasi-drugs" and cosmetics for external applications.
USA	Not approved for food, drugs and cosmetics.

For acceptance of this colorant in other countries, based on above mentioned approvals, see also 9.1.8.

C.I.15620

Name	EU-No.	C.I. No.	Class	Chemical name/ formula
Lissamine Red J C.I. Acid Red 88 Red # 506 (Japan) CAS # 1658-56-6 EINECS # unknown		15620	Monoazo	Naphthoic acid → 2-Naphthol, Sodium salt
Color	Red solution in water			
Solubility	Soluble in water and ethanol			
Chromatography DC Carrier	Source : Communication XVII DFG Farbstoff-Kommission Kieselgel Acetic acid ester 11 ml + Pyridine 5 ml + Water 4 ml			

Spectral photometry	Source : Communication XVII DFG Farbstoff-Kommission
Solvent	Water
Absorption maximum	505 nm

Main applications	No information available

Toxicological and dermatological data		Source
LD50 tested on rats	> 3600 mg/kg	Kosmetische Färbemittel 3. ed., 1991
Skin compatibility tested on rabbits	slightly irritant	
Mucous membrane compatibility tested on a rabbit eye	non-irritant	

Certification status

European Union	Approved for the coloration of cosmetics of group 4 (only for short residence time on the skin).
Hungary	Approved for the coloration of cosmetics of group 4 (only for short residence time on the skin).
Japan	Approved for drugs, "quasi-drugs" and cosmetics for external applications, but not on mucous membranes.
South Africa	Approved for the coloration of cosmetics of group 4 (only for short residence time on the skin).
Taiwan	Approved for facial toning masks, also in the form of Aluminum-lakes, but not for cosmetics.
Thailand	Approved for cosmetics.
Turkey	Approved for the coloration of cosmetics of group 4 (only for short residence time on the skin)
USA	Not approved for food, drugs and cosmetics.

For acceptance of this colorant in other countries, based on above mentioned approvals, see also 9.1.8.

C.I.15630

Name	EU-No.	C.I. No.	Class	Chemical name/ formula
Litholrot R C.I. Pigment Red 49 Red # 205 (Japan) CAS # 1248-18-6 EINECS # unknown		15630	Monoazo	Tobias-Acid → 2-Naphthol, Sodium salt (X)
C.I. Pigment Red 49:1 Red # 207 (Japan) CAS # 1103-38-4 Einecs # unknown		15630:1	Monoazo	-, Barium salt

C.I. Pigment Red 49:2 Red # 206 (Japan) CAS # 1103-38-4 EINECS # unknown	15630:2	Monoazo	-, Calcium salt
C.I. Pigment Red 49:3 Red # 208 (Japan) CAS # 6371-67-16 EINECS # unknown	15630:3	Monoazo	-, Strontium salt

Color	Red pigment
Solubility	Sodium salt very low solubility in hot water and ethanol, Barium-, Calcium- and Strontium salts insoluble in water
Chromatography DC Carrier	of the Barium salt Source : Communication XVII DFG Farbstoff-Kommission Kieselgel Acetic acid ester 11 ml + Pyridine 5 ml + Water 4 ml
Spectral photometry Solvent Absorption maximum	of the Barium salt Source : Communication XVII DFG Farbstoff-Kommission Dimethylformamide 490 nm
Main applications Cosmetics	 - lipstick, make-up - toilet soap

Toxicological and dermatological data		Source
1) C.I. 15630:1 (Barium salt)		
LD50 tested on rats	> 10000 mg/kg	Kosmetische Färbemittel 3. ed.,
Skin compatibility tested on rabbits	slightly irritant	1991
2) C.I. 15630:2 (Calcium salt)		
LD50 tested on rats	> 5000 mg/kg	Safety data sheet Sicomet-Rot
Skin compatibility tested on rabbits	non-irritant	P15630 Ca
Mucous membrane compatibility tested on a rabbit eye	non-irritant	

Data Sheets

Certification status

C.I.15630 to C.I.15630:3

European Union	Approved for the coloration of cosmetic preparations of group 1 (all cosmetic products). Maximum dosage in the finished product is 3%.
Argentina	Only the Sodium salt is approved for the coloration of soap.
Hungary	Approved for the coloration of cosmetic preparations of group 1 (all cosmetic products). Maximum dosage in the finished product is 3%.
Japan	Approved for drugs, "quasi-drugs" and cosmetics for external applications.
Korea (South)	Approved for cosmetics, but not for application in the eye and lip area.
Poland	Approved for cosmetics.
South Africa	Approved for the coloration of cosmetic preparations of group 1 (all cosmetic products). Maximum dosage in the finished product is 3%.
Switzerland	EU-approved cosmetic colorants are accepted.
Taiwan	All above mentioned salts are approved for cosmetics.
Thailand	Approved for cosmetics, maximum dosage in oral products 6%.
Turkey	Approved for the coloration of cosmetic preparations of group 1 (all cosmetic products). Maximum dosage in the finished product is 3%.
USA	Not approved for food, drugs and cosmetics.

For acceptance of this colorant in other countries, based on above mentioned approvals, see also 9.1.8.

C.I.15800

Name	EU-No.	C.I. No.	Class	Chemical name/ formula
C.I. Pigment Red 64 CAS # 16508-79-5 EINECS # unknown		15800	Monoazo	Aniline → 3-Hydroxy-2-naphthoic acid, Barium salt
C.I. Pigment Red 64:1 D&C Red # 31 (CTFA adopted name) Red # 219 (Japan) CAS # 1103-38-4 EINECS # unknown		15800:1	Monoazo	-, Calcium salt

C.I. Pigment Red 64:2   15800:2   Monoazo   -, Copper salt
CAS # unknown
EINECS # unknown

Color	Red pigment

Solubility	Calcium salt low solubility in Dimethylformamid, insoluble in water.

Chromatography	Source : Communication XVII DFG Farbstoff-Kommission
DC	Kieselgel
Carrier	Chloroform 90 ml + Ethanol 10 ml + Formic Acid 98% 6 ml

Spectral photometry	Source : Communication XVII DFG Farbstoff-Kommission
Solvent	Dimethylformamide
Absorption maximum	417, 500, 568 nm

Main applications	No information available

Toxicological and dermatological data   Source

1) C.I.15800:1 (Calcium salt)

LD50 tested on rats	> 10000 mg/kg	Kosmetische Färbemittel 3. ed., 1991
Skin compatibility tested on rabbits	slightly irritating	
Mucous membrane compatibility tested on a rabbit eye	non-irritant	

Certification status

1) C.I. 15800:1 (Calcium salt)

European Union	Approved for the coloration of cosmetic preparations of group 3 (not on mucous membranes).
Argentina	Approved for cosmetics for external applications.
Brazil	Approved for cosmetics for external applications.
Hungary	Approved for the coloration of cosmetic preparations of group 3 (not on mucous membranes).
Japan	Approved for drugs, "quasi-drugs" and cosmetics for external applications.
Korea (South)	Approved for cosmetics (Calcium salt).
Philippines	Approved for cosmetics for external applications.
South Africa	Approved for the coloration of cosmetic preparations of group 3 (not on mucous membranes).
Switzerland	EU-approved cosmetic colorants are accepted.
Taiwan	Approved for cosmetics (Calcium salt).
Thailand	Approved for cosmetics.
Turkey	Approved for the coloration of cosmetic preparations of group

USA		3 (not on mucous membranes). Approved for drugs and cosmetics for external applications, but not for the eye area. Utilization requires FDA certificate.
Venezuela		Approved for cosmetics for external application.

For acceptance of this colorant in other countries, based on above mentioned approvals, see also 9.1.8.

C.I.15850

Name	EU-No.	C.I. No.	Class	Chemical name/ formula
Litholrubin BN C.I. Pigment Red 57 D&C Red # 6 (CTFA adopted name) CAS # 5858-81-15 EINECS # unknown		15850	Monoazo	6-Amino-m-toluol-sulfo acid → 3-Hydroxy-2-naphthoic acid, Sodium salt
Litholrubin BK C.I. Pigment Red 57:1 D&C Red # 7 (CTFA adopted name) Red # 202 (Japan) CAS # 5281-04-9 EINECS # 226-109-5	E 180	15850:1	Monoazo	-, Calcium salt
C.I. Pigment Red 57:2 CAS # 7538-59-2 EINECS # unknown		15850:2	Monoazo	-, Barium salt
Color	Red pigment			
Solubility	Sodium salt soluble in hot water, Calcium- and Barium salt practically insoluble in water, low solubility in Dimethyl formamide.			
Chromatography DC Carrier	Source : Communication XVII DFG Farbstoff-Kommission Kieselgel Acetic acid ester 11 ml + Pyridine 5 ml + Water 4 ml			
Spectral photometry Solvent	of the Calcium salt Source : Communication XVII DFG Farbstoff-Kommission Dimethylformamide			

Absorption maximum	350, 445 nm
Solvent	50% ethanol (source: Kosmetische Färbemittel, 3.ed., 1991)
Absorption maximum	516 nm

Main applications

Food	- cheese wrappings
Cosmetics	- lipstick, make-up
	- toilet soap

Toxicological and dermatological data		Source

1) C.I.15850:1 (Calcium salt)

LD50 tested on rats	> 9800 mg/kg	Kosmetische Färbemittel 3. ed., 1991
Skin compatibility tested on rabbits	non-irritant	
Mucous membrane compatibility tested on a rabbit eye	very slight irritation, reversible within 24 hours	
ADI-value	0-1.5 mg/kg	

Certification status

1) C.I. 15850:1 (Calcium salt)

European Union	Approved for the coloration of cosmetic preparations of group 1 (all cosmetic products). Within the EU, the Calcium salt is approved for the coloration of cheese wrappings.
Argentina	Approved for cosmetics, but not for application in the eye area.
Brazil	Approved for cosmetics, but not for application in the eye area.
Hungary	Approved for the coloration of cosmetic preparations of group 1 (all cosmetic products).
Israel	Approved for drugs and cosmetics.
Japan	Red # 201 and # 202 are approved for drugs, "quasi-drugs" and cosmetics for external applications.
Korea (South)	Approved for cosmetics (Sodium- and Calcium salt).
Malta	Approved for the coloration of cheese wrappings.
Philippines	Approved for cosmetics, but not for application in the eye area.
Poland	Approved for cosmetics.
South Africa	Approved for the coloration of cheese wrappings. Approved for the coloration of cosmetic preparations of group 1 (all cosmetic products).
Taiwan	Approved for cosmetics (Sodium-, Calcium-, Barium salt and Aluminum compounds).
Thailand	Approved for cosmetics.
Turkey	Approved for the coloration of cosmetic preparations of group 1 (all cosmetic products).

Data Sheets

USA	D&C Red # 6 and # 7 are approved for drugs. The maximum daily dosage is (alone or in combination) 5 mg. Utilization requires FDA certificate. Both colorants are approved for cosmetics, but not for application in the eye area. Utilization requires FDA certificate.
Venezuela	Approved for cosmetics, but not for application in the eye area.

For acceptance of this colorant in other countries, based on above mentioned approvals, see also 9.1.8.

C.I.15865

Name	EU-No.	C.I. No.	Class	Chemical name/ formula
C.I. Pigment Red 48 CAS # 3564-21-45 EINECS # unknown		15865	Monoazo	6-Amino-4-chlor-m-toluol-sulfo acid → 3-Hydroxy-2-naphthoic acid, Sodium salt, (X)
C.I.Pigment Red 48:1 CAS # 7585-41-3 EINECS # 226-109-5		15865:1	Monoazo	-, Barium salt
Permanentrot BB C.I.Pigment Red 48:2 Red # 405 (Japan) CAS # 7023-61-2 EINECS # unknown		15865:2	Monoazo	-, Calcium salt
C.I.Pigment Red 48:3 CAS # 15782-05-5 EINECS # unknown		15865:3	Monoazo	-, Strontium salt

Color	Red pigment
Solubility	Calcium salt soluble in Dimethyl formamide, insoluble in water and ethanol.
Chromatography DC Carrier	of the Calcium salt Source : Communication XVII DFG Farbstoff-Kommission Kieselgel Acetic acid ester 11 ml + Pyridine 5 ml + Water 4 ml

Spectral photometry	of the Calcium salt
	Source : Communication XVII DFG Farbstoff-Kommission
Solvent	Dimethyl formamide
Absorption maximum	355, 450 nm

Main applications
Cosmetics
- lipstick, make-up
- toilet soap

Toxicological and dermatological data		Source
LD50 tested on rats	> 8000 mg/kg	Kosmetische Färbemittel 3. ed., 1991
Skin compatibility tested on rabbits	non-irritant	
Skin compatibility tested on humans	non-irritant	
Mucous membrane compatibility tested on a rabbit eye	slight irritation, reversible within 24 hours	

Certification status	
European Union	Approved for the coloration of cosmetic preparations of group 1 (all cosmetic products).
Bulgaria	Not approved for cosmetics.
Hungary	Approved for the coloration of cosmetic preparations of group 1 (all cosmetic products).
Japan	Red # 405 approved for drugs, "quasi-drugs" and cosmetics for external applications, but not on mucous membranes.
Korea (South)	Approved for cosmetics (Sodium salt).
Poland	Not approved for cosmetics.
South Africa	Approved for the coloration of cosmetic preparations of group 1 (all cosmetic products).
Taiwan	Approved for facial toning masks, but not for cosmetics (Calcium salt).
Thailand	Approved for cosmetics.
Turkey	Approved for the coloration of cosmetic preparations of group 1 (all cosmetic products).
USA	Not approved for food, drugs and cosmetics.

For acceptance of this colorant in other countries, based on above mentioned approvals, see also 9.1.8.

C.I.15880

Name	EU-No.	C.I. No.	Class	Chemical name/formula
C.I. Pigment Red 63 CAS # 5858-84-4 EINECS # unknown		15880	Monoazo	Tobias Acid → 3-Hydroxy-2-naphthoic acid, Sodium salt, (X)

Lackbordo BN 15880:1 Monoazo -, Calcium salt
C.I.Pigment Red 63:1
D&C Red # 34
 (CTFA adopted name)
Red # 220 (Japan)
CAS # 6417-83-0
EINECS # 229-142-3

Color	Red pigment
Solubility	Calcium salt soluble in Dimethyl formamide, insoluble in water and ethanol.
Chromatography DC Carrier	of the Calcium salt Source : Communication XVII DFG Farbstoff-Kommission Kieselgel Acetic acid ester 11 ml + Pyridine 5 ml + Water 4 ml
Spectral photometry Solvent Absorption maximum	of the Calcium salt Source : Communication XVII DFG Farbstoff-Kommission Dimethyl formamide 355, 450 nm
Main applications Cosmetics	- lipstick, make-up - toilet soap

Toxicological and dermatological data		Source
LD50 tested on rats	> 5000 mg/kg	Kosmetische Färbemittel 3. ed., 1991
Skin compatibility tested on rabbits	non-irritant	
Mucous membrane compatibility tested on a rabbit eye	non-irritant	

Certification status

European Union	Approved for the coloration of cosmetic preparations of group 1 (all cosmetic products).
Argentina	Approved for cosmetics, but not for application on mucous membranes.
Brazil	Approved for cosmetics, but not for application on mucous membranes.
Hungary	Approved for the coloration of cosmetic preparations of group 1 (all cosmetic products).
Japan	Red # 220 approved for drugs, "quasi-drugs" and cosmetics for external applications.
Korea (South)	Approved for cosmetics (Calcium salt).

Philippines	Approved for cosmetics, but not for application on mucous membranes.
Poland	Not approved for cosmetics.
South Africa	Approved for the coloration of cosmetic preparations of group 1 (all cosmetic products).
Taiwan	Approved for cosmetics (Calcium salt).
Thailand	Approved for cosmetics.
Turkey	Approved for the coloration of cosmetic preparations of group 1 (all cosmetic products).
USA	D&C # 34 approved for externally applied drugs and cosmetics, but not on mucous membranes. Utilization requires FDA certificate.

For acceptance of this colorant in other countries, based on above mentioned approvals, see also 9.1.8.

C.I.15980

Name	EU-No.	C.I. No.	Class	Chemical name/ formula
Orange GGN C.I. Food Orange 2 CAS # 2347-72-0 EINECS # unknown	Previously E 111	15980	Monoazo	Metanil acid → Schaeffer's acid, Sodium salt
Color	Yellow orange solution in water			
Solubility	Soluble in water, low solubility in ethanol			
Chromatography DC Carrier	Source : Communication XVII DFG Farbstoff-Kommission Kieselgel Acetic acid ester 11 ml + Pyridine 5 ml + Water 4 ml			
Spectral photometry Solvent Absorption maximum	Source : Communication XVII DFG Farbstoff-Kommission Water 480 nm			
Main applications	Not manufactured any more, chemically very similar to and replaced by C.I.15985.			

Toxicological and dermatological data		Source
LD50 tested on rats	> 5000 mg/kg	Kosmetische Färbemittel 3. ed., 1991
Skin compatibility tested on guinea pigs	non-irritant	

Certification status

European Union	Approved for the coloration of cosmetics of group 1 (all cosmetic products).
Brazil	Not approved for food and cosmetics.
Hungary	Approved for the coloration of cosmetics of group 1 (all cosmetic products).
Iran	Approved for food.
Japan	Not approved for food, drugs and cosmetics.
South Africa	Approved for the coloration of cosmetics of group 1 (all cosmetic products).
Thailand	Approved for cosmetics.
Turkey	Approved for the coloration of cosmetics of group 1 (all cosmetic products).
USA	Not approved for food, drugs and cosmetics.

For acceptance of this colorant in other countries, based on above mentioned approvals, see also 9.1.8.

C.I.15985

Name	EU-No.	C.I. No.	Class	Chemical name/formula
Gelborange S C.I. Food Yellow 3 FD&C Yellow # 6 (CTFA adopted name) Yellow # 5 (Japan) CAS # 2783-94-0 EINECS # 220-491-7	E 110	15985	Monoazo	Sulfanil acid → Schaeffer's acid, Sodium salt, (X)
Gelborange-Lack C.I.Pigment Yellow 104 CAS # 15790-07-5 EINECS # 239-888-1		15985:1	Monoazo	-, Aluminum lake
Color	Sodium salt yellow-orange solution in water, Aluminum lake yellow-orange powder.			
Solubility	Sodium salt soluble in water (at 20 °C about 70 g/l), Aluminum lake insoluble in water, soluble in diluted hydrochloric acid			

Chromatography	Source : own assay
DC	Schleicher & Schüll 2043 b Mgl
Carrier	Acetic acid ester 11 ml + Pyridine 5 ml + Water 4 ml

Spectral photometry	Source : Kosmetische Färbemittel, 3.ed., 1991
Solvent	Water
Absorption maximum	480 nm

Main applications	
Food	- Beverages, candies, dessert products, artificial honey, artificial ice-cream, fruit preserves, fish products.
Drugs	- General utilization, Aluminum lake used for the coloration of capsules.
Cosmetics	- Alcohol-based perfumes, insufficient light stability in products containing tensides.

Toxicological and dermatological data		Source
LD50 tested on rats	> 10000 mg/kg	Kosmetische Färbemittel 3. ed., 1991
Skin compatibility tested on rabbit's	non-irritant	
Mucous membrane compatibility tested on rabbit's eye	non-irritant	
ADI-value (SCF 1975)	0-2.5 mg/kg	

Certification status

European Union	Approved for defined food products (see 2.4.1.) and for the coloration of drugs and cosmetic preparations of group 1 (all cosmetic products).
Argentina	Approved for food.
	Approved for cosmetics, but not for application in the eye area.
Australia	Approved for defined food products.
Austria	Approved for defined food products.
Brazil	Approved for food.
	Approved for cosmetics, but not for application in the eye area.
Canada	Approved for defined food products.
Chile	Approved for food.
Colombia	Approved for food.
Cyprus	Approved for defined food products.
Dominican Republic	Approved for food.
Egypt	Approved for food.
Finland	Not approved for food and drugs.
Hungary	Approved for defined food products.
	Approved for the coloration of cosmetic preparations of group 1 (all cosmetic products).

India	Approved for food.
Indonesia	Approved for food.
Iran	Approved for food.
Israel	Approved for food.
Japan	Approved for defined food products, also in the form of Aluminum lakes.
	Approved for drugs, "quasi-drugs" and cosmetics for external applications, also in the form of Aluminum-, Barium- and Zirconium lakes.
Kenya	Approved for food.
Korea (South)	Approved for food and cosmetics.
Kuwait	Approved for food.
Malaysia	Approved for defined food products.
Malta	Approved for food.
Mexico	Approved for defined food products.
New Zealand	Approved for defined food products.
Peru	Approved for food.
Philippines	Approved for cosmetics, but not for application in the eye area.
Poland	Approved for food and cosmetics.
Saudi Arabia	Approved for food.
Singapore	Approved for food.
South Africa	Approved for the coloration of defined food products.
	Approved for the coloration of cosmetics of group 1 (all cosmetic products).
Sudan	Approved for food.
Sweden	Approved for defined food products.
Switzerland	Approved for defined food products and drugs.
Syria	Approved for food.
Taiwan	Approved for defined food products.
	Approved for cosmetics, also in the form of Aluminum-, Barium- and Zirconium lakes.
Thailand	Approved for food, approval status for cosmetics not clear.
Tunisia	Approved for defined food products.
Turkey	Approved for defined food products.
	Approved for the coloration of cosmetic preparations of group 1 (all cosmetic products).
Uruguay	Approved for food.
United Arab Emirates	Approved for food.
USA	Approved for defined food products, drugs and cosmetics, but not for application in the eye area.
	Utilization requires FDA certificate.
Venezuela	Approved for food.
	Approved for cosmetics, but not for application in the eye area.
Zambia	Approved for food.

For acceptance of this colorant in other countries, based on above mentioned approvals, see also 9.1.8.

C.I.16035

Name	EU-No.	C.I. No.	Class	Chemical name/ formula
Allura Rot C.I. Food Red 17 FD&C Red # 40 (CTFA adopted name) CAS # 25956-17-6 EINECS # 247-368-0	E 129	16035	Monoazo	4-Amino-5-methoxy-o-toluol sulfo acid → Schaeffer's acid, Sodium salt
Color	Red solution in water			
Solubility	Soluble in water (at 20 °C about 200 g/l and in glycerin (at 20 °C about 30 g/l), low solubility in ethanol (< 1 g/l)			
Chromatography DC Carrier	Source : Communication XVII DFG Farbstoff-Kommission Kieselgel Acetic acid ester 11 ml + Pyridine 5 ml + Water 4 ml			
Spectral photometry Solvent Absorption maximum	Source : Ringbook Kosmetische Färbemittel, 3.ed., 1991 Water 497 nm			
Main applications Food Cosmetics	- Candies, dessert products, beverages - Shampoos, foam bath, shower gel - Liquid soap - Alcohol-based perfumes			

Toxicological and dermatological data		Source
LD50 tested on rats	> 10000 mg/kg	Kosmetische Färbemittel 3. ed., 1991
Skin compatibility tested on rabbits	non-irritant	
Mucous membrane compatibility tested on a rabbit eye	non-irritant	
ADI-value (SCF 1975)	0-7 mg/kg	

Certification status	
European Union	Approved for the coloration of defined food products (see 2.4.1.) and for the coloration of cosmetic preparations of group 1 (all cosmetic products).
Argentina	Approved for cosmetics, but not for application in the eye area.
Australia	Approved for defined food products.

Brazil	Approved for defined food products.
	Approved for cosmetics, but not for application in the eye area.
Bulgaria	Not approved for food, drugs and cosmetics.
Canada	Approved for defined food products.
Chile	Approved for food.
Hungary	Approved for the coloration of cosmetic preparations of group 1 (all cosmetic products).
Japan	Not approved for food, drugs and cosmetics.
Korea (South)	Approved for food and cosmetics.
Kuwait	Approved for food.
New Zealand	Approved for defined food products.
Philippines	Approved not for food.
	Approved for cosmetics, but not for application in the eye area.
Poland	Approved for food and cosmetics.
Saudi Arabia	Approved for food.
Singapore	Approved for food.
South Africa	Approved for defined food products.
	Approved for the coloration of cosmetic preparations of group 1 (all cosmetic products).
Taiwan	Approved for defined food products and for cosmetics.
Turkey	Approved for the coloration of cosmetic preparations of group 1 (all cosmetic products).
United Arab Emirates	Approved for food.
USA	Approved for defined food products, drugs and cosmetics, but not for application in the eye area.
	Utilization requires FDA certificate.
Venezuela	Approved for cosmetics, but not for application in the eye area.

For acceptance of this colorant in other countries, based on above mentioned approvals, see also 9.1.8.

C.I.16045

Name	EU-No.	C.I. No.	Class	Chemical name/ formula
Echtrot E C.I. Food Red 4 C.I. Acid Red 13 CAS # unknown EINECS # unknown		16045	Monoazo	Naphthion-acid → Schaeffer's acid. Sodium salt
Color	Red solution in water			
Solubility	Soluble in water (at 20 °C about 70 g/l). Low solubility in ethanol. Very low solubility in acetone.			

Chromatography	No information available.
Spectral photometry	No information available.
Main applications	Utilized in Europe before 1963 as a food colorant

Toxicological and dermatological data	Source
No information available.	

Certification status

European Union	Not approved for food, drugs and cosmetics.
Japan	Not approved for food, drugs and cosmetics.
Taiwan	Approved for cosmetics.
USA	Not approved for food, drugs and cosmetics.

This colorant is not included in other positive lists of other nations.

C.I.16150

Name	EU-No.	C.I. No.	Class	Chemical name/ formula
Ponceau MX C.I. Acid Red 26 C.I. Food Red 5 Red # 503 (Japan) CAS # 3761-53-3 EINECS # unknown		16150	Monoazo	2,4-Xylidine → R-acid, Sodium salt
Color	Red solution in water.			
Solubility	Soluble in water. Low solubility in ethanol and acetone, insoluble in other organic solvents.			
Chromatography	No information available.			
Spectral photometry	No information available.			
Main applications	No information available.			

Toxicological and dermatological data	Source
No information available.	

Data Sheets

Certification status

European Union	Not approved for food, drugs and cosmetics.
Japan	Approved for drugs, "quasi-drugs" and cosmetics for external applications, also in the form of Aluminum lake, but not on mucous membranes.
Korea (South)	Approved for cosmetics.
Taiwan	Approved for facial toning masks, also in the form of Aluminum lake, but not for cosmetics.
USA	Not approved for food, drugs and cosmetics.

For acceptance of this colorant in other countries, based on above mentioned approvals, see 9.1.8.

C.I.16155

Name	EU-No.	C.I. No.	Class	Chemical name/formula
Ponceau 3R C.I. Acid Dye Red # 502 (Japan) CAS # 3564-09-8 EINECS # unknown		16155	Monoazo	2,4,5 Trimethylaniline → R-acid, Sodium salt

Color	Red solution in water.
Solubility	Soluble in water, low solubility in ethanol.
Chromatography	No information available.
Spectral photometry	No information available.
Main applications	No information available.

Toxicological and dermatological data	Source
No information available.	

Certification status

European Union	Not approved for food, drugs and cosmetics.
Japan	Approved for drugs, "quasi-drugs" and cosmetics for external applications, also in the form of Aluminum lake, but not on mucous membranes.
Korea (South)	Not approved for food, drugs and cosmetics.

Taiwan Approved for facial toning masks, also in the form of Aluminum lake, but not for cosmetics.
USA Not approved for food, drugs and cosmetics.
For acceptance of this colorant in other countries, based on above mentioned approvals, see 9.1.8.

C.I.16185

Name	EU-No.	C.I. No.	Class	Chemical name/formula
Amaranth C.I. Food Red 6 C.I. Acid Red 27 Red # 2 (Japan) CAS # 915-67-30 EINECS # 213-022-2	E 110	16185	Monoazo	Naphthion acid → R-acid, Sodium salt,
Amaranth-Lack CAS # unknown EINECS # unknown		16185:1	Monoazo	-, Aluminum lake
Color	Sodium salt red solution in water, Aluminum lake red powder.			
Solubility	Sodium salt soluble in water (at 20 °C about 70 g/l), low solubility in methanol. Aluminum lake insoluble in water, soluble in diluted hydrochloric acid.			
Chromatography DC Carrier	Source : own assay Schleicher & Schüll 2043 b Mgl Acetic acid ester 11 ml + Pyridine 5 ml + Water 4 ml			
Spectral photometry Solvent Absorption maximum	Source : own assay Water 520 nm			
Main applications Food Drugs Cosmetics	- Beverages, candies, dessert products, artificial honey, fruit preserves. - General utilization, Aluminum lake used for the coloration of capsules. - Shampoo, foam bath, shower gel. - Liquid soap.			

Data Sheets

Toxicological and dermatological data		Source
LD50 tested on rats	6000 mg/kg	Kosmetische Färbemittel 3. ed., 1991
Skin compatibility tested on rabbits	non-irritant	
Mucous membrane compatibility tested on rabbit's eye	non-irritant	
ADI-value (EEC Color Group 1983)	0-0.8 mg/kg	
(CIAA Liste Mouton)	0-0.5 mg/kg	

Certification status

European Union	Approved for defined food products (see 2.4.1.) and for the coloration of drugs and cosmetic preparations of group 1 (all cosmetic products).
Argentina	Approved for food.
Australia	Approved for defined food products.
Austria	Not approved for food.
Brazil	Approved for defined food products.
Canada	Approved for defined food products.
Chile	Not approved any more for food.
Colombia	Approved for food.
Dominican Republic	Approved for food.
Egypt	Not approved any more for food.
Hungary	Approved for defined food products. Approved for the coloration of cosmetic preparations of group 1 (all cosmetic products).
India	Not approved any more for food.
Indonesia	Approved for food.
Iran	Approved for food.
Israel	Not approved for food, drugs and cosmetics.
Japan	Approved for defined food products, also in the form of Aluminum lakes. Approved for drugs, quasi-drugs and cosmetics for external applications, also in the form of Aluminum lake.
Korea (South)	Approved for cosmetics.
New Zealand	Approved for defined food products.
Peru	Approved for food.
Philippines	Approved for food and cosmetics.
Poland	Approved for cosmetics.
Singapore	Approved for food.
South Africa	Not approved for food. Approved for the coloration of cosmetic preparations of group 1 (all cosmetic products).
Sweden	Approved for defined food products.
Switzerland	Approved for food and drugs.
Syria	Approved for food.
Turkey	Approved for the coloration of cosmetic preparations of group 1 (all cosmetic products).

USA	Not approved for food, drugs and cosmetics.
Venezuela	Approved for food.
Zambia	Approved for food.

For acceptance of this colorant in other countries, based on above mentioned approvals, see also 9.1.8.

C.I.16230

Name	EU-No.	C.I. No.	Class	Chemical name/formula
Orange GG C.I. Food Orange 4 C.I. Acid Orange 10 CAS # 1936-15-8 EINECS # unknown		16230	Monoazo	Aniline → G-acid, Sodium salt,
Color	Orange solution in water			
Solubility	Soluble in water, low solubility in ethanol.			
Chromatography DC Carrier	Source : Communication XVII DFG Farbstoff-Kommission Kieselgel Acetic acid ester 11 ml + Pyridine 5 ml + Water 4 ml			
Spectral photometry Solvent Absorption maximum	Source : Communication XVII DFG Farbstoff-Kommission Water 470 nm			
Main applications	No information available.			

Toxicological and dermatological data		Source
LD50 tested on rats	>5000 mg/kg	Safety data sheet Sandolan Orange E-GL 150 %, SANDOZ (1984)
Skin compatibility tested on rabbits	slightly irritating	
Mucous membrane compatibility tested on a rabbit eye	non-irritant	

Certification status	
European Union	Approved for the coloration of cosmetics of group 3 (not on mucous membranes).
Hungary	Approved for the coloration of cosmetics of group 3 (not on mucous membranes).

Japan	Not approved for food, drugs and cosmetics.
South Africa	Approved for the coloration of cosmetics of group 3 (not on mucous membranes).
Turkey	Approved for the coloration of cosmetics of group 3 (not on mucous membranes).
USA	Not approved for food, drugs and cosmetics.

For acceptance of this colorant in other countries, based on above mentioned approvals, see also 9.1.8.

C.I.16255

Name	EU-No.	C.I. No.	Class	Chemical name/formula
Ponceau 4R C.I. Food Red 7 C.I. Acid Red 18 CAS # 2611-82-7 EINECS # 220-036-2	E 124	16255	Monoazo	Naphthion acid → G-acid, Sodium salt, (X)
Ponceau 4R lake CAS # 12227-64-4 EINECS # 235-438-3	E 124	16255:1	Monoazo	-, Aluminum lake

For this colorant the term "Cochenillerot A" is used sometimes which can lead to confusion with the natural cochineal (C.I.75470).

Color	Sodium salt red solution in water, Aluminum lake red powder.
Solubility	Sodium salt soluble in water (at 20 °C about 100 g/l), low solubility in methanol. Aluminum lake insoluble in water, soluble in diluted hydrochloric acid.
Chromatography DC Carrier	Source : own assay Schleicher & Schüll 2043 b Mgl Acetic acid ester 11 ml + Pyridine 5 ml + Water 4 ml
Spectral photometry Solvent Absorption maximum	Source : own assay Water 510 nm
Main applications Food	- Beverages, candies, dessert products, artificial honey, fish products.

Drugs	- General utilization, Aluminum lake used for the coloration of capsules.	
Cosmetics	- Shampoo, foam bath, shower gel. - Liquid soap. - Alcohol-based perfumes.	

Toxicological and dermatological data		Source
LD50 tested on rats	> 8000mg/kg	Ringbook Kosmetische Färbemittel 3. ed., 1991
Skin compatibility tested on rabbits	non-irritant	
Mucous membrane compatibility tested on a rabbit eye	non-irritant	
ADI-value (EEC Color Group 1983)	0-4.0 mg/kg	

Certification status

European Union	Approved for defined food products (see 2.4.1.) and for the coloration of drugs and cosmetic preparations of group 1 (all cosmetic products).
Australia	Approved for food products.
Austria	Approved for defined food products.
Brazil	Approved for defined food products.
Chile	Approved for food.
Colombia	Approved for food.
Cyprus	Approved for defined food products.
Egypt	Approved for food.
Finland	Not approved for food and drugs.
Hungary	Approved for the coloration of cosmetics of group 1 (all cosmetic products).
India	Approved for food.
Indonesia	Approved for food.
Iran	Approved for food.
Israel	Approved for food, drugs and cosmetics.
Japan	Approved for defined food products, but not in the form of Aluminum lake. Approved for drugs, "quasi-drugs" and cosmetics for external applications, also in the form of Aluminum lake.
Kenya	Approved for food.
Korea (South)	Approved for cosmetics.
Kuwait	Approved for food.
Malaysia	Approved for defined food products.
Malta	Approved for food. Approved for cosmetics, but only for rinse-off products.
Mexico	Approved for defined food products.
New Zealand	Approved for defined food products.
Norway	EU-approved cosmetic colorants are accepted.
Poland	Approved for food and cosmetics.
Saudi Arabia	Approved for food.
Singapore	Approved for food.

South Africa	Approved for defined food products.
	Approved for the coloration of cosmetics of group 1 (all cosmetic products).
Sudan	Approved for food.
Sweden	Approved for defined food products.
Syria	Approved for food.
Taiwan	Approved for defined food products, but not as lakes.
	Approved for cosmetics, also in the form of Aluminum lakes.
Thailand	Approved for food and cosmetics.
Tunisia	Approved for defined food products.
Turkey	Approved for defined food products.
	Approved for the coloration of cosmetic preparations of group 1 (all cosmetic products).
Uruguay	Approved for food.
United Arab Emirates	Approved for food.
USA	Not approved for food, drugs and cosmetics.
Zambia	Approved for food.

For acceptance of this colorant in other countries, based on above mentioned approvals, see also 9.1.8.

C.I.16290

Name	EU-No.	C.I. No.	Class	Chemical name/ formula
Ponceau 6R C.I. Food Red 8 C.I. Acid Red 41 CAS # 5850-44-2 EINECS # unknown	previously E 126	16290	Monoazo	Naphthion acid → 2-Naphthol 3,6,8-trisulfo acid, Sodium salt
Color	Red solution in water			
Solubility	Soluble in water, low solubility in methanol.			
Chromatography DC Carrier	Source : Communication XVII DFG Farbstoff-Kommission Cellulose Chloroform 50 ml + Acetone 50 ml + Glacial acetic acid 1 ml			
Spectral photometry Solvent Absorption maximum	Source : Communication XVII DFG Farbstoff-Kommission Water 515 nm (own assay 520 nm)			
Main applications	No information available.			
Toxicological and dermatological data				Source

LD50 tested on rats	> 2.0 g/kg	Ringbook Kosmetische Färbemittel 1984 Kosmetische Färbemittel 3. ed., 1991.
Sensitivity tested on guinea pigs	non-sensitizing	

Certification status

European Union	Approved for the coloration of cosmetics of group 1 (all cosmetic products).
Hungary	Approved for the coloration of cosmetics of group 1 (all cosmetic products).
Iran	Approved for food.
Japan	Not approved for food, drugs and cosmetics.
South Africa	Approved for the coloration of cosmetics of group 1 (all cosmetic products).
Thailand	Approved for cosmetics.
Turkey	Approved for the coloration of cosmetics of group 1 (all cosmetic products).
USA	Not approved for food, drugs and cosmetics.

For acceptance of this colorant in other countries, based on above mentioned approvals, see also 9.1.8.

C.I.17200

Name	EU-No.	C.I. No.	Class	Chemical name/formula
Säurefuchsin B C.I. Food Red 12 C.I. Acid Red 33 D&C Red # 33 (CTFA adopted name) Red # 227 (Japan) CAS # 3567-66-6 EINECS # 222-656-9		17200	Monoazo	Aniline → (alkaline) H-acid, Sodium salt, (X)
Color	Blue-reddish solution in water.			
Solubility	Soluble in water, low solubility in ethanol.			
Chromatography DC Carrier	Source : Communication XVII DFG Farbstoff-Kommission Kieselgel Acetic acid ester 11 ml + Pyridine 5 ml + Water 4 ml			

Spectral photometry	Source : Communication XVII DFG Farbstoff-Kommission
Solvent	Water
Absorption maximum	470 nm

Spectral photometry	Source : own assay
Solvent	Water
Absorption maximum	530 nm

Main applications

Cosmetics — Alcohol-based perfumes.

Toxicological and dermatological data		Source
LD50 tested on rats	> 3600 mg/kg	Kosmetische Färbemittel 3. ed., 1991
Skin compatibility tested on rabbits	non-irritant	
Mucous membrane compatibility tested on a rabbit eye	non-irritant	

Certification status

European Union	Approved for the coloration of cosmetics of group 1 (all cosmetic products).
Argentina	Approved for cosmetics, but not for application in the eye area. Maximum dosage level in products for the lip area 3%, in tooth care products max. 0.1 %.
Brazil	Approved for cosmetics, but not for application in the eye area.
Bulgaria	Not approved for cosmetics.
China (People's Republic)	US-approved colorants for cosmetics are accepted. This colorant is not approved for eye-care products. Maximum dosage level in products for application on lips is 6 %.
Finland	EU-approved colorants for cosmetics are accepted. This colorant is not approved in the form of Barium, Strontium and Zirconium lake.
Hungary	Approved for the coloration of cosmetics of group 1 (all cosmetic products).
Japan	Approved for cosmetics.
Korea (South)	Approved for cosmetics.
Malta	Not approved for cosmetics.
Philippines	Approved for cosmetics for external applications, but not on eyes.
Poland	Not approved for cosmetics.
South Africa	Approved for the coloration of cosmetics of group 1 (all cosmetic products).
Taiwan	Approved for cosmetics, also in the form of Aluminum lake.
Thailand	Approved for cosmetics.
Turkey	Approved for the coloration of cosmetic of group 1 (all cosmetic products). Approved for oral drugs (maximum dosage per day 0.75 mg).

USA Approved for mouth wash water and tooth-care products as well as for externally applied drugs and cosmetics, but not for the eye area.

Venezuela Approved for cosmetics, but not for application in the eye area.

For acceptance of this colorant in other countries, based on above mentioned approvals, see also 9.1.8.

C.I.18050

Name	EU-No.	C.I. No.	Class	Chemical name/ formula
Rot 2G C.I. Food Red 10 C.I. Acid Red 1 CAS # 3734-67-6 EINECS # 223-098-9	E 128	18050	Monoazo	Aniline → N-Acetyl-H-acid, Sodium salt
Color	Red solution in water.			
Solubility	Soluble in water (at 20 °C about 100 g/l), low solubility in ethanol.			
Chromatography DC Carrier	Source : Communication XVII DFG Farbstoff-Kommission Kieselgel Petrol ether (100-160 °C) 50 ml + Petrol ether (40-60 °C) 50 ml + Isopropanol 10 ml			
Spectral photometry Solvent Absorption maximum	Source : Communication XVII DFG Farbstoff-Kommission Water 504, 532 nm			
Main applications Food Cosmetics	- Some meat- and sausage products. - Shampoo, foam bath, shower gel. - Liquid soap, toilet soap.			

Toxicological and dermatological data		Source
LD50 tested on rats	11400 mg/kg	Kosmetische Färbemittel 3. ed., 1991
Skin compatibility tested on rabbits	slight irritation	
Mucous membrane compatibility tested on a rabbit eye	minor irritation	
ADI-value (CIAA Liste Mouton)	0-0.1 mg/kg	

Certification status

European Union	Approved for defined food products (see 2.4.1.) and for the coloration of drugs and cosmetics of group 3 (not on mucous membranes).
Bulgaria	Not approved for cosmetics.
Hungary	Approved for the coloration of cosmetics of group 3 (not on mucous membranes).
Indonesia	Approved for drugs.
Japan	Not approved for food, drugs and cosmetics.
Kuwait	Approved for food.
Lebanon	Approved for drugs.
Malta	Not approved for cosmetics.
Poland	Not approved for cosmetics.
Saudi Arabia	Approved for food.
South Africa	Approved for defined food products and for drugs. Approved for the coloration of cosmetics of group 3 (not on mucous membranes).
Turkey	Approved for the coloration of cosmetics of group 3 (not on mucous membranes). Approved for the coloration of cosmetics of group 4 (only for a short residence time on skin).
Uruguay	Approved for drugs.
United Arab Emirates	Approved for food.
USA	Not approved for food, drugs and cosmetics.

For acceptance of this colorant in other countries, based on above mentioned approvals, see also 9.1.8.

C.I.18130

Name	EU-No.	C.I. No.	Class	Chemical name / formula
Supranolbrillantrot 3B C.I. Acid Red 155 CAS # 8004-53-3 EINECS # unknown		18130	Monoazo	4-Cyclohexyl-o-toluidine → N-Phenylsulfonyl-H-acid, Sodium salt
Color	Red solution in water.			
Solubility	Soluble in water and ethanol.			
Spectral photometry Solvent Absorption maximum	Source : Communication XVII DFG Farbstoff-Kommission Water 470 nm			

Spectral photometry	Source : own assay
Solvent	Water
Absorption maximum	530, 562 nm

Main applications No information available.

Toxicological and dermatological data		Source
LD50 tested on rats	> 5000 mg/kg	Kosmetische Färbemittel 3. ed., 1991
Skin compatibility tested on rabbits	non-irritant	
Mucous membrane compatibility tested on a rabbit eye	slight irritation, reversible within 6 hours	

Certification status

European Union	Approved for the coloration of cosmetics of group 4 (only for a short residence time on skin).
Bulgaria	Not approved for cosmetics.
Hungary	Approved for the coloration of cosmetics of group 4 (only for a short residence time on skin).
Japan	Not approved for food, drugs and cosmetics.
South Africa	Approved for the coloration of cosmetics of group 4 (only for a short residence time on skin).
Turkey	Approved for the coloration of cosmetics of group 4 (only for a short residence time on skin).
USA	Not approved for food, drugs and cosmetics.

For acceptance of this colorant in other countries, based on above mentioned approvals, see also 9.1.8.

C.I.18690

Name	EU-No.	C.I. No.	Class	Chemical name / formula
Zaponechtgelb R C.I. Acid Yellow 121 C.I. Solvent Yellow 21 CAS # 5601-29-6 EINECS # unknown		18690	Monoazo	Anthranil acid → 3-Methyl-1-p-5-pyrazolon, Chromium complex
Color	Yellow solution in water.			
Solubility	Soluble in water and methanol, insoluble in chloroform.			

Data Sheets

Chromatography DC Carrier	Source : Communication XVII DFG Farbstoff-Kommission Kieselgel n-Butanol 40 ml + Ethanol 40 ml + Ammonia 25 % 10 ml + Water 40 ml
Spectral photometry Solvent Absorption maximum	Source : Communication XVII DFG Farbstoff-Kommission Water 411 nm
Main applications	No information available.

Toxicological and dermatological data		Source
LD50 tested on rats	> 15000 mg/kg	Kosmetische Färbemittel 3. ed., 1991
Skin compatibility tested on guinea pigs	non-irritant	
Mucous membrane compatibility tested on a guinea pig eye	non-irritant	

Certification status

European Union	Approved for the coloration of cosmetics of group 4 (only for a short residence time on skin).
Bulgaria	Not approved for cosmetics.
Hungary	Approved for the coloration of cosmetics of group 4 (only for a short residence time on skin).
Japan	Not approved for food, drugs and cosmetics.
Malta	Not approved for cosmetics.
Poland	Not approved for cosmetics.
South Africa	Approved for the coloration of cosmetics of group 4 (only for a short residence time on skin).
Turkey	Approved for the coloration of cosmetics of group 4 (only for a short residence time on skin).
USA	Not approved for food, drugs and cosmetics.

For acceptance of this colorant in other countries, based on above mentioned approvals, see also 9.1.8.

C.I. 18736

Name	EU-No.	C.I. No.	Class	Chemical name / formula
Palatinechtrot RN C.I. Acid Red 180 CAS # 6408-26-0 EINECS # unknown		18736	Monoazo	6-Amino-4-chloro-1-phenol-2-sulfo acid → 3-Methyl-1-phenyl-5-pyrazolon, Chromium complex, Sodium salt

Color	Red solution in water.
Solubility	Soluble in water, ethanol and acetone.
Chromatography DC Carrier	Source : Communication XVII DFG Farbstoff-Kommission Kieselgel Acetic acid ester 11 ml + Pyridine 5 ml + Water 4 ml
Spectral photometry Solvent Absorption maximum	Source : Communication XVII DFG Farbstoff-Kommission Water 495 nm
Main applications	No information available.

Toxicological and dermatological data		Source
LD50 tested on rats	> 15000 mg/kg	Kosmetische Färbemittel 3. ed., 1991
Skin compatibility tested on guinea pigs	non-irritant	
Mucous membrane compatibility tested on a guinea pig eye	non-irritant	

Certification status	
European Union	Approved for the coloration of cosmetics of group 4 (only for a short residence time on skin).
Bulgaria	Not approved for cosmetics.
Hungary	Approved for the coloration of cosmetics of group 4 (only for a short residence time on skin).
Japan	Not approved for food, drugs and cosmetics.
Malta	Not approved for cosmetics.
Poland	Not approved for cosmetics.
South Africa	Approved for the coloration of cosmetics of group 4 (only for a short residence time on skin).
Turkey	Approved for the coloration of cosmetics of group 4 (only for a short residence time on skin).
USA	Not approved for food, drugs and cosmetics.

For acceptance of this colorant in other countries, based on above mentioned approvals, see also 9.1.8.

C.I.18820

Name	EU-No.	C.I. No.	Class	Chemical name / formula
Flavazin L C.I. Acid Yellow 11 Yellow # 407 (Japan) CAS # 6359-82-6 EINECS # unknown		18820	Monoazo	Aniline → 3-Methyl-1-(p-sulfo-phenyl)-5-pyrazolon, Sodium salt

Color	Yellow solution in water.
Solubility	Soluble in water, methanol and acetone, low solubility in chloroform.
Chromatography DC Carrier	Source : Communication XVII DFG Farbstoff-Kommission Kieselgel Isobutanol 60 ml + Ethanol 20 ml + Water 2 ml + Ammonia 25% 1 ml
Spectral photometry Solvent Absorption maximum	Source : Communication XVII DFG Farbstoff-Kommission Water 390 nm
Main applications	No information available.

Toxicological and dermatological data		Source
LD50 tested on rats	10120 mg/kg	Kosmetische Färbemittel 3. ed., 1991
Skin compatibility tested on rabbits	non-irritant	
Mucous membrane compatibility tested on a rabbit eye	reversible irritation	

Certification status

European Union	Approved for the coloration of cosmetics of group 4 (only for a short residence time on skin).
Bulgaria	Not approved for cosmetics.
Hungary	Approved for the coloration of cosmetics of group 4 (only for a short residence time on skin).
Japan	Approved for drugs, "quasi-drugs" and cosmetics for external applications, also in the form of Aluminum-lakes, but not on mucous membranes.
Korea (South)	Approved for cosmetics.
Poland	Not approved for cosmetics.
South Africa	Approved for the coloration of cosmetics of group 4 (only for a short residence time on skin).
Taiwan	Approved for facial toning masks, also in the form of Aluminum-lakes, but not for cosmetics.
Turkey	Approved for the coloration of cosmetics of group 4 (only for a short residence time on skin).
USA	Not approved for food, drugs and cosmetics.

For acceptance of this colorant in other countries, based on above mentioned approvals, see also 9.1.8.

C.I.18950

Name	EU-No.	C.I. No.	Class	Chemical name / formula
C.I. Acid Yellow 40 Yellow # 402 (Japan) CAS # 6372-96-9 EINECS # unknown		18950	Monoazo	p-Aminophenol → 1-(4-Chloro-2-sulfophenyl-3-methyl-5-pyrazolon and esterification of the phenolic hydroxy group with p-toluol-sulfonyl chloride, Sodium salt

Color	Yellow solution in water.
Solubility	Soluble in water, low solubility in ethanol and acetone.
Chromatography	No information available.
Spectral photometry	No information available.
Main applications	No information available.

Toxicological and dermatological data	Source
No information available.	

Certification status

European Union	Not approved for food, drugs and cosmetics.
Japan	Approved for drugs, "quasi-drugs" and cosmetics for external applications, also in the form of Aluminum-lakes, but not on mucous membranes.
Taiwan	Approved for facial toning masks, also in the form of Aluminum-lakes, but not for cosmetics.
USA	Not approved for food, drugs and cosmetics.

For acceptance of this colorant in other countries, based on above mentioned approvals, see also 9.1.8.

C.I. 18965

Name	EU-No.	C.I. No.	Class	Chemical name / formula
Sandolangelb E-2GL C.I. Food Yellow 5 C.I. Acid Yellow 17 CAS # 6359-98-4 EINECS # 228-819-0		18965	Monoazo	Sulfanil acid → 1-(2,5-Dichloro-4- sulfophenyl)-3- methyl-5-pyrazolon, Sodium salt

Color	Yellow solution in water.
Solubility	Soluble in water (at 20 °C about 80 g/l), low solubility in ethanol(< 1 g/l).
Chromatography DC Carrier	Source : own assay Schleicher & Schüll 2043 b Mgl Acetic acid ester 11 ml + Pyridine 5 ml + Water 4 ml
Spectral photometry Solvent Absorption maximum	Source : own assay Water 406 nm
Main applications Cosmetics	- Shampoo, foam bath, shower gel. - Liquid soap, toilet soap.

Toxicological and dermatological data		Source
LD50 tested on rats	> 5000 mg/kg	Kosmetische Färbemittel 3. ed., 1991
Skin compatibility tested on rabbits	slight irritation	
Mucous membrane compatibility tested on a rabbit eye	slight irritation	

Certification status

European Union	Approved for the coloration of cosmetics of group 1 (all cosmetic products).
Argentina	Approved only for soap.
Bulgaria	Not approved for cosmetics
Hungary	Approved for the coloration of cosmetics of group 1 (all cosmetic products).
Japan	Not approved for food, drugs and cosmetics.
Kuwait	Approved for food.
Poland	Not approved for cosmetics.
South Africa	Approved for the coloration of cosmetics of group 1 (all cosmetic products).

Turkey	Approved for the coloration of cosmetic of group 1 (all cosmetic products).
USA	Not approved for food, drugs and cosmetics.

For acceptance of this colorant in other countries, based on above mentioned approvals, see also 9.1.8.

C.I.19120

Name	EU-No.	C.I. No.	Class	Chemical name / formula
Echtlichtgelb 3G C.I. Acid Yellow 13 CAS # 1934-25-4 EINECS # unknown		19120	Monoazo	o-Aminobenzoyl-sulfo acid → 3-Carboxy-1-(o-sulfophenyl)-5-pyrazolon, Sodium salt
Color	Yellow solution in water.			
Solubility	Soluble in water.			
Chromatography DC Carrier	Source : Communication XVII DFG Farbstoff-Kommission Kieselgel Acetic acid ester 11 ml + Pyridine 5 ml + Water 4 ml			
Spectral photometry Solvent Absorption maximum	Source : Communication XVII DFG Farbstoff-Kommission Water 420 nm			
Main applications	No information available. The chemical structure is only marginally different to the one of Tartrazine C.I.19410. Tartrazine is therefore used as a substitute.			

Toxicological and dermatological data	Source
No information available.	

Certification status

European Union	Not approved for the coloration of cosmetics.
Japan	Not approved for food, drugs and cosmetics.
USA	Not approved for food, drugs and cosmetics.

For acceptance of this colorant in other countries, based on above mentioned approvals, see also 9.1.8.

C.I.19140

Name	EU-No.	C.I. No.	Class	Chemical name / formula
Tartrazin C.I. Food Yellow 4 C.I. Acid Yellow 23 FD&C Yellow # 5 (CTFA adopted name) Yellow # 4 (Japan) CAS # 1934-21-0 EINECS # 217-699-5	E 102	19140	Monoazo	Sulfanil acid → 3-Carboxy-1-(p-sulfophenyl)-5-pyrazolon, Sodium salt
Tartrazin Lack C.I.Pigment Yellow 100 CAS # 12225-21-7 EINECS # 235-428-9	E 102	19140:1	Monoazo	-, Aluminum lake

Color	Sodium salt yellow solution in water, Aluminum lake yellow powder.
Solubility	Sodium salt soluble in water (at 20 °C about 70 g/l), low solubility in ethanol. Aluminum lake insoluble in water, soluble in diluted hydrochloric acid.
Chromatography DC Carrier	Source : Communication XVII DFG Farbstoff-Kommission Cellulose trt. Sodium citrate solution 2.5% 80 ml + Ammonia 25% 20 ml + Methanol 12 ml
Spectral photometry Solvent Absorption maximum	Source : Communication XVII DFG Farbstoff-Kommission Water 420 nm
Main applications Food Drugs Cosmetics	 - Beverages, candies, dessert products, pudding powder, artificial ice-cream, carbonated beverage powder. - General utilization, Aluminum lake used for the coloration of capsules. - Shampoo, foam bath, shower gel. - Liquid soap.

Toxicological and dermatological data		Source
LD50 tested on rats	> 12750 mg/kg	Kosmetische Färbemittel
Skin compatibility tested on rabbits	non-irritant	3. ed., 1991

Mucous membrane compatibility tested on a rabbit eye	non-irritant	
ADI-value (WHO 1966, SCF 1975)	0-7.5 mg/kg	Ringbook Colorants for food 1978

Certification status

European Union	Approved for defined food products (see 2.4.1.) and for the coloration of drugs and cosmetic preparations of group 1 (all cosmetic products).
Argentina	Approved for food. Approved for cosmetics for external applications, but not on eyes and lips.
Australia	Approved for defined food products.
Austria	Not approved for food.
Brazil	Approved for defined food products. Approved for cosmetics, but not for application in the eye area.
Canada	Approved for defined food products.
Chile	Approved for food.
Colombia	Approved for food.
Cyprus	Approved for defined food products.
Dominican Republic	Approved for food.
Egypt	Approved for food.
Hungary	Approved for defined food products. Approved for the coloration of cosmetics of group 1 (all cosmetic products).
India	Approved for food.
Indonesia	Approved for food.
Iran	Approved for food.
Israel	Approved for food and cosmetics. Warning sticker "Contains Tartrzine" must be attached.
Japan	Approved for defined food products, also in the form of Aluminum lakes. Approved for drugs, "quasi-drugs" and cosmetics for external applications, also in the form of Aluminum-, Barium- and Zirconium lakes.
Kenya	Approved for food.
Korea (South)	Approved for cosmetics.
Malaysia	Approved for defined food products.
Malta	Approved for food.
Mexico	Approved for defined food products.
New Zealand	Approved for defined food products.
Peru	Approved for food.
Philippines	Approved for food. Approved for cosmetics, but not for application in the eye area.
Poland	Approved for defined food products. Approved for cosmetics.
Saudi Arabia	Approved for food.
Singapore	Approved for food.

South Africa	Approved for defined food products, but not any more in liquor products.
	Approved for the coloration of cosmetics of group 1 (all cosmetic products).
Sudan	Approved for food.
Sweden	Approved only for alcoholic beverages.
Switzerland	Not approved any more for food.
Syria	Approved for food.
Taiwan	Approved for defined food products.
	Approved for cosmetics, also in the form of Aluminum-, Barium- and Zirconium lakes.
Thailand	Approved for food.
Tunisia	Not approved any more for food.
Turkey	Approved for defined food products.
	Approved for the coloration of cosmetics of group 1 (all cosmetic products).
Uruguay	Approved for food.
United Arab Emirates	Approved for food.
USA	Approved for defined food products.
	Approved drugs and cosmetics, but not for application in the eye area.
	Utilization requires FDA certificate.
Venezuela	Approved for food.
	Approved for cosmetics, but not for application in the eye area.
Zambia	Approved for food.

For acceptance of this colorant in other countries, based on above mentioned approvals, see also 9.1.8.

C.I.19235

Name	EU-No.	C.I. No.	Class	Chemical name / formula
C.I. Acid Orange 137 Orange B (CFR21) CAS # unknown EINECS # unknown		19235	Monoazo	Naphthion acid → R-acid, Sodium salt
Color	Yellow-orange solution in water.			
Solubility	Soluble in water.			
Chromatography	No information available.			
Spectral photometry Solvent Absorption maximum	Source : Marmion, Handbook of U.S. Colorants Water 437 nm			

Main applications
Food   - Coloration of sausages.

Toxicological and dermatological data	Source
No information available.	

Certification status

European Union	Not approved for food, drugs and cosmetics.
Japan	Not approved for food, drugs and cosmetics.
USA	Approved for surface coloration of "frankfurter" and sausages. Maximum dosage 150 ppm based on finished product. Utilization requires FDA certificate.

This colorant is not included in other national positive lists.

C.I.20040

Name	EU-No.	C.I. No.	Class	Chemical name / formula
Permanentgelb NGG C.I. Pigment Yellow 16 CAS # 5979-28-2 EINECS # unknown		20040	Bisazo	2 Mol 2,4-Dichloroaniline → 4,4'-Bi-o-aceto-acet-anilide
Color	Yellow pigment.			
Solubility	Insoluble in water.			
Chromatography	No information available.			
Spectral photometry	No information available.			
Main applications	No information available.			

Toxicological and dermatological data		Source
LD50 tested on rats	> 15000 mg/kg	Kosmetische Färbemittel 3. ed., 1991
Skin compatibility tested on rabbits	non-irritant	
Mucous membrane compatibility tested on a rabbit eye	non-irritant	

Data Sheets 177

Certification status

European Union	Approved for the coloration of cosmetics of group 4 (only for a short residence time on skin).
Bulgaria	Not approved for cosmetics.
Hungary	Approved for the coloration of cosmetics of group 4 (only for a short residence time on skin).
Japan	Not approved for food, drugs and cosmetics.
Poland	Not approved for cosmetics.
South Africa	Approved for the coloration of cosmetics of group 4 (only for a short residence time on skin).
Turkey	Approved for the coloration of cosmetics of group 4 (only for a short residence time on skin).
USA	Not approved for food, drugs and cosmetics.

For acceptance of this colorant in other countries, based on above mentioned approvals, see also 9.1.8.

C.I.20170

Name	EU-No.	C.I. No.	Class	Chemical name / formula
Resorcinbraun C.I. Acid Orange D&C Brown #1 (CTFA adopted name) Brown # 201 (Japan) CAS # 1320-07-6 EINECS # unknown		20170	Bisazo	Sulfanil acid (1) → Resorcin ← (2) Xylidine, Sodium salt
Color	Yellow-brown solution in water.			
Solubility	Soluble in water and ethanol.			
Chromatography DC Carrier	Source : Communication XVII DFG Farbstoff-Kommission Kieselgel Acetic acid ester 11 ml + Pyridine 5 ml + Water 4 ml			
Spectral photometry Solvent Absorption maximum	Source : Communication XVII DFG Farbstoff-Kommission Water 425 nm (own assay : 430 nm)			
Main applications Cosmetics	 - Shampoo, foam bath, shower gel. - Liquid soap.			

Toxicological and dermatological data		Source
LD50 tested on rats	> 15000 mg/kg	Kosmetische Färbemittel
Skin compatibility tested on rabbits	non-irritant	3. ed., 1991
Mucous membrane compatibility tested on a rabbit eye	minor irritation	

Certification status

European Union	Approved for the coloration of cosmetics of group 3 (not on mucous membranes.
Argentina	Approved for cosmetics for external applications, but not on eyes and lips.
Brazil	Approved for cosmetics for external applications, but not on eyes and lips.
Hungary	Approved for the coloration of cosmetics of group 1 (all cosmetic products).
Japan	Approved for drugs, "quasi-drugs" and cosmetics for external applications, also in the form of Aluminum-lakes, but not on mucous membranes.
Korea (South)	Approved for cosmetics.
Philippines	Approved for cosmetics for external applications, but not on eyes and lips.
South Africa	Approved for the coloration of cosmetics of group 3 (not on mucous membranes).
Taiwan	Approved for cosmetics.
Thailand	Approved for cosmetics.
Turkey	Approved for the coloration of cosmetics of group 3 (not on mucous membranes.
USA	Approved for cosmetics, but not for application in the eye and lip area. Utilization requires FDA certificate.
Venezuela	Approved for cosmetics, but not for application in the eye and lip area.

For acceptance of this colorant in other countries, based on above mentioned approvals, see also 9.1.8.

C.I.20470

Name	EU-No.	C.I. No.	Class	Chemical name / formula
Amidoschwarz 10B C.I. Acid Black 1 Black # 401 (Japan) CAS # 1046-48-8 EINECS # 213-903-1		20470	Bisazo	p-Nitroaniline (H+) (1) → H-acid ← (2)(OH)-Aniline, Sodium salt

Color	Blue-black solution in water, dark blue in ethanol.
Solubility	Soluble in water (at 20 °C about 20 g/l) and ethanol.
Chromatography DC Carrier	Source : Communication XVII DFG Farbstoff-Kommission Kieselgel Acetic acid ester 11 ml + Pyridine 5 ml + Water 4 ml
Spectral photometry Solvent Absorption maximum	Source : Communication XVII DFG Farbstoff-Kommission Water 613 nm

Main applications
Cosmetics
- Shampoo, shower gel.
- Liquid soap, toilet soap.

Toxicological and dermatological data		Source
LD50 tested on rats	> 13915 mg/kg	Kosmetische Färbemittel 3. ed., 1991
Skin compatibility tested on rabbits	non-irritant	
Mucous membrane compatibility tested on a rabbit eye	non-irritant	

Certification status

European Union	Approved for the coloration of cosmetics of group 4 (only for a short residence time on skin).
Bulgaria	Not approved for cosmetics.
Hungary	Approved for the coloration of cosmetics of group 1 (all cosmetic products).
Japan	Approved for drugs, "quasi-drugs" and cosmetics for external applications, but not on mucous membranes.
South Africa	Approved for the coloration of cosmetics of group 4 (only for a short residence time on skin).
Taiwan	Approved for facial toning masks, also in the form of Aluminum-lakes, but not for cosmetics.
Turkey	Approved for the coloration of cosmetics of group 4 (only for a short residence time on skin).
USA	Not approved for food, drugs and cosmetics.

For acceptance of this colorant in other countries, based on above mentioned approvals, see also 9.1.8.

C.I.21090

Name	EU-No.	C.I. No.	Class	Chemical name / formula
C.I. Pigment Yellow 12 Yellow # 205 (Japan) CAS # 6358-85-6 EINECS # unknown		21090	Bisazo	3,3'-Dichloro-benzidine → Acetoacetanilide (2 Mol)

Color	Yellow pigment.
Solubility	Insoluble in water, low solubility in ethanol.
Chromatography	No information available.
Spectral photometry	No information available.
Main applications	No information available.

Toxicological and dermatological data	Source
No information available.	

Certification status

European Union	Not approved for food, drugs and cosmetics.
Japan	Approved for drugs, "quasi-drugs" and cosmetics for external applications, also in the form of Aluminum-lakes, but not on mucous membranes.
Korea (South)	Approved for cosmetics.
Taiwan	Approved for cosmetics.
USA	Not approved for food, drugs and cosmetics.

For acceptance of this colorant in other countries, based on above mentioned approvals, see also 9.1.8.

C.I.21100

Name	EU-No.	C.I. No.	Class	Chemical name / formula
Vulcanechtgelb C.I. Pigment Yellow 13 CAS # 5102-83-0 EINECS # unknown		21100	Bisazo	3,3'-Dichlorobenzidine → 2mol 2,4-Acet-acetoxylidide

Color	Yellow pigment.
Solubility	Insoluble in water.
Chromatography	No information available.
Spectral photometry	No information available.

Main applications
Cosmetics   - Toilet soap.

Toxicological and dermatological data	**Source**
No information available.	

Certification status

European Union	Approved for the coloration of cosmetics of group 4 (only for a short residence time on skin).
Bulgaria	Not approved for cosmetics.
Hungary	Approved for the coloration of cosmetics of group 1 (all cosmetic products).
Japan	Not approved for food, drugs and cosmetics.
Poland	Not approved for cosmetics.
South Africa	Approved for the coloration of cosmetics of group 4 (only for a short residence time on skin).
Turkey	Approved for the coloration of cosmetics of group 4 (only for a short residence time on skin).
USA	Not approved for food, drugs and cosmetics.

For acceptance of this colorant in other countries, based on above mentioned approvals, see also 9.1.8.

C.I.21108

Name	EU-No.	C.I. No.	Class	Chemical name / formula
Graphtol Gelb RCL C.I. Pigment Yellow 83 CAS # 5567-15-7 EINECS # unknown		21108	Bisazo	3,3'-Dichlorobenzidine → 2mol 4-Chlor-2',5'-dimethoxyacetanilide
Color	Yellow pigment.			
Solubility	Insoluble in water.			

Chromatography	No information available.
Spectral photometry	No information available.
Main applications Cosmetics	- Toilet soap.

Toxicological and dermatological data		Source
LD50 tested on rats	> 16000 mg/kg	Kosmetische Färbemittel
Skin compatibility tested on rabbits	non- to slightly irritating	3. ed., 1991
Mucous membrane compatibility tested on a rabbit eye	slightly irritating	

Certification status	
European Union	Approved for the coloration of cosmetics of group 4 (only for a short residence time on skin).
Bulgaria	Not approved for cosmetics.
Hungary	Approved for the coloration of cosmetics of group 1 (all cosmetic products).
Japan	Not approved for food, drugs and cosmetics.
Poland	Not approved for cosmetics.
South Africa	Approved for the coloration of cosmetics of group 4 (only for a short residence time on skin).
Turkey	Approved for the coloration of cosmetics of group 4 (only for a short residence time on skin).
USA	Not approved for food, drugs and cosmetics.

For acceptance of this colorant in other countries, based on above mentioned approvals, see also 9.1.8.

C.I.21110

Name	EU-No.	C.I. No.	Class	Chemical name / formula
Permanentorange G C.I. Pigment Orange 13 Orange # 204 (Japan) CAS # 3520-72-7 EINECS # unknown		21110	Bisazo	3,3'-Dichlorobenzidine → 2mol 3-Methyl-1-phenyl-5-pyrazolon
Color		Orange pigment.		

Data Sheets

Solubility	Insoluble in water.
Chromatography	No information available.
Spectral photometry	No information available.
Main applications	No information available.
Main applications Cosmetics	- Toilet soap.

Toxicological and dermatological data		**Source**
No information available		
LD50 tested on rats	> 5000 mg/kg	Safety data sheet Graphtol Orange GPS Sandoz (1983)
Skin compatibility tested on rabbits	non-irritant	
Mucous membrane compatibility tested on a rabbit eye	non-irritant	

Certification status

European Union	Not approved for cosmetics.
Japan	Approved for drugs, "quasi-drugs" and cosmetics for external applications.
Korea (South)	Approved for cosmetics.
Taiwan	Approved for cosmetics.
USA	Not approved for food, drugs and cosmetics.

For acceptance of this colorant in other countries, based on above mentioned approvals, see also 9.1.8.

C.I.21115

Name	EU-No.	C.I. No.	Class	Chemical name / formula
C.I. Pigment Orange 34 CAS # 15793-73-4 EINECS # unknown		21115	Bisazo	3,3'-Dichlorobenzidine →2mol 3-Methyl-1-p-tolyl-5-pyrazolon
Color	Orange pigment.			
Solubility	Insoluble in water.			
Chromatography	No information available.			

Spectral photometry	No information available.

Main applications	
Cosmetics	- Toilet soap.

Toxicological and dermatological data	**Source**
No information available.	

Certification status

European Union	Not approved for cosmetics.
Japan	Not approved for food, drugs and cosmetics.
USA	Not approved for food, drugs and cosmetics.

For acceptance of this colorant in other countries, based on above mentioned approvals, see also 9.1.8.

C.I.21230

Name	EU-No.	C.I. No.	Class	Chemical name / formula
Sudangelb GRN C.I. Solvent Yellow 29 CAS # 6706-82-7 EINECS # unknown	C 9	21230	Bisazo	4,4'-Cyclohexyl-iden-di-o-toluidine→ 2mol p=Cyclo-hexylphenol
Color	Yellow solution in chloroform.			
Solubility	Soluble in methanol, acetone, chloroform, insoluble in water.			
Chromatography DC Carrier	Source : Communication XVII DFG Farbstoff-Kommission Cellulose Gasoline 40 ml + Benzole 20 ml + Methylethylketone 4ml + acetic acid ester 16 ml			
Spectral photometry Solvent Absorption maximum	Source : Communication XVII DFG Farbstoff-Kommission Dimethylformamide (own assay :1,1,1-Trichloroethane) 350 nm (own assay: 350 m, shoulder at 400 nm)			
Main applications Cosmetics	- Oil products.			

Data Sheets

Toxicological and dermatological data		Source
LD50 tested on rats	> 15000 mg/kg	Kosmetische Färbemittel 3. ed., 1991
Skin compatibility tested on rabbits	non-irritant	
Mucous membrane compatibility tested on a rabbit eye	non-irritant	

Certification status

European Union	Approved for the coloration of cosmetics of group 3 (not on mucous membranes). According to Colorant Guideline 94/36/EU not approved anymore for food surface stamps and for the coloration of egg shells as of June 30, 1996.
Bulgaria	Not approved for cosmetics.
Hungary	Approved for the coloration of cosmetics of group 1 (all cosmetic products).
Japan	Not approved for food, drugs and cosmetics.
Malta	Not approved for cosmetics.
Poland	Not approved for cosmetics.
South Africa	Approved for the coloration of cosmetics of group 3 (not on mucous membranes).
Turkey	Approved for the coloration of cosmetics of group 3 (not on mucous membranes).
USA	Not approved for food, drugs and cosmetics.

For acceptance of this colorant in other countries, based on above mentioned approvals, see also 9.1.8.

C.I.24790

Name	EU-No.	C.I. No.	Class	Chemical name / formula
Supranolrot BR C.I. Acid Red 163 CAS # 13421-53-9 EINECS # unknown		24790	Bisazo	4,4'-Cyclohexyl-iden-di-aniline→ 2mol 4,6-Dihydroxy-naphthalin-2-sulfo acid esterized with 1 mol Benzol sulfonic acid chloride, sodium salt
Color	Red solution in water.			
Solubility	Soluble in water, low solubility in ethanol.			

Chromatography DC Carrier	Source : Communication XVII DFG Farbstoff-Kommission Kieselgel Acetic acid ester 11 ml + Pyridine 5 ml + Water 4ml
Spectral photometry Solvent Absorption maximum	Source : Communication XVII DFG Farbstoff-Kommission Water 510 nm
Main applications	No information available.

Toxicological and dermatological data		Source
LD50 tested on rats	> 5000 mg/kg	Kosmetische Färbemittel
Skin compatibility tested on rabbits	non-irritant	3. ed., 1991
Mucous membrane compatibility tested on a rabbit eye	non-irritant	

Certification status

European Union	Approved for the coloration of cosmetics of group 4 (only for a short residence time on the skin).
Japan	Not approved for food, drugs and cosmetics.
Poland	Not approved for cosmetics.
South Africa	Approved for the coloration of cosmetics of group 4 (only for a short residence time on the skin).
Turkey	Approved for the coloration of cosmetics of group 4 (only for a short residence time on the skin).
USA	Not approved for food, drugs and cosmetics.

For acceptance of this colorant in other countries, based on above mentioned approvals, see also 9.1.8.

C.I.26100

Name	EU-No.	C.I. No.	Class	Chemical name / formula
Sudan Rot BK C.I. Solvent Red 23 D&C Red # 17 (CTFA adopted name) Red # 225 (Japan) CAS # 85-86-9 EINECS # 201-638-4		26100	Bisazo	p-Phenylazoaniline → 2-Naphthol

Color	Red solution in chloroform or 1,1,1-Trichlorethane.
Solubility	Soluble in chlorocarbon hydrogen and galcial acetic acid, low solubitlity in ethanol, ether and acetone, insoluble in water.
Chromatography DC Carrier	Source : Communication XVII DFG Farbstoff-Kommission Kieselgel Benzol 90 ml + Acetone 10 ml
Spectral photometry Solvent Absorption maximum	Source : Communication XVII DFG Farbstoff-Kommission Dichloromethane 352, 515 nm

Main applications
Cosmetics   - Oil products.

Toxicological and dermatological data		Source
No information available		
LD50 tested on rats	> 16000 mg/kg	Kosmetische Färbemittel
Skin compatibility tested on rabbits	non-irritant	3. ed., 1991
Mucous membrane compatibility tested on a rabbit eye	non-irritant	

Certification status

European Union	Approved for the coloration of cosmetics of group 3 (not on mucous membranes).
Argentina	Approved for cosmetics for external applications.
Brazil	Approved for cosmetics for external applications.
Hungary	Not approved for cosmetics.
Japan	Approved for drugs, "quasi-drugs" and cosmetics for external applications.
Korea (South)	Approved for cosmetics.
Philippines	Approved for cosmetics for external applications.
Poland	Approved for cosmetics.
South Africa	Approved for the coloration of cosmetics of group 3 (not on mucous membranes).
Taiwan	Approved for cosmetics.
Thailand	Approved for cosmetics, but not for application in the eye area and on mucous membranes.
Turkey	Approved for the coloration of cosmetics of group 3 (not on mucous membranes.
USA	Approved for drugs and cosmetics for external applications, but not for the eye and lip area. Utilization requires FDA certificate.

For acceptance of this colorant in other countries, based on above mentioned approvals, see also 9.1.8.

C.I.26105

Name	EU-No.	C.I. No.	Class	Chemical name / formula
Sudanrot BB C.I. Solvent Red 24 Red # 501 (Japan) CAS # 85-83-6 EINECS # 201-635-8		26105	Bisazo	4-o-Tolylazo-o-toluidine → 2-Naphthol

Color	Red solution in oranic solutions.
Solubility	Soluble in ethanol, acetone and 1,1,1-Trichloroethane.
Chromatography DC Carrier	Source : own assay Kieselgel Toluol
Spectral photometry Solvent Absorption maximum	Source : own assay 1,1,1-Trichloroethane 518 nm
Main applications	No information available.

Toxicological and dermatological data		Source
No information available		
LD50 tested on rats	ca. 3600 mg/kg	Safety data sheet Basaacid Gelb 230 Bayer 1981
Skin compatibility tested on rabbits	non-irritant	
Mucous membrane compatibility tested on a rabbit eye	slight irritant	

Certification status

European Union	Not approved for food, drugs and cosmetics.
Israel	Not approved for food, drugs and cosmetics.
Japan	Approved for drugs, "quasi-drugs" and cosmetics for external applications, but not on mucous membranes.
Taiwan	Approved for facial toning masks, not for cosmetics.
USA	Not approved for food, drugs and cosmetics.

For acceptance of this colorant in other countries, based on above mentioned approvals, see also 9.1.8.

C.I.27290

Name	EU-No.	C.I. No.	Class	Chemical name / formula
Brillantcrocein C.I. Acid Red 73 CAS # 5413-75- EINECS # unknown		27290	Bisazo	p-Phenylazoaniline→ G-acid, Sodium salt, (X)

Color	Red solution in water.
Solubility	Soluble in water and ethanol.
Chromatography Paper Carrier	Source : (own assay) Schleicher& Schüll 2043b Mgl Acetic acid ester 11 ml + Pyridine 5 ml + Water 4 ml
Spectral photometry Solvent Absorption maximum	Source : (own assay) Water 510 nm
Main applications	No information available.

Toxicological and dermatological data		Source
LD50 tested on rats	> 5000 mg/kg	Kosmetische Färbemittel 3. ed., 1991
Skin compatibility tested on rabbits	non-irritant	
Mucous membrane compatibility tested on a rabbit eye	non-irritant	

Certification status	
European Union	Approved for the coloration of cosmetics of group 4 (only for a short residence time on the skin).
Bulgaria	Not approved for cosmetics.
Hungary	Approved for the coloration of cosmetics of group 1 (all cosmetic products).
Japan	Not approved for food, drugs and cosmetics.
Poland	Approved for cosmetics.
South Africa	Approved for the coloration of cosmetics of group 4 (only for a short residence time on the skin).
Turkey	Approved for the coloration of cosmetics of group 4 (only for a short residence time on the skin).
USA	Not approved for food, drugs and cosmetics.

For acceptance of this colorant in other countries, based on above mentioned approvals, see also 9.1.8.

C.I.27755

Name	EU-No.	C.I. No.	Class	Chemical name / formula
Schwarz 7984 C.I. Food Black 2 CAS # 2118-39-0 EINECS # unknown	previously E 152	27755	Bisazo	Sulfanil acid→ 1,7-Cleve"s acid →(alkyl.) 2R-acid, Sodium salt
Color	Blue-black solution in water.			
Solubility	Soluble in water.			
Chromatography DC Carrier	Source : Communication XVII DFG Farbstoff-Kommission Kieselgel Acetic acid ester 11 ml + Pyridine 5 ml + Water 4 ml			
Spectral photometry Solvent Absorption maximum	Source : Communication XVII DFG Farbstoff-Kommission Water 445, 582 nm			
Main applications	No information available, can be replaced by C.I.28440.			

Toxicological and dermatological data		Source
LD50 tested on rats	> 5000 mg/kg	Kosmetische Färbemittel 3. ed., 1991
Skin compatibility tested on rabbits	non-irritant	
Mucous membrane compatibility tested on a rabbit eye	non-irritant	

Certification status

European Union	Not approved any more for food. Approved for the coloration of cosmetics of group 1 (all cosmetic products).
Bulgaria	Not approved for cosmetics.
Hungary	Approved for the coloration of cosmetics of group 1 (all cosmetic products).
Iran	Approved for food.
Japan	Not approved for food, drugs and cosmetics.
Poland	Approved for cosmetics.
South Africa	Approved for the coloration of cosmetics of group 1 (all cosmetic products).
Turkey	Approved for the coloration of cosmetic of group 1 (all cosmetic products).
USA	Not approved for food, drugs and cosmetics.

For acceptance of this colorant in other countries, based on above mentioned approvals, see also 9.1.8.

C.I.28440

Name	EU-No.	C.I. No.	Class	Chemical name / formula
Brillantschwarz BN C.I. Food Black 1 CAS # 2519-30-4 EINECS # 219-746-5	E 151	28440	Bisazo	Sulfanil acid → 1,7-Cleve's acid → N-Acetyl-K-Acid, Sodium salt

Color	Blue-violet solution in water.
Solubility	Sodium salt soluble in water (at 20 °C about 100 g/l), low solubility in ethanol.
Chromatography DC Carrier	Source : own assay Schleicher & Schüll 2043 b Mgl Acetic acid ester 11 ml + Pyridine 5 ml + Water 4 ml
Spectral photometry Solvent Absorption maximum	Source : own assay Water 410, 575 nm
Main applications Food Drugs Cosmetics	 - Candies, fish roe products. - General utilization, Aluminum lake for coloration of capsules. - Shampoo, foam bath, shower gel. - Liquid soap.

Toxicological and dermatological data		Source
LD50 tested on rats	>5000 mg/kg	Kosmetische Färbemittel 3. ed., 1991

ADI-value (EEC Color Group 1983 .
    EU- document III/9280/90)
    (CIAA Liste Mouton)
	
	0-5.0 mg/kg
	0-1.0 mg/kg	

Certification status

European Union	Approved for defined food products (see 2.4.1.) and for the coloration of drugs and cosmetic preparations of group 1 (all cosmetic products).
Australia	Approved for defined food products.
Austria	Approved Caviar substitute products.
Cyprus	Approved for defined food products.
Egypt	Approved for food.
Hungary	Approved for the coloration of cosmetics of group 1 (all cosmetic products).

Iran	Approved for food.
Kuwait	Approved for food.
Malta	Approved for food.
New Zealand	Approved for defined food products.
Philippines	Approved for food.
Poland	Approved for defined food products. Approved for cosmetics.
Saudi Arabia	Approved for food.
Singapore	Approved for food.
South Africa	Approved for defined food products. Approved for the coloration of cosmetics of group 1 (all cosmetic products).
Switzerland	Approved for defined food products and drugs.
Syria	Approved for food.
Tunisia	Approved for defined food products.
Turkey	Approved for the coloration of cosmetic of group 1 (all cosmetic products).
United Arab Emirates	Approved for food.
USA	Not approved for food, drugs and cosmetics.

For acceptance of this colorant in other countries, based on above mentioned approvals, see also 9.1.8.

C.I.40215

Name	EU-No.	C.I. No.	Class	Chemical name / formula
Siriuslichtorange 2GL C.I. Direct Orange 34,39 CAS # 1325-54-8 EINECS # 215-397-8		40215	Stilbene/ Monoazo	Product of the alkaline condensation of 4,4'-Di-nitro-2,2'-stilbendisulfoacid with 4-Amino-azobenzol-4'-sulfoacid, Sodium salt
Color	Orange solution in water.			
Solubility	Soluble in water, insoluble in methanol and Dichloromethane.			
Chromatography DC Carrier	Source : Communication XVII DFG Farbstoff-Kommission Kieselgel n-Butanol 40 ml + Ethanol 40 ml + Ammonia 25% 10 ml + Water 30 ml			

Spectral photometry	Source : Communication XVII DFG Farbstoff-Kommission
Solvent	Water
Absorption maximum	410 nm (own assay : 422 nm)

Main applications	
Cosmetics	Basically suitable for shampoo, shower gel, liquid soap and toilet soap. Utilization cannot be recommended, as the colorant can migrate from the cosmetic products directly onto textiles.

Toxicological and dermatological data		Source
LD50 tested on rats	6836 mg/kg	Kosmetische Färbemittel
Skin compatibility tested on rabbits	non-irritant	3. ed., 1991
Mucous membrane compatibility tested on a rabbit eye	slightly irritating	

Certification status

European Union	Approved for the coloration of cosmetics of group 4 (only for a short residence time on skin).
Bulgaria	Not approved for cosmetics.
Hungary	Approved for the coloration of cosmetics of group 1 (all cosmetic products).
Japan	Not approved for food, drugs and cosmetics.
Poland	Not approved for cosmetics.
South Africa	Approved for the coloration of cosmetics of group 4 (only for a short residence time on skin).
Turkey	Approved for the coloration of cosmetics of group 4 (only for a short residence time on skin).
USA	Not approved for food, drugs and cosmetics.

For acceptance of this colorant in other countries, based on above mentioned approvals, see also 9.1.8.

C.I.40800

Name	EU-No.	C.I. No.	Class	Chemical name / formula
beta-Carotene C.I. Food Orange 5 beta-carotene (CTFA adopted name) β-carotene Japan) CAS # 7235-40-7 EINECS # 230-636-6	E 160a	40800	Carotenoide	β,β carotene

Color	Yellow-orange solution in cyclohexane.
Solubility	Soluble in chloroform, cyclohexane and fatty oils, low solubility in ethanol, insoluble in water. Also commercially available as a water-dispersible product.
Chromatography DC Carrier	Source : Communication XVII DFG Farbstoff-Kommission Kieselgel Cyclohexane 100 ml + Acetic acid ester 50 ml
Spectral photometry Solvent Absorption maximum	Source : Kosmetische Färbemittel 1984 Cyclohexane 453-456 nm
Main applications	see C.I.75130

Toxicological and dermatological data		Source
LD50 tested on dogs	> 8000 mg/kg	Kosmetische Färbemittel 3. ed., 1991
Mucous membrane compatibility tested on a rabbit eye	non-irritant	
ADI-value (WHO 1974, SCF 1975) in the form of total carotenoids such as β-carotene, β-Apo-8'-carotenal and β-Apo-8'-carotene acid ethyl ester.	0-5.0 mg/kg	

Certification status

see C.I.75130

C.I.40820

Name	EU-No.	C.I. No.	Class	Chemical name / formula
beta-Apo-8'-carotenal C.I. Food Orange 6 beta-Apo-8'-carotenal (CFR21) CAS # 1107-26-2 EINECS # 214-171-6	E 160e	40820	Carotenoide	β-Carotene-aldehyde
Color		Orange solution in water.		

Data Sheets

Solubility	Soluble in chloroform, cyclohexane and fatty oils, low solubility in ethanol, insoluble in water. Also commercially available as a water-dispersible product.
Chromatography DC Carrier	Source : Communication XVII DFG Farbstoff-Kommission Kieselgel Gasoline 40 ml + Benzol 20 ml + Methylethylketone 4 ml + Acetic acid ester 16 ml.
Spectral photometry	Source : Communication XVII DFG Farbstoff-Kommission and Kosmetische Färbemittel 3. ed., 1991)
Solvent Absorption maximum	Water-Methanol 1:1 330, 462 nm
Solvent Absorption maximum	Cyclohexane 460-462 nm

Main applications
Food — cream and sauce products, water-dispersible products for candies and beverages.

Toxicological and dermatological data		Source
LD50 tested on mice	>10000 mg/kg	Kosmetische Färbemittel 3. ed., 1991
ADI-value (WHO 1974, SCF 1975) in the form of total carotenoids such as β-carotene, β-Apo-8'-carotenal and β-Apo-8'-carotene acid ethyl ester.	0-5.0 mg/kg	

Certification status

European Union	Approved for defined food products (see 2.4.1.) and for the coloration of drugs and cosmetic preparations of group 1 (all cosmetic products).
Argentina	Approved for food.
Australia	Approved for defined food products.
Austria	Approved for defined food products.
Brazil	Approved for defined food products.
Canada	Approved for defined food products.
Chile	Approved for food.
Colombia	Approved for food.
Costa Rica	Approved for food.
Cyprus	Approved for defined food products.
Egypt	Approved for food.
Finland	Approved for defined food products.
Hungary	Approved for the coloration of cosmetics of group 1 (all cosmetic products).
India	Approved for food.

Indonesia	Approved for food.
Iran	Approved for food.
Israel	Approved for food.
Japan	Not approved for food, drugs and cosmetics.
Kenya	Approved for food.
Kuwait	Approved for food.
Malaysia	Approved for defined food products.
Malta	Approved for food.
New Zealand	Approved for defined food products.
Philippines	Approved for food.
Saudi Arabia	Approved for food.
South Africa	Approved for defined food products. Approved for the coloration of cosmetics of group 1 (all cosmetic products).
Sweden	Approved for defined food products.
Switzerland	Approved for defined food products.
Syria	Approved for food.
Taiwan	Approved for defined food products.
Thailand	Approved for food.
Turkey	Approved for defined food products. Approved for the coloration of cosmetics of group 1 (all cosmetic products).
United Arab Emirates	Approved for food.
USA	Approved for defined food products. Utilization requires FDA certificate. Not approved for drugs and cosmetics.
Zambia	Approved for food.

For acceptance of this colorant in other countries, based on above mentioned approvals, see also 9.1.8.

C.I.40825

Name	EU-No.	C.I. No.	Class	Chemical name / formula
beta-Apo-8'-carotene acid ethyl ester C.I. Food Orange 7 CAS # 1109-11-1 EINECS # 214-173-7	E 160f	40825	Carotenoide	Carotene acid ethyl ester
Color	Orange solution in water.			
Solubility	Soluble in ethanol, chloroform, cyclohexane and fatty oils, insoluble in water. Also commercially available as a water-dispersible product.			

Chromatography DC Carrier	Source : Communication XVII DFG Farbstoff-Kommission Kieselgel Cyclohexane 40 ml + Acetic acid ester 10 ml.

Spectral photometry	Source : Kosmetische Färbemittel 3. ed., 1991)
Solvent Absorption maximum	Cyclohexane 449 nm

Main applications	Feed additive for egg yolk pigmentation.

Toxicological and dermatological data		Source
LD50 tested on mice	>10000 mg/kg	Kosmetische Färbemittel 3. ed., 1991
ADI-value (WHO 1974, SCF 1975) in the form of total carotenoids such as β-carotene, β-Apo-8'-carotenal and β-Apo-8'-carotene acid ethyl ester.	0-5.0 mg/kg	Ringbook Colorants for food, 1978

Certification status

European Union	Approved for defined food products (see 2.4.1.) and for the coloration of drugs and cosmetic preparations of group 1 (all cosmetic products).
Argentina	Approved for food.
Australia	Approved for defined food products.
Austria	Approved for defined food products.
Brazil	Approved for defined food products.
Canada	Approved for defined food products.
Chile	Approved for food.
Cyprus	Approved for defined food products.
Egypt	Approved for food.
Finland	Approved for defined food products.
Hungary	Approved for the coloration of cosmetics of group 1 (all cosmetic products).
India	Approved for food.
Iran	Approved for food.
Israel	Approved for food.
Japan	Not approved for food, drugs and cosmetics.
Kenya	Approved for food.
Kuwait	Approved for food.
Malaysia	Approved for defined food products.
Malta	Approved for food.
New Zealand	Approved for defined food products.
Norway	Approved for defined food products.
Philippines	Approved for food.

South Africa	Approved for defined food products.
	Approved for the coloration of cosmetics of group 1 (all cosmetic products).
Switzerland	Approved for defined food products.
Syria	Approved for food.
Taiwan	Approved for defined food products.
Thailand	Approved for defined food products.
Turkey	Approved for defined food products.
	Approved for the coloration of cosmetics of group 1 (all cosmetic products).
United Arab Emirates	Approved for food.
USA	Not approved for food, drugs and cosmetics.
Zambia	Approved for food.

For acceptance of this colorant in other countries, based on above mentioned approvals, see also 9.1.8.

C.I.40850

Name	EU-No.	C.I. No.	Class	Chemical name / formula
beta-Apo-8'-carotene acid ethyl ester C.I. Food Orange 7 CAS # 1109-11-1 EINECS # 214-173-7	E 161g	40850	Carotenoide (Xanthophyll)	Carotene acid ethyl ester

Color	Yellow-orange to yellow in oil.
Solubility	Soluble in chloroform and oils, insoluble in water and ethanol. Also commercially available as a water-dispersible products.
Chromatography DC Carrier	Source : Ringbook Colorants for food, (1978) Kieselgel Petrol ether (100-160 °C) 50 ml + Petrol ether (40-60 °C) 50 ml + Isopropanol 10 ml
Spectral photometry	Source : Ringbook Colorants for food, (1978)
Solvent Absorption maximum	Chloroform 485 nm
Main applications Food	- Beverages, tomato products, candies, salmon subtitute products.

Data Sheets

Toxicological and dermatological data		Source
LD50 tested on rats	>10000 mg/kg	Kosmetische Färbemittel 3. ed., 1991
Skin compatibility tested on guinea pigs	non-irritant	
Mucous membrane compatibility tested on a rabbit eye	minimal irritation on	
ADI-value (WHO 1974, SCF 1975)	0-25.0 mg/kg	
ADI-value (SCF 1987)	0-0.05 mg/kg	

Certification status

European Union	Approved for defined food products (see 2.4.1.) and for the coloration of drugs and cosmetic preparations of group 1 (all cosmetic products).
Argentina	Approved for food.
Australia	Approved for defined food products.
Austria	Approved for defined food products.
Brazil	Approved for defined food products.
Canada	Approved for defined food products.
Chile	Approved for food.
Cyprus	Approved for defined food products.
Egypt	Approved for food.
Hungary	Approved for the coloration of cosmetics of group 1 (all cosmetic products).
India	Approved for food.
Indonesia	Approved for food.
Iran	Approved for food.
Israel	Approved for food.
Japan	Approved for food. Not approved for cosmetics.
Kenya	Approved for food.
Kuwait	Approved for food.
Malaysia	Approved for defined food products.
Malta	Approved for food.
New Zealand	Approved for defined food products.
Saudi Arabia	Approved for food.
South Africa	Approved for defined food products. Approved for the coloration of cosmetics of group 1 (all cosmetic products).
Sweden	Approved for defined food products.
Switzerland	Approved for defined food products.
Syria	Approved for food.
Taiwan	Approved for defined food products.
Thailand	Approved for defined food products.
Turkey	Approved for defined food products. Approved for the coloration of cosmetics of group 1 (all cosmetic products).
United Arab Emirates	Approved for food.

USA	Approved for defined food products and feed additive for broilers: see restrictions (CFR 21, § 73.85) Approved for orally applied drugs. FDA certificate not required. Not approved for cosmetics.
Zambia	Approved for food.

For acceptance of this colorant in other countries, based on above mentioned approvals, see also 9.1.8.

C.I.42045

Name	EU-No.	C.I. No.	Class	Chemical name / formula
Patentblau VF C.I. Food Blue 3 C.I. Acid Blue 1 CAS # 129-17-9 EINECS # 204-934-1		42045	Triaryl-methane	4,4'-Bis(N-diethyl-amino)-triphenyl-carbinol-anhydride-2'',4''-disulfoacid, Sodium salt
Color	Blue solution in water.			
Solubility	Soluble in water (at 20 °C about 100 g/l), methanol, chloroform and dichloromethane.			
Chromatography DC Carrier	Source : Communication XVII DFG Farbstoff-Kommission Kieselgel Acetic acid ester 11 ml + Pyridine 5 ml + Water 4 ml			
Spectral photometry Solvent Absorption maximum	Source : Communication XVII DFG Farbstoff-Kommission Water 407, 635 nm			
Main applications Cosmetics	- Shampoo, foam bath, shower gel. - Liquid soap.			

Toxicological and dermatological data		Source
LD50 tested on rats	> 10000 mg/kg	Kosmetische Färbemittel 3. ed., 1991
Skin compatibility tested on rabbits	non-irritant	
Mucous membrane compatibility tested on a rabbit eye	non-irritant	

Data Sheets

Certification status

European Union	Approved for the coloration of cosmetics of group 3 (not on mucous membranes).
Hungary	Approved for the coloration of cosmetics of group 2 (not on eyes).
Japan	Not approved for food, drugs and cosmetics.
Poland	Approved for cosmetics.
South Africa	Approved for the coloration of cosmetics of group 3 (not on mucous membranes).
Turkey	Approved for the coloration of cosmetics of group 3 (not on mucous membranes).
USA	Not approved for food, drugs and cosmetics.

For acceptance of this colorant in other countries, based on above mentioned approvals, see also 9.1.8.

C.I.42052

Name	EU-No.	C.I. No.	Class	Chemical name / formula
C.I. Acid Blue 5 Blue # 203 (Japan) CAS # 3374-30-9 EINECS # unknown		42052	Triaryl-methane	2,4-Disulfo-5-hydroxy-4',4''-bis(N-ethyl-N-benzyl-amino)-triphenylcarbinol-anhydride, Calcium salt
Blue # 202 (Japan) CAS # unknown EINECS # unknown		42052:1	Triaryl-methane	-, Sodium salt

Color	Green-blue solution in water.
Solubility	Soluble in water and ethanol.
Chromatography	No information available.
Spectral photometry	No information available.

Toxicological and dermatological data	**Source**
No information available.	

Certification status

European Union	Not approved for food, drugs and cosmetics.
Argentina	Approved for cosmetics (Sodium salt) but not for application in the eye, mouth and lip areas.
Japan	Approved for drugs, quasi-drugs and cosmetics for external applications. Blue # 202 also in the form of Barium-lake.
Korea (South)	Approved for cosmetics (Sodium- and Calcium salt).
Taiwan	Approved for cosmetics (Calcium salt).
USA	Not approved for food, drugs and cosmetics.

For acceptance of this colorant in other countries, based on above mentioned approvals, see also 9.1.8.

C.I.42053

Name	EU-No.	C.I. No.	Class	Chemical name / formula
Echtgrün FCF C.I. Food Green 3 FD&C Green # 3 (CTFA adopted name) Green # 3 (Japan) CAS # 2353-45-9 EINECS # 219-091-5		42053	Triaryl-methane	2-Sulfo-4-hydroxy-4',4''-bis(N-ethyl-m-sulfo-benzyl-amino)-triphenylcarbinol-anhydride, Sodium salt
Color	Blue-green solution in water.			
Solubility	Soluble in water (ca. 20 g/l), in ethanol (< 1 g/l) and in glycerin (ca. 20 g/l).			
Chromatography DC Carrier	Source : Communication XVII DFG Farbstoff-Kommission Cellulose tert. Sodiumtricitrate solution 2.5 % 80 ml + Ammonia 25% 20 ml + Methanol 12 ml			
Spectral photometry Solvent Absorption maximum	Source : Communication XVII DFG Farbstoff-Kommission Water 420, 627 nm			
Main applications Cosmetics	- Mouthwash products.			

Toxicological and dermatological data		Source
LD50 tested on rats	> 2000 mg/kg	Kosmetische Färbemittel 3. ed., 1991

Data Sheets

Skin compatibility tested on rabbits	non-irritant
Mucous membrane compatibility tested on a rabbit eye	non-irritant
ADI-value (WHO 1986)	0-25 mg/kg

Certification status

European Union	Approved for the coloration of cosmetics of group 1 (all cosmetic products). Recommendation of the DFG Farbstoff-Kommission (1984) : Not to be used for application in the eye area.
Argentina	Approved for cosmetics, but not on eyes
Brazil	Approved for cosmetics, but not on eyes.
Canada	Approved for defined food products.
Hungary	Approved for the coloration of cosmetics of group 2 (not on eyes).
India	Approved for food.
Indonesia	Approved for food.
Iran	Approved for food.
Israel	Approved for drugs and cosmetics.
Japan	Approved for defined food products, also in the form of Aluminum lakes. Approved for drugs, "quasi-drugs" and cosmetics for external applications, also in the form of Aluminum lake.
Korea (South)	Approved for cosmetics.
Kuwait	Approved for food.
Philippines	Approved for food and cosmetics, but not on eyes.
Poland	Approved for cosmetics.
Saudi Arabia	Approved for food.
Singapore	Approved for food.
South Africa	Approved for the coloration of cosmetics of group 1 (all cosmetic products).
Sweden	Approved for defined food products.
Syria	Approved for food.
Taiwan	Approved for defined food products. Approved for cosmetics, also in the form of Aluminum-lakes.
Thailand	Approved for food.
Turkey	Approved for defined food products. Approved for the coloration of cosmetics of group 1 (all cosmetic products).
United Arab Emirates	Approved for food.
USA	Approved for defined food products. Approved for drugs and cosmetics, but not for application in the eye area. Utilization requires FDA certificate.
Venezuela	Approved for cosmetics, but not for application in the eye area.

For acceptance of this colorant in other countries, based on above mentioned approvals, see also 9.1.8.

C.I.42080

Name	EU-No.	C.I. No.	Class	Chemical name / formula
Amidoblau A C.I. Acid Blue 7 CAS # 3486-30-4 EINECS # 220-476-0		42080	Triaryl-methane	2,4-Disulfo-4',4''-bis(N-ethyl-benzyl-amino)-triphenyl-carbinol-anhydride, Sodium salt

Color	Blue solution in water.
Solubility	Soluble in water, ethanol and dichloromethane.
Chromatography DC Carrier	Source : Communication XVII DFG Farbstoff-Kommission Kieselgel Acetic acid ester 50 ml + Ammonia 25% 10 ml + Methanol 20 ml
Spectral photometry Solvent Absorption maximum	Source : Communication XVII DFG Farbstoff-Kommission Water 437, 633 nm (own assay : 412, 638 nm)
Main applications Cosmetics	- Shampoo, shower gel. - Liquid soap.

Toxicological and dermatological data		Source
LD50 tested on rats	11400 mg/kg	Kosmetische Färbemittel 3. ed., 1991
Skin compatibility tested on rabbits	non-irritant	
Mucous membrane compatibility tested on a rabbit eye	non-irritant	

Certification status

European Union	Approved for the coloration of cosmetics of group 4 (only for a short residence time on skin).
Hungary	Approved for the coloration of cosmetics of group 2 (not on eyes).
Israel	Approved for drugs and cosmetics.
Japan	Not approved for food, drugs and cosmetics.
Poland	Approved for cosmetics.
South Africa	Approved for the coloration of cosmetics of group 4 (only for a short residence time on skin).

| Turkey | Approved for the coloration of cosmetics of group 4 (only for a short residence time on skin). |
| USA | Not approved for food, drugs and cosmetics. |

For acceptance of this colorant in other countries, based on above mentioned approvals, see also 9.1.8.

C.I.42085

Name	EU-No.	C.I. No.	Class	Chemical name / formula
Guineagrün B C.I. Acid Green 3 C.I. Food Green 1 Green # 402 (Japan) CAS # 4680-78-8 EINECS # unknown		42085	Triaryl-methane	4',4''-Bis(N-ethyl-m-sulfo-benzyl-amino)-triphenylcarbinol-anhydride, Sodium salt

Color	Green solution in water.
Solubility	Soluble in water (green) and in ethanol (blue-green).
Chromatography	No information available.
Spectral photometry Solvent Absorption maximum	Source : own assay Water 428, 618 nm
Main applications	No information available.

Toxicological and dermatological data		Source
No information available.		

Certification status

European Union	Not approved for food, drugs and cosmetics.
Japan	Approved for the coloration of cosmetics of group 3 (not on mucous membranes), also in the form of Aluminum- and Barium lake.
Taiwan	Approved for facial toning masks, also in the form of aluminum-lakes, but not for cosmetics.
USA	Not approved for food, drugs and cosmetics.

For acceptance of this colorant in other countries, based on above mentioned approvals, see also 9.1.8.

C.I. 42090

Name	EU-No.	C.I. No.	Class	Chemical name / formula
Brillantblau FCF Patentblau AE C.I. Food Blue 2 C.I. Acid Blue 9 FD&C Blue # 1 (CTFA adopted name) Blue # 1 (Japan) CAS # 3844-45-9 EINECS # 223-339-8		42090	Triaryl-methane	2,4-Sulfo-4',4''-bis(N-ethyl-m-sulfo-benzyl-amino)-triphenyl-carbinol-anhydride, Sodium salt

D&C Blue # 4
  (CTFA adopted name)
Blue # 205 (Japan)
CAS # 2650-18-2;
     # 6371-85-3;
     # 3703-56-5
EINECS # 220-168-0
		42090	Triaryl-methane	-, Ammonium salt

Synonym unknown CAS # unknown EINECS # unknown		42090:1	Triaryl-methane	-, Barium salt
FD&C Blue # 1 lake CAS # 53026-57-6 EINECS # unknown		42090:2	Triaryl-methane	-, Aluminum lake

Color	Sodium- and ammonium salt result in a blue aqueous solution. Aluminum lake is a blue powder.
Solubility	Sodium salt soluble in water (at 20 °C ca. 70 g/l). Aluminum lake insoluble in water.
Chromatography DC Carrier	Source : Communication XVII DFG Farbstoff-Kommission Kieselgel Acetic acid ester 11 ml + Pyridine 5 ml + Water 4 ml
Spectral photometry Solvent Absorption maximum	Source : Communication XVII DFG Farbstoff-Kommission Water 405, 632 nm
Main applications Food Cosmetics Remark :	 - Beverages, candies. - Shampoo, foam bath, shower gel. - Liquid soap. - Toothpaste gels. In acidic media the color changes to green.

Toxicological and dermatological data		Source
LD50 tested on rats	>20400 mg/kg	Kosmetische Färbemittel 3. ed., 1991
Skin compatibility tested on rabbits	non-irritant	
Mucous membrane compatibility tested on a rabbit eye	non-irritant	
ADI-value (SCF 1975)	0-2.5 mg/kg	
(FDA 1982)	0-12 mg/kg	
(CIAA-liste Mouton)	0-12.5 mg/kg	
(EU document III/9280/90)	0-10 mg/kg	

Certification status

European Union	Approved for defined food products (see 2.4.1.) and for the coloration of drugs and cosmetic preparations of group 1 (all cosmetic products).
Argentina	Approved for cosmetics, but not on eyes.
Australia	Approved for defined food products.
Brazil	Approved for defined food products. Approved for cosmetics, but not for application in the eye area.
Canada	Approved for defined food products.
Chile	Approved for food.
Cyprus	Approved for defined food products.
Egypt	Approved for food.
Hungary	Approved for the coloration of cosmetics of group 2 (not on eyes).
India	Approved for food.
Indonesia	Approved for food.
Iran	Approved for food.
Israel	Approved for food, drugs and cosmetics.
Japan	Blue # 1 (Sodium salt). Approved for defined food products, also in the form of Aluminum lake. Approved for all drugs, "quasi-drugs" and cosmetics, also in the form of Aluminum-, Barium- and Zirconium lake. Blue # 205 (Ammonium salt). Approved for all drugs, "quasi-drugs" and cosmetics, also in the form of Aluminum-, Barium- and Zirconium lake.
Kenya	Approved for defined food products.
Korea (South)	Approved for food (Sodium salt). Approved for cosmetics (Sodium- and Ammonium salt).
Kuwait	Approved for food.
Malaysia	Approved for defined food products.
Malta	Approved for food.
Mexico	Approved for defined food products.
New Zealand	Approved for defined food products.
Philippines	Approved for food. Approved for cosmetics, but not in the eye area.
Poland	Approved for cosmetics.

Saudi Arabia	Approved for food.
Singapore	Approved for food.
South Africa	Approved for defined food products.
	Approved for the coloration of cosmetics of group 1 (all cosmetic products).
Switzerland	Approved for drugs.
Syria	Approved for food.
Taiwan	Approved for defined food products.
	Approved for cosmetics (Sodium salt), also in the form of Aluminum-, Barium- and Zirconium lakes. Ammonium salt approved for cosmetics, also in the form of Aluminum lake.
Thailand	Approved for food and cosmetics.
Turkey	Approved for the coloration of cosmetic of group 1 (all cosmetic products).
Uruguay	Approved for food.
United Arab Emirates	Approved for food.
USA	FD&C Blue # 1 (Sodium salt)
	Approved for defined food products, drugs and cosmetics (also in the form of Aluminum lake), but not for application in the eye area.
	Utilization requires FDA certificate.
	D&C Blue # 4 (Ammonium salt).
	Approved for cosmetics (also in the form of Aluminum lake), but not for application in the eye and lip area.
	Utilization requires FDA certificate.
Venezuela	Approved for food.
	Approved for cosmetics, but not for application in the eye area.
Zambia	Approved for food.

For acceptance of this colorant in other countries, based on above mentioned approvals, see also 9.1.8.

C.I.42095

Name	EU-No.	C.I. No.	Class	Chemical name / formula
Säuregrün F C.I. Food Green 2 C.I. Acid Green 5 CAS # 5141-20-8 EINECS # unknown		42095	Triaryl-methane	4,4''-bis (N-ethyl-N-m-sulfo-benzyl)-triphenyl-carbinol-anhydride, Sodium salt
Color	Blue-green solution in water.			
Solubility	Soluble in water. Nearly insoluble in ethanol.			

Chromatography	No information available.
Spectral photometry	No information available.
Main applications	No information available.
Toxicological and dermatological data	**Source**

No information available.

Certification status

European Union	Not approved for food, drugs and cosmetics.
Argentina	Approved only for soap.
Japan	Approved for drugs, "quasi-drugs" and cosmetics for external applications (group 3), also in the form of Aluminum- and Zirconium lakes.
Korea (South)	Approved for cosmetics.
Taiwan	Approved for cosmetics, also in the form of Aluminum- and Zirconium lakes.
USA	Not approved for food, drugs and cosmetics.

For acceptance of this colorant in other countries, based on above mentioned approvals, see also 9.1.8.

C.I.42100

Name	EU-No.	C.I. No.	Class	Chemical name / formula
Neptungrün SGX C.I. Acid Green 9 CAS # 4857-8-2 EINECS # unknown		42100	Triaryl-methane	2-Chloro-4,4''-bis (N-ethyl-m-sulfo-benzylamino)-triphenyl-carbinol-anhydride, Sodium salt

Color	Green solution in water.
Chromatography DC Carrier	Source : Communication XVII DFG Farbstoff-Kommission Kieselgel Petrolether (100-160 °C) 50 ml + petrolether (40-60 °C) 50 ml + isopropanol 10 ml

Spectral photometry	Source : Communication XVII DFG Farbstoff-Kommission
Solvent	Water
Absorption maximum	416, 638 nm

Main applications	No information available.

Toxicological and dermatological data		**Source**
LD50 tested on rats	> 11500 mg/kg	Kosmetische Färbemittel 3. ed., 1991
Skin compatibility tested on rabbits	non irritating	
Mucous membrane compatibility tested on a rabbit eye	temporary irritations	

Certification status

European Union	Approved for the coloration of cosmetics of group 4 (only for a short residence time on skin).
Bulgaria	Not approved for cosmetics.
Hungary	Approved for the coloration of cosmetics of group 2 (not on eyes).
Japan	Not approved for food, drugs and cosmetics.
Poland	Not approved for cosmetics.
South Africa	Approved for the coloration of cosmetics of group 4 (only for a short residence time on skin).
Turkey	Approved for the coloration of cosmetics of group 4 (only for a short residence time on skin).
USA	Not approved for food, drugs and cosmetics.

For acceptance of this colorant in other countries, based on above mentioned approvals, see also 9.1.8.

C.I.42170

Name	**EU-No.**	**C.I. No.**	**Class**	**Chemical name / formula**
Acilanechtgrün 10G C.I. Acid Green 22 CAS # 5863-51-4 EINECS # unknown		42170	Triaryl-methane	2-Chloro-2',2''-dimethyl-4',4''-bis (N-methyl-m-sulfobenzylamino)-triphenylcarbinol-anhydride, Sodium salt
Color	Green solution in water.			

Solubility	Soluble in water, ethanol and dichloromethane.
Chromatography DC Carrier	Source : Communication XVII DFG Farbstoff-Kommission Kieselgel Acetic acid ester 11 ml + Pyridine 5 ml + Water 4 ml
Spectral photometry Solvent Absorption maximum	Source : Communication XVII DFG Farbstoff-Kommission Water 435, 663 nm
Main applications Food	Painting, lacquering and coloration of egg shells. As well as for the coloration of Easter grass (wood shavings for bunny nests).

Toxicological and dermatological data		Source
LD50 tested on rats	> 8500 mg/kg	Kosmetische Färbemittel 3. ed., 1991
Skin compatibility tested on rabbits	slightly irritating temporary irritations	
Mucous membrane compatibility tested on a rabbit eye		

Certification status

European Union	According to Colorant Guideline 94/36/EU, not approved any more after June 30, 1996 for food surface stamps and for the coloration of egg shells. Approved for the coloration of cosmetics of group 4 (only for a short residence time on skin).
Bulgaria	Not approved for cosmetics.
Hungary	Approved for the coloration of cosmetics of group 2 (not on eyes).
Japan	Not approved for food, drugs and cosmetics.
Poland	Not approved for cosmetics.
South Africa	Approved for the coloration of cosmetics of group 4 (only for a short residence time on skin).
Thailand	Approved for cosmetics.
Turkey	Approved for the coloration of cosmetics of group 4 (only for a short residence time on skin).
USA	Not approved for food, drugs and cosmetics.

For acceptance of this colorant in other countries, based on above mentioned approvals, see also 9.1.8.

C.I.42510

Name	EU-No.	C.I. No.	Class	Chemical name / formula
Fuchsin C.I. Basic Violet 14 CAS # 632-99-50 EINECS # unknown		42510	Triaryl-methane	4,4',4''-Triamino-3-methyl-triphenyl-carbinol-anhydride, Sodium salt
Color	Red-violet solution in water.			
Solubility	Insoluble in water, ethanol and dichloromethane.			
Chromatography DC Carrier	Source : Communication XVII DFG Farbstoff-Kommission Kieselgel Benzol 90 ml + Acetone 10 ml			
Spectral photometry Solvent Absorption maximum	Source : Communication XVII DFG Farbstoff-Kommission Water 546 nm			
Main applications	No information available.			

Toxicological and dermatological data		Source
No information available		
LD50 tested on rats	> 12000 mg/kg	Kosmetische Färbemittel 3. ed., 1991
Skin compatibility tested on rabbits	non-irritant	
Mucous membrane compatibility tested on a rabbit eye	non-irritant	

Certification status

European Union	Approved for the coloration of cosmetics of group 3 (not on mucous membranes).
Bulgaria	Not approved for cosmetics.
Hungary	Approved for the coloration of cosmetics of group 2 (not on eyes).
Indonesia	Approved for food.
Japan	Not approved for food, drugs and cosmetics.
Malta	Approved for cosmetics, but only for rinse-off products.
Poland	Not approved for cosmetics.
South Africa	Approved for the coloration of cosmetics of group 3 (not on mucous membranes).
Turkey	Approved for the coloration of cosmetics of group 3 (not on mucous membranes).
USA	Not approved for food, drugs and cosmetics.

For acceptance of this colorant in other countries, based on above mentioned approvals, see also 9.1.8.

C.I.42520

Name	EU-No.	C.I. No.	Class	Chemical name / formula
Neufuchsin C.I. Basic Violet 2 CAS # 3248-91-7 EINECS # unknown		42520	Triaryl- methane	4,4',4''-Triamino- 3,3',3''-trimethyl- triphenylcarbinol- anhydride, Chloride
Color	Red-violet solution in water.			
Solubility	Soluble in water and ethanol.			
Chromatography DC Carrier	Source : own assay Schleicher & Schüll 2043 b Mgl Acetic acid ester 11 ml + Pyridine 5 ml + Water 4 ml			
Spectral photometry Solvent Absorption maximum	Source : own assay Water 542 nm			
Main applications	No information available.			

Toxicological and dermatological data		Source
LD50 tested on rats	> 200 mg/kg (?)	Kosmetische Färbemittel
Skin compatibility tested on rabbits	non-irritant	3. ed., 1991
Mucous membrane compatibility tested on a rabbit eye	reversible ... within 9 days	

Certification status

European Union	Approved for the coloration of cosmetics of group 4 (only for a short residence time on skin).
Bulgaria	Not approved for cosmetics.
Hungary	Approved for the coloration of cosmetics of group 1 (all cosmetic products, max. level not more than 5 ppm).
Japan	Not approved for food, drugs and cosmetics.
Poland	Not approved for cosmetics.
South Africa	Approved for the coloration of cosmetics of group 4 (only for a short residence time on skin).
Turkey	Approved for the coloration of cosmetics of group 4 (only for a short residence time on skin).
USA	Not approved any more for cosmetics.

For acceptance of this colorant in other countries, based on above mentioned approvals, see also 9.1.8.

C.I.42535

Name	EU-No.	C.I. No.	Class	Chemical name / formula
Methyl Violet B C.I. Basic Violet 1 CAS # 8004-87-3 EINECS # unknown		42535	Triaryl- methane	4-Methylamino- 4',4''-bis (dimethyl- amino)-triphenyl- carbinol-anhydride, Chloride, isomere blend

Color	Red-violet solution in water.
Solubility	Soluble in water (at 20° C ca. 50 g/l), ethanol, methanol and dichloromethane.
Chromatography DC Carrier	Source : Communication DFG Farbstoff-Kommission Cellulose tert. Butanol 40 ml + Methylethylketone 25 ml + Water 25 ml
Spectral photometry Solvent Absorption maximum	Source : Communication DFG Farbstoff-Kommission Water 584 nm (own assay : 584 nm)
Main applications Food	stamp color for food products.

Toxicological and dermatological data		Source
LD50 tested on rats	> 460 / < 680 mg/kg	Safety Data Sheet Basonyl Violett 600 BASF (1982)
Skin compatibility tested on rabbits	slightly irritating	
Mucous membrane compatibility tested on a rabbit eye	slightly irritating	

Certification status	
European Union	Not approved for cosmetics. According to Colorant Guideline 94/36/EU not approved any-more as food surface stamp and for the coloration of egg shells.
Japan	Not approved for food, drugs and cosmetics.
Malta	Approved for food.
Poland	Not approved for cosmetics.
South Africa	Approved for the declaration of meat. Not approved for cosmetics.
Switzerland	Approved as a food surface stamp and for the coloration of egg shells.
USA	Not approved any more for cosmetics.

For acceptance of this colorant in other countries, based on above mentioned approvals, see also 9.1.8.

Data Sheets

C.I.42640

Name	EU-No.	C.I. No.	Class	Chemical name / formula
Formylviolett S4BN C.I. Food Red 6 C.I. Acid Red 27 Red # 2 (Japan) CAS # 915-67-30 EINECS # 213-022-2		42640	Triaryl-methane	4-N-Dimethylamino-4',4''-bis (N-ethyl-m-sulfobenzyl-amino)-triphenyl-carbinol-anhydride, Sodium salt

Color	Violet solution in water.
Solubility	Soluble in water, ethanol, methanol.
Chromatography DC Carrier	Source : Communication XVII DFG Farbstoff-Kommission Kieselgel n-Butanol 40 ml + Acetone 40 ml + Ammonia 25% 10 ml + Water 30 ml
Spectral photometry Solvent Absorption maximum	Source : Communication XVII DFG Farbstoff-Kommission Water 543 nm
Solvent Absorption maximum	Methanol (own assay) 586 nm
Solvent Absorption maximum	Ethanol 590 nm
Main applications Cosmetics	- Shampoo, foam bath, shower gel. - Not suitable for toilet soap.

Toxicological and dermatological data	Source
No information available.	

Certification status

European Union	Not approved for cosmetics.
Hungary	Not approved for cosmetics.
Japan	Not approved for food, drugs and cosmetics.
Poland	Approved for cosmetics.
South Africa	Not approved for cosmetics.
Thailand	Approved for cosmetics.
USA	Not approved for food, drugs and cosmetics.

For acceptance of this colorant in other countries, based on above mentioned approvals, see also 9.1.8.

C.I.42735

Name	EU-No.	C.I. No.	Class	Chemical name / formula
Acilanbrillantblau FFR C.I. Acid Blue 104 CAS # 6505-30-2 EINECS # not known		42735	Triaryl-methane	2,2'-Dimethyl-4,4'-bis (N-ethyl-m-sulfobenzyl)-4''-diethylamino-tri-phenylcarbinol-anhydride, Sodium salt

Color	Blue solution in water.
Solubility	Soluble in water (ca. 10g/l at 20 °C), methanol and dichloromethane.
Chromatography DC Carrier	Source : Communication XVII DFG Farbstoff-Kommission Kieselgel Acetic acid ester 11 ml + Pyridine 5 ml + Water 40 ml
Spectral photometry Solvent Absorption maximum	Source : Communication XVII DFG Farbstoff-Kommission Methanol 604 nm (own assay)
Main applications Food Cosmetics	- Stamping of food surfaces and packaging material, painting and coloring of egg shells. - Shampoo, foam bath, shower gel. - Liquid soap.

Toxicological and dermatological data		Source
LD50 tested on rats	> 8000 mg/kg	Kosmetische Färbemittel 3. ed., 1991
Skin compatibility tested on rabbits	non-irritant	
Mucous membrane compatibility tested on a rabbit eye	non-irritant	

Certification status	
European Union	According to Colorant Guideline 94/36/EU not approved anymore as food surface stamp and for the coloration of egg shells. Approved for the coloration of cosmetics of group 3 (not on mucous membranes).
Bulgaria	Not approved for cosmetics.
Hungary	Approved for the coloration of cosmetics of group 2 (not on eyes).

Japan	Not approved for food, drugs and cosmetics.
Malta	Not approved for cosmetics.
Poland	Not approved for cosmetics.
South Africa	Approved for the coloration of cosmetics of group 3 (not on mucous membranes).
Thailand	Approved for cosmetics.
Turkey	Approved for the coloration of cosmetics of group 3 (not on mucous membranes).
USA	Not approved for food, drugs and cosmetics.

For acceptance of this colorant in other countries, based on above mentioned approvals, see also 9.1.8.

C.I.44025

Name	EU-No.	C.I. No.	Class	Chemical name / formula
Naphtalingrün V C.I. Acid Green 16 CAS # unknown EINECS # unknown		44025	Triaryl-methane	3,6-Disulfo-naphthyl-4',4''=bis (dimethylamino)-diphenylmethane, Sodium salt
Color	Blue-green solution in water.			
Solubility	Soluble in water.			
Chromatography DC Carrier	Source : own assay Schleicher & Schüll 2043 b Mgl Acetic acid ester 11 ml + Pyridine 5 ml + Water 4 ml			
Spectral photometry Solvent Absorption maximum	Source : own assay Water 426, 640 nm			
Main applications Cosmetics	- Shampoo, shower gel. - Liquid soap.			

Toxicological and dermatological data		Source
LD50 tested on rats	> 5000 mg/kg	Safety data sheet Sandolan Brillant-grün EB 400%, Sandoz 10/77
Skin compatibility tested on rabbits	slightly irritating	
Mucous membrane compatibility tested on a rabbit eye	slightly irritating	

Certification status

European Union	Not approved for cosmetics.
Hungary	Not approved for cosmetics.
Japan	Not approved for food, drugs and cosmetics.
South Africa	Not approved for cosmetics.
USA	Not approved for food, drugs and cosmetics.

For acceptance of this colorant in other countries, based on above mentioned approvals, see also 9.1.8.

C.I.44040

Name	EU-No.	C.I. No.	Class	Chemical name / formula
Viktoriablau R C.I. Basic Blue 11 CAS # unknown EINECS # unknown	C 3	44040	Triaryl-methane	4-Ethylamino-naphthyl-4',4''bis(dimethylamino)-diphenylmethane, Chloride
Color	Blue solution in water.			
Solubility	Soluble in water.			
Chromatography DC Carrier	Source : Communication XVII DFG Farbstoff-Kommission Kieselgel Acetic acid ester 11 ml + Pyridine 5 ml + Water 4 ml			
Spectral photometry Solvent Absorption maximum	Source : Communication XVII DFG Farbstoff-Kommission Dimethylformamide 610 nm			
Main applications	No information available.			

Toxicological and dermatological data

No information available.

Certification status

European Union	According to Colorant Guideline 94/36/EU not approved anymore as food surface stamp and for the coloration of egg shells. Not approved for cosmetics.
Hungary	Not approved for cosmetics.
Japan	Not approved for food, drugs and cosmetics.

Data Sheets

South Africa   Not approved for cosmetics.
USA   Not approved for food, drugs and cosmetics.
For acceptance of this colorant in other countries, based on above mentioned approvals, see also 9.1.8.

C.I.44045

Name	EU-No.	C.I. No.	Class	Chemical name / formula
Viktoriablau B C.I. Basic Blue 26 CAS # 2580-56-5 EINECS # unknown	C 4	44045	Triaryl-methane	4-Anilino-naphthyl-4',4''-bis(dimethylamino)-diphenyl-methane, Chloride
Color	Blue solution in water.			
Solubility	Soluble in water.			
Chromatography DC Carrier	Source : Communication XVII DFG Farbstoff-Kommission Kieselgel Acetic acid ester 11 ml + Pyridine 5 ml + Water 4 ml			
Spectral photometry Solvent Absorption maximum	Source : Communication XVII DFG Farbstoff-Kommission Dimethylformamide 612 nm			
Main applications	No information available.			

Toxicological and dermatological data

LD50 tested on rats	1037 mg/kg	Kosmetische Färbemittel 3. ed., 1991
Skin compatibility tested on rabbits	non-irritant	
Mucous membrane compatibility tested on a rabbit eye	strong irritation after 7 days	

Certification status

European Union	Approved for the coloration of cosmetics of group 3 (not on mucous membranes). According to Colorant Guideline 94/36/EU not approved as food surface stamp and for the coloration of egg shells. Not approved for cosmetics.
Argentina	Approved only for soap.

Hungary	Approved for the coloration of cosmetics of group 2 (not on eyes).
Japan	Not approved for food, drugs and cosmetics.
South Africa	Approved for the coloration of cosmetics of group 3 (not on mucous membranes).
Turkey	Approved for the coloration of cosmetics of group 3 (not on mucous membranes).
USA	Not approved for food, drugs and cosmetics.

For acceptance of this colorant in other countries, based on above mentioned approvals, see also 9.1.8.

C.I.44090

Name	EU-No.	C.I. No.	Class	Chemical name / formula
Brillantsäuregrün BS C.I. Food Green 4 C.I. Acid Green 50 CAS # 3087-16-9 EINECS # 221-409-2	E 142	44090	Triaryl-methane	2-Hydroxy-3,6-di-sulfo-naphthyl-4',4''-bis (dimethylamino)-diphenylmethane, Sodium salt
Color	Blue-green solution in water.			
Solubility	Soluble in water (ca. 80 g/l at 20 °C), and ethanol (ca. 10 g/l), insoluble in oil.			
Chromatography DC Carrier	Source : Communication XVII DFG Farbstoff-Kommission Kieselgel Acetic acid ester 11 ml + Pyridine 5 ml + Water 4 ml			
Spectral photometry Solvent Absorption maximum	Source : Communication XVII DFG Farbstoff-Kommission Water 543 nm			
Main applications Food Cosmetics	 - Candies. - Poor light stability in products containing tensides.			

Toxicological and dermatological data		Source
LD50 tested on rats	>2000 mg/kg	Kosmetische Färbemittel 3. ed., 1991
ADI-value (EEC Color Group 1983):	0-5.0 mg/kg	

Data Sheets

Certification status

European Union	Not approved for cosmetics.
Argentina	Approved for food products.
Australia	Approved only for defined food products.
Austria	Approved only for defined food products.
Bulgaria	Not approved for cosmetics.
Chile	Approved for food products.
Cyprus	Approved for defined food products.
Hungary	Approved for the coloration of cosmetics of group 2 (not on eyes).
India	Not approved for food products.
Indonesia	Approved for food products.
Japan	Not approved for food, drugs and cosmetics.
Malta	Approved for food products.
New Zealand	Approved only for defined food products.
Poland	Not approved for cosmetics.
Singapore	Approved for food products.
South Africa	Approved only for defined food products.
	Approved for the coloration of cosmetics of group 1 (all cosmetic products).
Switzerland	Approved only for defined food products.
Thailand	Approved for cosmetics.
Tunisia	Approved for food products.
Turkey	Approved for the coloration of cosmetics of group 1 (all cosmetic products).
USA	Not approved for food, drugs and cosmetics.
Zambia	Approved for food products.

For acceptance of this colorant in other countries, based on above mentioned approvals, see also 9.1.8.

C.I. 45100

Name	EU-No.	C.I. No.	Class	Chemical name / formula
Sulforhodamin B C.I. Acid Red 52 Red # 102 (Japan) CAS # 3520-42-1 EINECS # 222-529-8		45100	Xanthene	3,6-Bis (diethylamino)-9-(2,4-disulfophenyl)-xanthyl-immonium, Sodium salt
Color	Red fluorescent solution in water.			
Solubility	Soluble in water and ethanol.			
Chromatography DC Carrier	Source : own assay Schleicher & Schüll 2043 b Mgl Acetic acid ester 11 ml + Pyridine 5 ml + Water 4 ml			

Spectral photometry	Source : own assay
Solvent	Water
Absorption maximum	566 nm, shoulder at 530 nm

Main applications
Cosmetics
- Shampoo, foam bath.
- Liquid soap.
- Can be used as substitute for the disapproved Rhodamin C.I.45170.

Toxicological and dermatological data		Source
LD50 tested on rats	> 10000 mg/kg	Kosmetische Färbemittel
Skin compatibility tested on rabbits	non-irritant	3. ed., 1991
Mucous membrane compatibility tested on a rabbit eye	non-irritant	

Certification status	
European Union	Approved for the coloration of cosmetics of group 4 (only for a short residence time on skin).
Hungary	Approved for the coloration of cosmetics of group 1 (all cosmetic products).
Indonesia	Not approved for cosmetics.
Japan	Approved for defined food products. Approved for drugs, "quasi-drugs" and cosmetics for external applications, also in the form of aluminum-lakes.
Korea (South)	Approved for cosmetics, but not for application in the eye and lip area.
South Africa	Approved for the coloration of cosmetics of group 4 (only for a short residence time on skin).
Turkey	Approved for the coloration of cosmetics of group 4 (only for a short residence time on skin)
USA	Not approved for food, drugs and cosmetics.

For acceptance of this colorant in other countries, based on above mentioned approvals, see also 9.1.8.

C.I.45170

Name	EU-No.	C.I. No.	Class	Chemical name / formula
Rhodamin B C.I. Basic Violet 10 CAS # 81-88-930 EINECS # unknown		45170	Xanthene	3,6-Bis (diethyl-amino)-9-(2'-benzoic acid)-xanthyl-immonium, Chloride (X)

Data Sheets

Solvent Red 49 45170:1 Xanthene -, free base
CAS # unknown
EINECS # unknown

Erroneously called "stearate" in the literature, previously called D&C Red # 37

Color	Red violet fluorescent solution in water.
Solubility	Soluble in water and ethanol.
Chromatography	No information available.
Chromatography DC Carrier	Source : Communication XVII DFG Farbstoff-Kommission Kieselgel Acetic acid ester 11 ml + Pyridine 5 ml + Water 4 ml
Spectral photometry Solvent Absorption maximum	Source : Communication XVII DFG Farbstoff-Kommission Methanol 470 nm
Solvent Absorption maximum	Water (own assay) 350, 554 nm

Main applications
Cosmetics
- Shampoo, foam bath, shower gel.
- Liquid soap, toilet soap.
- Can be replaced by Sulforhodamin C.I.45100.

Toxicological and dermatological data		Source
LD50 tested on rats	> 2000 mg/kg	Safety data sheet Sicomet Rot B
Skin compatibility tested on rabbits	non-irritant	45170 BASF
Mucous membrane compatibility tested on a rabbit eye	strong irritation	

Certification status

European Union	Not approved for cosmetics.
Hungary	Not approved for cosmetics.
Japan	Not approved for food, drugs and cosmetics.
Korea (South)	Approved for cosmetics (chloride, stearate and acetate).
South Africa	Not approved for cosmetics.
Taiwan	Approved for cosmetics (in the form of chloride, stearate and acetate. Chloride also in the form of Aluminum lake.
USA	Not approved for drugs and cosmetics.

For acceptance of this colorant in other countries, based on above mentioned approvals, see also 9.1.8.

C.I.45190

Name	EU-No.	C.I. No.	Class	Chemical name / formula
Echtsäureviolett ARR C.I. Acid Violet 9 Red # 401 (Japan) CAS # 6252-76-2 EINECS # unknown	C 17	45190	Xanthene	3-m-Toluidine-6-m-toluidine-p-sulfo acid-9-(2-benzoic acid)-xanthyl-immonium, Sodium salt

Color	Red violet solution in water.
Solubility	Soluble in water (at 20 °C about 40 g/l).
Chromatography DC Carrier	Source : Communication XVII DFG Farbstoff-Kommission Kieselgel tert. Butanol 40 ml + Methylethylketone 25 ml + Water 25 ml
Spectral photometry Solvent Absorption maximum	Source : Communication XVII DFG Farbstoff-Kommission Water 350, 527 nm
Main applications Cosmetics	- Shampoo, shower gel. - Liquid soap, toilet soap.

Toxicological and dermatological data		Source
LD50 tested on rats	> 5000 mg/kg	Kosmetische Färbemittel 3. ed., 1991
Skin compatibility tested on rabbits	slightly irritating	
Mucous membrane compatibility tested on a rabbit eye	minor irritation	

Certification status	
European Union	Approved for the coloration of cosmetics of group 4 (only for a short residence time on skin). According to Colorant Guideline 94/36/EU not approved after June 30, 1996 as food surface stamp and for coloration of egg shells.
Bulgaria	Approved for cosmetics.
Hungary	Approved for the coloration of cosmetics of group 1 (all cosmetic products).
Japan	Approved for drugs, "quasi-drugs" and cosmetics for external applications, but not on mucous membranes.

Korea (South)	Approved for cosmetics.
South Africa	Approved for the coloration of cosmetics of group 4 (only for a short residence time on skin).
Taiwan	Approved for facial toning masks, also in the form of aluminum-lakes, but not for cosmetics.
Turkey	Approved for the coloration of cosmetics of group 4 (only for a short residence time on skin).
USA	Not approved for food, drugs and cosmetics.

For acceptance of this colorant in other countries, based on above mentioned approvals, see also 9.1.8.

C.I. 45220

Name	EU-No.	C.I. No.	Class	Chemical name / formula
Sulforhodamin G C.I. Acid Red 50 CAS # 5873-16-5 EINECS # unknown		45220	Xanthene	3,6-Bis(ethylamino)-2,7-dimethyl-9-(2,4-disulfophenyl)-xanthylimmonium, Sodium salt
Color	Red solution in water.			
Solubility	Soluble in water.			
Chromatography DC Carrier	Source : Communication XVII DFG Farbstoff-Kommission Kieselgel n-Butanol 40 ml + Acetone 40 ml + Ammonia 25% 10 ml + Water 30 ml			
Spectral photometry Solvent Absorption maximum	Source : Communication XVII DFG Farbstoff-Kommission Water 530 nm			
Main applications	No information available.			

Toxicological and dermatological data		Source
LD50 tested on rats	> 10000 mg/kg	Kosmetische Färbemittel 3. ed., 1991
Skin compatibility tested on rabbits	non-irritating	
Mucous membrane compatibility tested on a rabbit eye	non-irritating	

Certification status

European Union	Approved for the coloration of cosmetics of group 4 (only for a short residence time on skin).
Hungary	Approved for the coloration of cosmetics of group 1 (all cosmetic products).
Japan	Not approved for food, drugs and cosmetics.
South Africa	Approved for the coloration of cosmetics of group 4 (only for a short residence time on skin).
Turkey	Approved for the coloration of cosmetics of group 4 (only for a short residence time on skin).
USA	Not approved for food, drugs and cosmetics.

For acceptance of this colorant in other countries, based on above mentioned approvals, see also 9.1.8.

C.I.45350

Name	EU-No.	C.I. No.	Class	Chemical name / formula
Uranin C.I. Acid Yellow 73 C-ext. Gelb 16 Gelb-10, III, 2 D&C Yellow # 8 (CTFA adopted name) Yellow # 202 (Japan) CAS # 518-47-80 EINECS # 208-253-0		45350	Xanthene	Fluorescin, Sodium salt
Yellow # 2 (Japan) CAS # 6417-85-2 EINECS # unknown		45350	Xanthene	-, Potassium salt
Fluorescin C.I. solvent Yellow 94 D&C Yellow # 7 (CTFA adopted name) Yellow # 203 (Japan) CAS # 2321-07-5 EINECS # unknown		45350:1	Xanthene	-, free acid
Color	Sodium salt : yellow fluorescent solution in water. Free acid : yellow fluorescent solution in oil.			
Solubility	Sodium salt soluble in water (at 20 °C about 100 g/l), low solubility in alcohol. Free acids soluble in oils.			

Chromatography	Source : Communication XVII DFG Farbstoff-Kommission
DC	Cellulose
Carrier	tert. Sodium citrate solution 2.5 % 80 ml + Ammonia 25% 20 ml + Methanol 12 ml

Spectral photometry	Of the Sodium salt : Source : Communication XVII DFG Farbstoff-Kommission
Solvent	Water
Absorption maximum	485 nm 490 nm (own assay in diluted ammonia)

Main applications	
Cosmetics	- Shampoo, foam bath, shower gel, bathing salt, liquid soap (due to poor light stability not recommended for toilet soap).

Toxicological and dermatological data		Source
Sodium salt		
LD50 tested on rats	6721 / 9300 mg/kg	Kosmetische Färbemittel 3. ed., 1991
Skin compatibility tested on rabbits	non-irritant	
Mucous membrane compatibility tested on a rabbit eye	non-irritant	

Certification status

European Union	Approved for the coloration of cosmetics of group 1 (all cosmetic products, max. level not more than 6% of total mass).
Argentina	Approved for cosmetics for external applications, but not on mucous membranes.
Brazil	Approved for cosmetics for external applications, but not on mucous membranes.
Bulgaria	Approved for cosmetics, but not in the eye area.
Hungary	Approved for the coloration of cosmetics of group 1 (all cosmetic products, max. level not more than 6% of total mass).
Israel	Approved for drugs and cosmetics.
Japan	Yellow # 202(1) and (2) (Sodium- and Potassium salt), also in the form of Aluminum lake : Approved for drugs, "quasi-drugs" and cosmetics for external applications. Yellow # 201 (free acid), but not in the form of paint : Approved for drugs, "quasi-drugs" and cosmetics for external applications.
Korea (South)	Approved for cosmetics, but not for application in the eye area.
Philippines	Approved for cosmetics but only for external applications.
Poland	Approved for cosmetics, but not for application in the eye area.
South Africa	Approved for the coloration of cosmetics of group 1 (all cosmetic products, max. level not more than 6% of total mass).
Taiwan	Approved for cosmetics (all compounds and also in the form of Aluminum lake).

Thailand	Approved for cosmetics.
Turkey	Approved for the coloration of cosmetics of group 1 (all cosmetic products, max. level not more than 6% of total mass).
USA	Approved for drugs and cosmetics, but not for application in the eye area. Utilization requires FDA certificate.
Venezuela	Approved for cosmetics but not for application on mucous membranes.

For acceptance of this colorant in other countries, based on above mentioned approvals, see also 9.1.8.

C.I.45370

Name	EU-No.	C.I. No.	Class	Chemical name / formula
Eosin H8G C.I. Acid Orange 11 CAS # unknown EINECS # unknown		45370	Xanthene	4,5-Dibrom-fluorescin, Sodium salt, (X)
C.I. solvent Red 72 D&C Orange # 5 (CTFA adopted name) Orange # 202 (Japan) CAS # 596-02-3 EINECS # unknown		45370:1	Xanthene	-, free acid

Color	of the free acid : Orange fluorescent solution in water or ethanol.
Solubility	of the free acid : Soluble in ethanol, acetone, glycol and oil, low solubility in water.
Chromatography DC Carrier	of the free acid : Source: Communication XVII DFG Farbstoff-Kommission Kieselgel Acetic acid ester 11 ml + Pyridine 5 ml + Water 4 ml
Spectral photometry Solvent Absorption maximum	of the free acid: Source: Communication XVII DFG Farbstoff-Kommission Methanol 510 nm
Main applications Cosmetics	 - Lipstick.

Data Sheets

Toxicological and dermatological data		Source
LD50 tested on rats	11300 mg/kg	Kosmetische Färbemittel 3. ed., 1991
Skin compatibility tested on rabbits	non-irritant	
Mucous membrane compatibility tested on a rabbit eye	temporary irritation	

Certification status

Note : All data are related to the free acid.
Literature data relating to C.I./CAS/Sodium salt/free acid are contradictory and sometimes incorrect.

European Union	Approved for the coloration of cosmetics of group 1 (all cosmetic products).
Hungary	Approved for the coloration of cosmetics of group 1 (all cosmetic products).
Japan	Approved for drugs, "quasi-drugs" and cosmetics for external applications.
Korea (South)	Approved for cosmetics (free acid).
South Africa	Approved for the coloration of cosmetics of group 1 (all cosmetic products).
Taiwan	Approved for cosmetics (free acid, Sodium and Potassium salt, Aluminum- and Zirconium lake).
Turkey	Approved for the coloration of cosmetic of group 1 (all cosmetic products).
USA	Approved for orally applied drugs including mouth wash water and tooth care products. Daily maximum dosage in orally applied drugs 5 mg. Approved for cosmetics, but not for application in the eye area. Maximum dosage in lipsticks 5%. Utilization requires FDA certificate.

For acceptance of this colorant in other countries, based on above mentioned approvals, see also 9.1.8.

C.I.45380

Name	EU-No.	C.I. No.	Class	Chemical name / formula
Eosin C.I. Acid Red 87 D&C Red # 22 (CTFA adopted name) Red # 230(1) (Japan) CAS # 17372-87-1 EINECS # unknown		45380	Xanthene	-, Sodium salt

Red # 230(2) Japan) CAS # 548-26-5 EINECS # unknown	45380	Xanthene	-, Potassium salt
C.I. solvent Red 43 D&C Red # 21 (CTFA adopted name) Red # 223 (Japan) CAS # 15086-94-9 EINECS # unknown	45380:1	Xanthene	-, free acid

Color	of the Sodium salt : Red fluorescent solution in water.
Solubility	of the Sodium salt : Soluble in water and ethanol, insoluble in ether.
Chromatography DC Carrier	of the Sodium salt : Source : Communication XVII DFG Farbstoff-Kommission Kieselgel Acetic acid ester 50 ml + Ammonia 25% 10 ml + Methanol 20 ml
Spectral photometry Solvent Absorption maximum Solvent Absorption maximum	of the Sodium salt : Source : Kosmetische Färbemittel, 3. ed., 1991 Water 518 nm Ethanol (own assay) 544 nm, shoulder at 506 nm
Spectral photometry Solvent Absorption maximum	of the free acid : Source : Kosmetische Färbemittel 3. ed., 1991 Water, pH > 7 518 nm
Main applications Cosmetics	- Lipsticks.

Toxicological and dermatological data		**Source**
LD50 tested on rats	13900 mg/kg	Kosmetische Färbemittel 3. ed., 1991
Skin compatibility tested on rabbits	non-irritant	
Mucous membrane compatibility tested on a rabbit eye	non-irritant	

Certification status	
European Union	Approved for the coloration of cosmetics of group 1 (all cosmetic products).

Argentina	Approved for cosmetics, but not for application in the eye area.
Brazil	Approved for cosmetics, but not for application in the eye area.
Hungary	Approved for the coloration of cosmetics of group 1 (all cosmetic products).
Japan	Red # 230 (1) and (2), also in the form of Aluminum lake : Approved for drugs, "quasi-drugs" and cosmetics for external applications. Red # 223, but not in the form of paint lacquer : Approved for drugs, "quasi-drugs" and cosmetics for external applications.
Korea (South)	Approved for cosmetics.
Philippines	Approved for cosmetics, but not for application in the eye area.
South Africa	Approved for the coloration of cosmetics of group 1 (all cosmetic products).
Taiwan	Approved for cosmetics (free acid, Potassium- and Sodium salt, Aluminum- and Zirconium lake).
Thailand	Approved for cosmetics.
Turkey	Approved for the coloration of cosmetic of group 1 (all cosmetic products).
USA	D&C Red # 21/22 are approved for drugs and cosmetics (D&C Red # 22 also in the form of paint lacquer), but not for application in the eye area. Utilization requires FDA certificate.
Venezuela	Approved for cosmetics, but not for application in the eye area.

For acceptance of this colorant in other countries, based on above mentioned approvals, see also 9.1.8.

C.I.45396

Name	EU-No.	C.I. No.	Class	Chemical name / formula
C.I. Solvent Orange 16 CAS # 2545-86-6 EINECS # unknown		45396	Xanthene	4,5-Dinitro-fluorescin, free acid
Color	Orange			
Solubility	No information available.			
Chromatography	No information available.			
Spectral photometry	No information available.			

Main applications
Cosmetics   - Lipstick.

Toxicological and dermatological data   **Source**

not mentioned in Kosmetische Färbemittel 3.ed., 1991

Certification status

European Union	Approved for the coloration of cosmetics of group 1 (all cosmetic products, in lipsticks only in the form of free acids, max. level not more than 1%)
Hungary	Approved for the coloration of cosmetics of group 1 (all cosmetic products, in lipsticks only in the form of free acids, max. level not more than 1%)
Japan	Not approved for food, drugs and cosmetics.
Malta	Not approved for cosmetics.
South Africa	Approved for the coloration of cosmetics of group 1 (all cosmetic products, in lipsticks only in the form of free acids, max. level not more than 1%)
Turkey	Approved for the coloration of cosmetics of group 1 (all cosmetic products, in lipsticks only in the form of free acids, max. level not more than 1%)
USA	Not approved for food, drugs and cosmetics.

For acceptance of this colorant in other countries, based on above mentioned approvals, see also 9.1.8.

C.I.45405

Name	EU-No.	C.I. No.	Class	Chemical name / formula
Phloxin C.I. Acid Red 98 CAS # 6441-77-6 EINECS # unknown		45405	Xanthene	2,4,5,7-Tetrabrom-3',6'-dichloro-fluorescin, Potassium salt
Color	Red fluorescent solution in water.			
Solubility	Soluble in water.			
Chromatography	No information available.			
Spectral photometry	No information available.			
Main applications	No information available.			

Data Sheets

Toxicological and dermatological data	Source

Not mentioned in Kosmetische Färbemittel 3.ed., 1991

Certification status

European Union	Approved for the coloration of cosmetics of group 2 (not on eyes).
Hungary	Approved for the coloration of cosmetics of group 1 (all cosmetic products).
Japan	Not approved for food, drugs and cosmetics.
South Africa	Approved for the coloration of cosmetics of group 2 (not on eyes).
Thailand	Approved for cosmetics.
Turkey	Approved for the coloration of cosmetics of group 2 (not on eyes).
USA	Not approved for food, drugs and cosmetics.

For acceptance of this colorant in other countries, based on above mentioned approvals, see also 9.1.8.

C.I.45410

Name	EU-No.	C.I. No.	Class	Chemical name / formula
Phloxin B C.I. Acid Red 92 D&C Red # 28 (CTFA adopted name) Red # 104 (Japan) CAS # 18472-87-2 EINECS # 242-355-6		45410	Xanthene	2,4,56-Tetrabrom-3',4',5',6'-tetra-chloro-fluorescin, Sodium salt, (X)
Red # 231 (Japan) CAS # 13473-26-2 EINECS # unknown		45410	Xanthene	-, Potassium salt
C.I. Solvent Red 48 D&C Red # 27 (CTFA adopted name) Red # 218 (Japan) CAS # 13473-26-3 EINECS # unknown		45410:1	Monoazo	-, free acid
Color	Sodium salt : Blue-red solution in water. free acid : red solution in ethanol.			

Solubility	Sodium salt : soluble in water. free acid : soluble in ethanol and oil.

Chromatography	of the Sodium salt : Source : Communication XVII DFG Farbstoff-Kommission
DC	Kieselgel
Carrier	Acetic acid ester 50 ml + Ammonia 25% 10 ml + Methanol 20 ml

Spectral photometry	of the Sodium salt : Source : Communication XVII DFG Farbstoff-Kommission
Solvent	Water
Absorption maximum	537 nm

Main applications
Cosmetics — Lipstick.

Toxicological and dermatological data		Source
Sodium salt :		
LD50 tested on rats	8400 mg/kg	Kosmetische Färbemittel
Skin compatibility tested on rabbits	non-irritant	3. ed., 1991

Certification status

European Union	Approved for the coloration of cosmetics of group 1 (all cosmetic products).
Argentina	Approved for cosmetics, but not for application in the eye area.
Brazil	Approved for cosmetics, but not for application in the eye area.
Hungary	Approved for the coloration of cosmetics of group 1 (all cosmetic products).
Japan	Approved for defined food products, Red # 104 (1). Approved for drugs, "quasi-drugs" and cosmetics, also in the form of Aluminum- and Barium lake. Red # 231 : Approved for drugs, "quasi-drugs" and cosmetics for external applications, also in the form of Aluminum lake. Red # 218 : Approved for drugs, "quasi-drugs" and cosmetics for external application.
Korea (South)	Approved for cosmetics.
Philippines	Approved for cosmetics, but not for application in the eye area.
South Africa	Approved for the coloration of cosmetics of group 1 (all cosmetic products).
Taiwan	Sodium salt : Approved for cosmetics, also in the form of Aluminum- and Barium lakes. Potassium salt :

Data Sheets

Tiawan (continued)	Approved for cosmetics, also in the form of Aluminum lake. Free acid: Approved for cosmetics, also in the form of Aluminum- and Zirconium lake.
Tanzania	Approved for cosmetics.
Turkey	Approved for the coloration of cosmetic of group 1 (all cosmetic products).
USA	D&C Red # 27/28 are approved for drugs and cosmetics, but not for application in the eye area. Utilization requires FDA certificate.

For acceptance of this colorant in other countries, based on above mentioned approvals, see also 9.1.8.

C.I.45425

Name	EU-No.	C.I. No.	Class	Chemical name / formula
Erythrosin 6G C.I. Acid Red 95 D&C Orange # 11 (CTFA adopted name) Orange # 207 (Japan) CAS # 33239-19-9 EINECS # unknown		45425	Xanthene	2,4-Diiodide-fluorescin, Sodium salt
C.I. Solvent Red 73 D&C Orange # 10 (CTFA adopted name) Orange # 206 (Japan) CAS # 38577-97-8 EINECS # unknown		45425:1	Xanthene	-, free acid
C.I. Pigment Red 191 CAS # unknown EINECS # unknown		45425:2	Xanthene	-, Aluminum lake

Color	Red solution in water (Sodium salt) and in ethanol (free acid).
Solubility	Sodium salt soluble in water, free acid soluble in ethanol and oil.
Chromatography	of the Sodium salt: Source: Communication XVII DFG Farbstoff-Kommission
DC	Kieselgel
Carrier	Acetic acid ester 50 ml + Ammonia 25% 10 ml + Methanol 20 ml

Spectral photometry

	of the Sodium salt: Source : Communication XVII DFG Farbstoff-Kommission
Solvent	Water
Absorption maximum	507 nm

	of the free acid (own assay)
Solvent	Ethanol
Absorption maximum	390, 524 nm

Main applications

Cosmetics — Lipstick.

Toxicological and dermatological data | | **Source**

LD50 tested on rats	15400 mg/kg	Kosmetische Färbemittel 3. ed., 1991
Skin compatibility tested on rabbits	non-irritant	
Mucous membrane compatibility tested on a rabbit eye	temporary minor irritation	

Certification status

European Union	Approved for the coloration of cosmetics of group 1 (all cosmetic products).
Argentina	Approved for cosmetics, but not for application in the eye area.
Brazil	Approved for cosmetics, but not for application in the eye area.
Hungary	Approved for the coloration of cosmetics of group 1 (all cosmetic products).
Japan	Orange # 207 : Approved for drugs, "quasi-drugs" and cosmetics for external applications, also in the form of aluminum-lake. Orange # 206 : Approved for drugs, "quasi-drugs" and cosmetics for external applications, but approved as paint lacquer.
Korea (South)	Approved for cosmetics.
Philippines	Approved for cosmetics for external applications.
South Africa	Approved for the coloration of cosmetics of group 1 (all cosmetic products).
Taiwan	Approved for cosmetics (free acid, Sodium salt, Aluminum lake).
Thailand	Approved for cosmetics.
Turkey	Approved for the coloration of cosmetic of group 1 (all cosmetic products).
USA	D&C Orange # 10/11 are approved for drugs and cosmetics (also in the form of paint lacquer), but not for application in the eye and lip area.

For acceptance of this colorant in other countries, based on above mentioned approvals, see also 9.1.8.

C.I.45430

Name	EU-No.	C.I. No.	Class	Chemical name / formula
Erythrosin C.I. Food Red 14 C.I. Acid Red 51 FD&C Red # 3 (CTFA adopted name) Red # 3 (Japan) CAS # 16423-68-0 EINECS # 240-474-8	E 127	45430	Xanthene	2,4,5,7-Tetraiodide- fluorescin, Sodium salt
Erythrosin-Lack C.I. Pigment Red 172 CAS # 12227-78-0 EINECS # 235-440-4		45430:1	Xanthene	-, Aluminum lake
Erythrosin-Säure C.I. Solvent Red 140 CAS # unknown EINECS # unknown		45430:2	Xanthene	-, free acid

Color	Sodium salt : Red solution in water. Aluminum lake red powder.
Solubility	Sodium salt soluble in water (at 20 °C about 70 g/l), ethanol (ca. 10 g/l) and glycerin (ca. 35 g/l). Aluminum lake insoluble in water.
Chromatography DC Carrier	Source : Communication XVII DFG Farbstoff-Kommission Kieselgel Acetic acid ester 11 ml + Pyridine 5 ml + Water 4 ml
Spectral photometry Solvent Absorption maximum	Source : Communication XVII DFG Farbstoff-Kommission Water 416, 510, 544 nm (free acid) 528 nm (own assay of the Sodium salt)
Main applications Food Drugs	- Candies. - Fruit preserves (in solutions with a pH of 3-4, there is the formation of very low soluble erythrosinic acid, therefore erythrosinic acid is the only suitable dye for coloring cherries in fruit salad without coloring the fruit juice.) - Aluminum lake for the coloration of capsules.

Toxicological and dermatological data		Source
LD50 tested on rats	7100 mg/kg	Kosmetische Färbemittel 3. ed., 1991
Skin compatibility tested on rabbits	non-irritant	
Mucous membrane compatibility tested on a rabbit eye	non-irritant	
ADI-value (WHO 1986)	0-0.6 mg/kg	
(SCF 1987)	0-0.1 mg/kg	
(CIAA Liste Mouton)	0.05 mg/kg	

Certification status

European Union	Approved for defined food products (see 2.4.1.) and for the coloration of drugs and cosmetic preparations of group 1 (all cosmetic products).
Argentina	Approved for food. Approved for cosmetics, but not for application in the eye area.
Austria	Approved for defined food products.
Brazil	Approved for food and cosmetics.
Canada	Approved for defined food products.
Colombia	Approved for food.
Cyprus	Approved for defined food products.
Egypt	Approved for food.
Finland	Approved for defined food products.
Hungary	Approved for defined food products. Approved for the coloration of cosmetics of group 1 (all cosmetic products).
India	Not approved for food.
Indonesia	Approved for food. Not approved for cosmetics.
Iran	Approved for food.
Israel	Approved for food, drugs and cosmetics.
Japan	Approved for defined food products, also in the form of Aluminum lakes. Approved for drugs, quasi-drugs and cosmetics for external applications, also in the form of Aluminum lake.
Kenya	Approved for food.
Korea (South)	Approved for food and cosmetics.
Kuwait	Approved for food.
Malaysia	Approved for defined food products.
Malta	Approved for food.
Mexico	Approved for defined food products.
New Zealand	Approved for defined food products.
Peru	Approved for food.
Philippines	Approved for food and cosmetics.
Poland	Approved for cosmetics.
Saudi Arabia	Approved for food.
Singapore	Approved for food.
South Africa	Approved for the coloration of cosmetics of group 1 (all cosmetic products).

Sudan	Approved for food.
Sweden	Approved for defined food products.
Switzerland	Approved for defined food products and drugs.
Syria	Approved for food.
Taiwan	Approved for food and cosmetics, also in the form of Aluminum lake.
Thailand	Approved for food and cosmetics.
Tunisia	Approved for defined food products.
Turkey	Approved for defined food products. Approved for the coloration of cosmetics of group 1 (all cosmetic products).
United Arab Emirates	Approved for food.
USA	Not approved for food, drugs and cosmetics.
Venezuela	Not approved anymore for food and cosmetics.
Zambia	Approved for food.

For acceptance of this colorant in other countries, based on above mentioned approvals, see also 9.1.8.

C.I.45440

Name	EU-No.	C.I. No.	Class	Chemical name / formula
Rose Bengale C.I. Acid Red 94 Red # 105 (Japan) CAS # 632-69-90 EINECS # unknown		45440	Xanthene	2,4,5,7-Tetraiodide-3',4',5',6'-tetrachloro fluorescin, Sodium salt
Red # 232 (Japan) CAS # unknown EINECS # unknown		45440	Xanthene	-, Potassium salt
Color	Red, fluorescent solution in water.			
Solubility	Soluble in water.			
Chromatography	No information available.			
Spectral photometry Solvent Absorption maximum	Source : own assay Water 548 nm			
Main applications	No information available.			

Toxicological and dermatological data	Source
No information available.	

Certification status	
European Union	Not approved for food, drugs and cosmetics.
Japan	Approved for defined food products. Red # 105 (1) : Approved for drugs, "quasi-drugs" and cosmetics for external applications, also in the form of Aluminum lake. Red # 232 : Approved for drugs, "quasi-drugs" and cosmetics for external applications, also in the form of Aluminum lake.
Korea (South)	Approved for cosmetics.
Taiwan	Approved for cosmetics (Sodium- and Potassium salt), also in the form Aluminum lakes of these salts.
USA	Not approved for food, drugs and cosmetics.

For acceptance of this colorant in other countries, based on above mentioned approvals, see also 9.1.8.

C.I.47000

Name	EU-No.	C.I. No.	Class	Chemical name / formula
Chinolingelb A spritl. C.I. Solvent Yellow 33 D&C Yellow # 11 (CTFA adopted name) Yellow # 204 (Japan) CAS # 8003-22-3 EINECS # unknown		47000	Chino-phtalon	2-(2-Chinolyl)-1,3-indandion
Color	Yellow solution in ethanol.			
Solubility	Soluble in acetone, chloroform and benzol, low solubility in ethanol, insoluble in water.			
Chromatography DC Carrier	Source : Communication XVII DFG Farbstoff-Kommission Kieselgel Benzol 90 ml + Acetone 10 ml			
Spectral photometry Solvent Absorption maximum	Source : Communication XVII DFG Farbstoff-Kommission Ethanol 414, 436 nm			

Data Sheets

Main applications No information available.

Toxicological and dermatological data		Source
LD50 tested on rats	> 10000 mg/kg	Kosmetische Färbemittel
Skin compatibility tested on rabbits	minor irritation	3. ed., 1991
Mucous membrane compatibility tested on a rabbit eye	minor irritation of	

Certification status	
European Union	Approved for the coloration of cosmetics of group 3 (not on mucous membranes).
Argentina	Approved for cosmetics, but not for application on eyes and lips.
Brazil	Approved for cosmetics, but not for application on eyes and lips.
Hungary	Approved for the coloration of cosmetics of group 1 (all cosmetic products).
Japan	Approved for drugs, "quasi-drugs" and cosmetics for external applications, but not on mucous membranes.
Korea (South)	Approved for cosmetics.
Philippines	Approved for cosmetics for external applications, but not on eyes and lips.
South Africa	Approved for the coloration of cosmetics of group 3 (not on mucous membranes).
Taiwan	Approved for cosmetics.
Thailand	Approved for cosmetics for external applications, but not on eyes and lips.
Turkey	Approved for the coloration of cosmetics of group 3 (not on mucous membranes).
USA	Approved for drugs and cosmetics, but not for application in the eye and lip area. Utilization requires FDA certificate.
Venezuela	Approved for cosmetics, but not for application in the eye and lip area.

For acceptance of this colorant in other countries, based on above mentioned approvals, see also 9.1.8.

C.I.47005

Name	EU-No.	C.I. No.	Class	Chemical name / formula
Chinolingelb C.I. Food Yellow 13 C.I. Acid Yellow 3	E 104	47005	Chiniphthalon	2-(2-Chinolyl)-1,3-indandion-disulfo acid (with parts of

Red # 203 (Japan)
CAS # 95193-83-2
EINECS # 305-897-5

mono- and trisulfo acid), Sodium salt

Chinolingelb Lack   E 104   47005:1   Chino-   -, Aluminum lake
C.I. Pigment Yellow   phthalon
115
CAS # unknown
EINECS # unknown

D&C Yellow # 10   47005   Chino-   2-(2-Chinolyl)-1,3-
(CTFA adopted name)   phthalon   indadion-mono-sulfo-
CAS # 8004-92-0   acid (with parts of di-
EINECS # unknown   and tri-sulfo acid),
                                                                                                Sodium salt

Note :
Based on its percent composition of mono-, di- and trisulfo acid D&C Yellow # 10 is not a food colorant according to the FAO specification (Food and Nutrition Paper 31/1, 1984)

Color	Sodium salt : Yellow solution in water. Aluminum lake yellow powder.
Solubility	C.I. Food Yellow 13 soluble in water (at 20 °C about 50 g/l) and glycerin (ca. 20 g/l). D&C Yellow # 10 has a significant lower solubility in water due to its higher content of monosulfo acid (min. 75%) than C.I. Food Yellow 13 (level of di-sulfo acid ca. 80%, mono-sulfo acid ca. 5%).
Chromatography DC Carrier	Source : Communication XVII DFG Farbstoff-Kommission Kieselgel tert. Sodium citrate solution 2.5% 80 ml + Ammonia 25% 20 ml + Methanol 12 ml
Spectral photometry Solvent Absorption maximum Solvent Absorption maximum	for C.I. Food Yellow 13 Source : Communication XVII DFG Farbstoff-Kommission Water 418 nm of D&C Yellow # 10 (own assay) water 408 nm (different cube pattern than C.I. Food Yellow 13)
Main applications Food Drugs Cosmetics	 - Beverages, candies, dessert products, artificial ice-cream powdered carbonated beverages. - General utilization, paint lacquer for capsules. - Shampoo, foam bath, shower gel. - Liquid soap, toilet soap. - Hair care products (perms).

Data Sheets

Toxicological and dermatological data		Source
LD50 tested on rats	> 5000 mg/kg	Kosmetische Färbemittel 3. ed., 1991
Skin compatibility tested on rabbits	slightly irritating non-irritant	
Mucous membrane compatibility tested on a rabbit eye	0-0.5 mg/kg	
ADI-value (WHO 1974, SCF 1975) (EEC Color Group 1983)	0-10 mg/kg	

Certification status

If not indicated otherwise, all information is valid for C.I. Food Yellow 13.

European Union	Approved for defined food products (see 2.4.1.) and for the coloration of drugs and cosmetic preparations of group 1 (all cosmetic products).
Argentina	Approved for cosmetics, but not for application in the eye area. Maximum dosage level in products for the lip area 1.5%.
Austria	Approved for defined food products.
Brazil	Approved for cosmetics, but not for application in the eye area.
Chile	Approved for food.
Colombia	Approved for food.
Cyprus	Approved for defined food products.
Finland	Approved for defined food products.
Hungary	Approved for defined food products. Approved for the coloration of cosmetics of group 1 (all cosmetic products).
Indonesia	Approved for food.
Iran	Approved for food.
Israel	Approved for food and drugs.
Japan	Approved for drugs, "quasi-drugs" and cosmetics for external applications, also in the form of Aluminum-, Barium- and Zirconium lakes.
Korea (South)	Approved for cosmetics.
Kuwait	Approved for food.
Malta	Approved for food.
Philippines	Approved for cosmetics, but not for application in the eye area.
Poland	Approved for food and cosmetics.
Saudi Arabia	Approved for food.
South Africa	Approved for defined food products and drugs. Approved for the coloration of cosmetics of group 1 (all cosmetic products).
Sweden	Approved for defined food products.
Switzerland	Approved for defined food products.
Taiwan	Approved for cosmetics (Sodium salt, Aluminum-, Barium- and Zirconium lake).
Thailand	Approved for cosmetics.
Tunisia	Approved for defined food products.
Turkey	Approved for the coloration of cosmetic of group 1 (all cosmetic products).

United Arab Emirates	Approved for food.	
USA	D&C Yellow # 10	
	Approved for drugs and cosmetics (also in the form of paint lacquer), but not for application in the eye area.	
	Utilization requires FDA certificate.	
Zambia	Approved for food.	

For acceptance of this colorant in other countries, based on above mentioned approvals, see also 9.1.8.

C.I.50325

Name	EU-No.	C.I. No.	Class	Chemical name / formula
Wollechtviolett B C.I. Acid Violet 50 CAS # 6837-46-3 EINECS # unknown		50325	Phenazine	5-Aniline-9-(3-methoxy-aniline)-7-phenyl-10-sulfo-benzo(a)phenazine-4-sulfonate, Sodium salt
Color	Red-violet solution in water.			
Solubility	Soluble in water, low solubility in ethanol.			
Chromatography DC Carrier	Source : Communication XVII DFG Farbstoff-Kommission Kieselgel Acetic acid ester 11 ml + Pyridine 5 ml + Water 4 ml			
Spectral photometry Solvent Absorption maximum	Source : Communication XVII DFG Farbstoff-Kommission Water 560 nm			
Main applications	No information available.			

Toxicological and dermatological data		Source
LD50 tested on rats	> 10000 mg/kg	Kosmetische Färbemittel 3. ed., 1991
Skin compatibility tested on rabbits	non-irritant	
Mucous membrane compatibility tested on a rabbit eye	slight irritation	

Certification status	
European Union	Approved for the coloration of cosmetics of group 4 (only for a short residence time on skin).

Data Sheets

Hungary	Approved for the coloration of cosmetics of group 1 (all cosmetic products).
Japan	Not approved for food, drugs and cosmetics.
South Africa	Approved for the coloration of cosmetics of group 4 (only for a short residence time on skin).
Turkey	Approved for the coloration of cosmetics of group 4 (only for a short residence time on skin).
USA	Not approved for food, drugs and cosmetics.

For acceptance of this colorant in other countries, based on above mentioned approvals, see also 9.1.8.

C.I.50420

Name	EU-No.	C.I. No.	Class	Chemical name / formula
Nigrosin GF wasserl. C.I. Acid Black 2 CAS # 8005-03-6 EINECS # unknown		50420	Azine	Composition unknown

Color	Blue-violet solution in water.
Solubility	Soluble in water.
Chromatography	No information available.
Spectral photometry	No information available.
Main applications	No information available.

Toxicological and dermatological data		Source
LD50 tested on rats	> 4000 mg/kg	Kosmetische Färbemittel 3. ed., 1991
Skin compatibility tested on rabbits	non-irritant	
Mucous membrane compatibility tested on a rabbit eye	non-irritant	

Certification status

European Union	Approved for the coloration of cosmetics of group 3 (not on mucous membranes).
Hungary	Approved for the coloration of cosmetics of group 1 (all cosmetic products).
Japan	Not approved for food, drugs and cosmetics.

South Africa   Approved for the coloration of cosmetics of group 3 (not on mucous membranes).
Turkey   Approved for the coloration of cosmetics of group 3 (not on mucous membranes.
USA   Not approved for food, drugs and cosmetics.
For acceptance of this colorant in other countries, based on above mentioned approvals, see also 9.1.8.

C.I.53319

Name	EU-No.	C.I. No.	Class	Chemical name / formula
Hostaperm Violet RL C.I. Pigment Violet 23 CAS # 6358-30-1 EINECS # 228-767-9		53319	Dioxazine	8,18-Dichloro-5,15-Diethyl-carbazol0/3',2':5,6//1,4/oxa-zino-/2,3-b/indolo/2,3-I-/

Color	Violet pigment.
Solubility	Insoluble in all standard solvents, available commercially in a water-dispersible form.
Chromatography	Not applicable.
Spectral photometry	Not applicable.
Main applications Cosmetics	- Toilet soap.

Toxicological and dermatological data		Source
LD50 tested on rats	> 10000 mg/kg	Kosmetische Färbemittel
Skin compatibility tested on rabbits	non-irritant	3. ed., 1991
Mucous membrane compatibility tested on a rabbit eye	non-irritant	

Certification status	
European Union	Approved for the coloration of cosmetics of group 4 (only for a short residence time on skin).
Bulgaria	Not approved for cosmetics.
Hungary	Approved for the coloration of cosmetics of group 1 (all cosmetic products).
Japan	Not approved for food, drugs and cosmetics.

Malta	Not approved for cosmetics.	
Poland	Approved for cosmetics.	
South Africa	Approved for the coloration of cosmetics of group 4 (only for a short residence time on skin).	
Turkey	Approved for the coloration of cosmetics of group 4 (only for a short residence time on skin).	
USA	Not approved for food, drugs and cosmetics.	

For acceptance of this colorant in other countries, based on above mentioned approvals, see also 9.1.8.

C.I.56059

Name	EU-No.	C.I. No.	Class	Chemical name / formula
Arianor Steel Blue C.I. Basic Blue 99 C-ext. Blau 17 CAS # 93280-94-5 EINECS # unknown		56059	Naphtho-hinon	8-Amino-6-(amino-phenyl-m-trimethyl-ammonium chloride)-5-hydroxy-2-brom-1,4-naphthochinon-imine

Color	Blue solution in water.
Solubility	Soluble in water and alcohol.
Chromatography DC Carrier	Source : own assay Schleicher & Schüll 2043 b Mgl 2 g Tri-Sodium-citrate-2-hydrate in 100 ml Ammonia 5%
Spectral photometry Solvent Absorption maximum	Source : own assay Water 576, 618 nm
Main applications	Hair coloration

Toxicological and dermatological data		Source
LD50 tested on rats	1-2 g/kg	Ringbook Kosmetische Färbemittel 3. ed., 1991
Skin compatibility tested on rabbits Mucous membrane compatibility tested on a rabbit eye	minor irritation no irritation	

Certification status	
European Union	Not approved for food, drugs and cosmetics. Approved for hair dying.

Japan	Not approved for food, drugs and cosmetics. Approval status for hair dying not known.
USA	Not approved for food, drugs and cosmetics. Approval status for hair dying not known.

There is no information available from other countries, i.e., this colorant is not included in other national positive lists.

C.I.56238

Name	EU-No.	C.I. No.	Class	Chemical name / formula
Hostasolgelb 3G C.I. Solvent Yellow 98 CAS # 27870-92-4 EINECS # unknown		56238	Amino-ketone	Not listed in Kosmet. Färbemittel, 3.ed., 1991
Color	Yellow solution in chloroform.			
Solubility	Insoluble in water, low solubility in ethanol, soluble in chloroform and acetic acid ester.			
Chromatography	No information available.			
Spectral photometry Solvent Absorption maximum	Source : Kosmetische Färbemittel, 3.ed., 1991 Chloroform 258, 454 nm			
Main applications Cosmetics	- Nail polish.			

Toxicological and dermatological data		Source
LD50 tested on rats	> 15000 mg/kg	Ringbook Kosmetische Färbemittel 3. ed., 1991
Skin compatibility tested on rabbits	non-irritant	
Mucous membrane compatibility tested on a rabbit eye	non-irritant	

Certification status

European Union	Not approved for cosmetics. In Germany the preliminary approval for nail polish (cosmetic application group 5) has been rescinded in 1989.
Japan	Not approved for food, drugs and cosmetics.
USA	Not approved for food, drugs and cosmetics.

There is no additional information available from other countries, i.e., this colorant is not included in other national positive lists.

Data Sheets

C.I. 58000

Name	EU-No.	C.I. No.	Class	Chemical name / formula
Alizarin C.I. Mordant Red 11 CAS # 72-48-0 EINECS # unknown		58000	Anthra-quinone	1,2-Dihydro-9,10-anthraquinone, Calcium-Aluminum-complex
C.I. Pigment Red 83 CAS # unknown EINECS # unknown		58000:1	Anthra-quinone	-, metallic complex

Color	Red pigment.
Solubility	Soluble in acetone, hot ethanol, alkali, dimethylformamide, insoluble in water.
Chromatography DC Carrier	of the Calcium-Aluminum-complex : Source : Communication XVII DFG Farbstoff-Kommission Kieselgel Acetic acid ester 11 ml + Pyridine 5 ml + Water 4 ml
Spectral photometry Solvent Absorption maximum	of the Calcium-Aluminum-complex Source : Communication XVII DFG Farbstoff-Kommission Dimethylformamide 525 nm
Main applications Cosmetics	- Make-up, Rouge, lipstick (pigment). - Toilet soap.

Toxicological and dermatological data		Source
LD50 tested on rats	> 8000 mg/kg	Kosmetische Färbemittel 3. ed., 1991
Skin compatibility tested on rabbits	non-irritant	
Mucous membrane compatibility tested on a rabbit eye	non-irritant	

Certification status

European Union	Approved for the coloration of cosmetics of group 1 (all cosmetic products).
Hungary	Approved for the coloration of cosmetics of group 1 (all cosmetic products).
Japan	Not approved for food, drugs and cosmetics.
Poland	Approved for cosmetics.

South Africa	Approved for the coloration of cosmetics of group 1 (all cosmetic products).
Thailand	Approved for cosmetics.
Turkey	Approved for the coloration of cosmetic of group 1 (all cosmetic products).
USA	Not approved for food, drugs and cosmetics.

For acceptance of this colorant in other countries, based on above mentioned approvals, see also 9.1.8.

C.I.59040

Name	EU-No.	C.I. No.	Class	Chemical name / formula
Pyranin C.I. Solvent Green 7 D&C Green # 8 (CTFA adopted name) Green # 2o4 (Japan) CAS # 6358-69-6 EINECS # 228-783-6		59040	Pyrene	8-Hydroxy-1,3,6-pyrene-trisulfo acid, Sodium salt
Color	Yellow-green fluorescent solution in water.			
Solubility	Soluble in water and ethanol.			
Spectral photometry Solvent Absorption maximum	Source : Communication XVII DFG Farbstoff-Kommission Methanol 363, 400 nm			
Solvent Absorption maximum	Water (own assay) 370, 404 nm			
Main applications Cosmetics	- Shampoo, foam bath, shower gel. - Liquid soap, toilet soap.			

Toxicological and dermatological data		Source
LD50 tested on rats	16000 mg/kg	Kosmetische Färbemittel 3. ed., 1991
Skin compatibility tested on rabbits	non-irritant	
Mucous membrane compatibility tested on a rabbit eye	non-irritant	

Data Sheets

Certification status

European Union	Approved for the coloration of cosmetics of group 3 (not on mucous membranes).
Argentina	Approved for cosmetics, but not for application on mucous membranes.
Brazil	Approved for cosmetics, but not for application on mucous membranes.
Hungary	Approved for the coloration of cosmetics of group 2 (not on eyes).
Israel	Approved for drugs and cosmetics.
Japan	Approved for drugs, "quasi-drugs" and cosmetics for external applications, also in the form of aluminum-lakes.
Korea (South)	Approved for cosmetics.
Philippines	Approved for cosmetics, but not for application on mucous membranes.
South Africa	Approved for the coloration of cosmetics of group 3 (not on mucous membranes).
Taiwan	Approved for cosmetics, also in the form of Aluminum lake.
Thailand	Approved for cosmetics.
Turkey	Approved for the coloration of cosmetics of group 3 (not on mucous membranes).
USA	Approved for drugs and cosmetics (also in the form of paint lacquer), but not for application in the eye and lip area. Maximum dosage in the finished product 0.01%. Utilization requires FDA certificate.
Venezuela	Approved for cosmetics, but not for application on mucous membranes.

For acceptance of this colorant in other countries, based on above mentioned approvals, see also 9.1.8.

C.I.60724

Name	EU-No.	C.I. No.	Class	Chemical name / formula
Foron Brillantviolett E-BLN C.I. Disperse Violet 27 CAS # 19286-75-0 EINECS # unknown		60724	Anthraquinone	1-Hydroxy-4-N-phenylamino-anthraquinone
Color	Violet dispersion in water.			
Solubility	Dispersible in water.			

Chromatography	No information available.

Spectral photometry	Source : own assay
Solvent	Water (opaque)
Absorption maximum	598, 656 nm

Main applications	No information available.

Toxicological and dermatological data		Source
LD50 tested on rats	> 5000 mg/kg	Kosmetische Färbemittel 3. ed., 1991
Skin compatibility tested on rabbits	non-irritant	
Mucous membrane compatibility tested on a rabbit eye	non-irritant	

Certification status

European Union	Approved for the coloration of cosmetics of group 4 (only for a short residence time on skin).
Hungary	Approved for the coloration of cosmetics of group 1 (all cosmetic products).
Japan	Not approved for food, drugs and cosmetics.
Malta	Not approved for cosmetics.
South Africa	Approved for the coloration of cosmetics of group 4 (only for a short residence time on skin).
Turkey	Approved for the coloration of cosmetics of group 4 (only for a short residence time on skin).
USA	Not approved for food, drugs and cosmetics.

For acceptance of this colorant in other countries, based on above mentioned approvals, see also 9.1.8.

C.I.60725

Name	EU-No.	C.I. No.	Class	Chemical name / formula
Irisol spritl. C.I. Solvent Violet 13 D&C Violet # 2 (CTFA adopted name) Purple Violet # 201 (Japan) CAS # 81-48-1 EINECS # 201-353-5		60725	Anthra-quinone	1-Hydroxy-4-(4'-methyl-phenyl-amino)-anthraquinone

Color	Blue-violet solution in benzol.
Solubility	Soluble in benzol, 1,1,1-trichloroethane, dichloromethane, insoluble in water.
Chromatography DC Carrier	Source : Communication XVII DFG Farbstoff-Kommission Kieselgel Gasoline 40 ml + Benzol 20 ml + Methylethylketone 4 ml + Acetic acid ester 16 ml.
Spectral photometry Solvent Absorption maximum	Source : Communication XVII DFG Farbstoff-Kommission Dimethylformamide 577 nm
Solvent Absorption maximum	Toluol (Source Kosmetische Färbemittel, 3.ed., 1991) 580 nm
Main applications Cosmetics	- Oil products.

Toxicological and dermatological data		Source
LD50 tested on rats	> 16000 mg/kg	Kosmetische Färbemittel
Skin compatibility tested on rabbits	non-irritant	3. ed., 1991
Mucous membrane compatibility tested on a rabbit eye	non-irritant	

Certification status

European Union	Approved for the coloration of cosmetics of group 1 (all cosmetic products).
Argentina	Approved for cosmetics, but not for application on eyes and mucous membranes.
Brazil	Approved for cosmetics, but not for application on eyes and mucous membranes.
Bulgaria	Approved for cosmetics, but not for application on eyes and lips.
Hungary	Approved for the coloration of cosmetics of group 1 (all cosmetic products).
Japan	Approved for drugs, "quasi-drugs" and cosmetics for external applications.
Korea (South)	Approved for cosmetics.
Poland	Approved for cosmetics, but not for application in the eye and lip area.
South Africa	Approved for the coloration of cosmetics of group 1 (all cosmetic products).
Taiwan	Approved for cosmetics.
Thailand	Approved for cosmetics but not for application on eyes and lips.

Turkey	Approved for the coloration of cosmetics of group 1 (all cosmetic products).
USA	Approved for externally applied drugs and for cosmetics (also in the form of paint lacquer), but not for the eye and lip area. Utilization requires FDA certificate.
Venezuela	Approved for cosmetics, but not for application in the eye area and on mucous membranes.

For acceptance of this colorant in other countries, based on above mentioned approvals, see also 9.1.8.

C.I.60730

Name	EU-No.	C.I. No.	Class	Chemical name / formula
Anthralanviolet 3B. C.I. Acid Violet 43 Ext.D&C Violet # 2 (CTFA adopted name) Purple Violet # 401 (Japan) CAS # 4430-18-6 EINECS # 224-618-7		60730	Anthraquinone	1-Hydroxy-4-(4-methyl-2-sulfophenylamino)-anthraquinone, Sodium salt
Color	Violet solution in water.			
Solubility	Soluble in water.			
Chromatography DC Carrier	Source : Communication XVII DFG Farbstoff-Kommission Kieselgel Acetic acid ester 11 ml + Pyridine 5 ml + Water 4 ml.			
Spectral photometry Solvent Absorption maximum	Source : Communication XVII DFG Farbstoff-Kommission Water 580 nm			
Main applications Cosmetics	- Hair dying. - Alcohol-based perfumes.			
Toxicological and dermatological data			**Source**	
LD50 tested on rats		13000 mg/kg	Kosmetische Färbemittel 3. ed., 1991	
Skin compatibility tested on rabbits Mucous membrane compatibility tested on a rabbit eye		non-irritant non-irritant		

Data Sheets

Certification status

European Union	Approved for the coloration of cosmetics of group 3 (not on mucous membranes).
Argentina	Approved for cosmetics, but not for application on eyes and lips.
Brazil	Approved for cosmetics, but not for application on eyes and lips.
Hungary	Approved for the coloration of cosmetics of group 1 (all cosmetic products).
Japan	Approved for drugs, "quasi-drugs" and cosmetics for external applications, also in the form of aluminum lakes, but not on mucous membranes.
Korea (South)	Approved for cosmetics.
Malta	Approved only for rinse-off products.
Philippines	Approved for cosmetics, but not for application in the eye and lip area.
Poland	Approved for cosmetics, but not for application in the eye and lip area.
South Africa	Approved for the coloration of cosmetics of group 3 (not on mucous membranes).
Taiwan	Approved for facial toning masks, also in the form of aluminum lakes, but not for cosmetics.
Turkey	Approved for the coloration of cosmetics of group 3 (not on mucous membranes).
USA	Approved for externally applied drugs and for cosmetics (also in the form of paint lacquer), but not for the eye and lip area. Utilization requires FDA certificate.
Venezuela	Approved for cosmetics, but not for application in the eye or lip area.

For acceptance of this colorant in other countries, based on above mentioned approvals, see also 9.1.8.

C.I.61520

Name	EU-No.	C.I. No.	Class	Chemical name / formula
Sudanblau GN C.I. Solvent Blue 63 Blue # 403 (Japan) CAS # 64553-79-3 EINECS # unknown		61520	Anthra-quinone	1-Methylamino-4-m-toluidine-anthraquinone
Color		Blue solution in organic solvents.		

Solubility	Soluble in organic solvents.
Chromatography	No information available.
Spectral photometry Solvent Absorption maximum	Source : own assay 1,1,1-Trichloroethane 520 nm
Main applications	No information available.

Toxicological and dermatological data		Source
LD50 tested on rats	> 5000 mg/kg	Safety data sheet Ceresblau GN
Skin compatibility tested on rabbits	non-irritant	Bayer AG
Mucous membrane compatibility tested on a rabbit eye	non-irritant	

Certification status

European Union	Not approved for food, drugs and cosmetics.
Japan	Approved for drugs, "quasi-drugs" and cosmetics for external applications.
Korea (South)	Approved for cosmetics.
Taiwan	Approved for facial toning masks, not for cosmetics.
USA	Not approved for food, drugs and cosmetics.

For acceptance of this colorant in other countries, based on above mentioned approvals, see also 9.1.8.

C.I.61554

Name	EU-No.	C.I. No.	Class	Chemical name / formula
Sudanblau II C.I. Solvent Blue 35 CAS # 17354-14-2 EINECS # unknown		61554	Anthra-quinone	1,4-Bis (butylamino)-anthraquinone
Color	Blue solution in halogenated hydrocarbons.			
Solubility	Soluble in oil, fat and organic solvents.			
Chromatography DC Carrier	Source : Communication XVII DFG Farbstoff-Kommission Kieselgel Acetic acid ester 11 ml + Pyridine 5 ml + Water 4 ml			

Data Sheets

Spectral photometry	Source : Communication XVII DFG Farbstoff-Kommission
Solvent	Methanol
Absorption maximum	592, 639 nm
Solvent	1,1,1-Trichloroethane (own assay)
Absorption maximum	600, 650 nm

Main applications	
Cosmetics	- Oil products.

Toxicological and dermatological data		Source
LD50 tested on rats	> 6400 mg/kg	Safety data sheet Fettblau B, Hoechst 1981
Skin compatibility tested on rabbits	non-irritant	
Mucous membrane compatibility tested on a rabbit eye	slight irritant	

Certification status

European Union	Not approved for food, drugs and cosmetics. According to Colorant Guideline 94/36/EU not approved after June 30, 1996 as a food surface stamp and for coloration of egg shells.
Japan	Not approved for food, drugs and cosmetics.
USA	Not approved for food, drugs and cosmetics.

There is no information available from other countries, i.e., this colorant is not included in other national positive lists.

C.I.61565

Name	EU-No.	C.I. No.	Class	Chemical name / formula
Alizarincyaningrün fttl. D&C Green # 6 (CTFA adopted name) Green # 202 (Japan) CAS # 128-80-30 EINECS # 204-909-5		61565	Anthra-quinone	1,4-Bis (p-toluidine)-anthraquinone
Color		Blue-green solution in benzol.		
Solubility		Soluble in benzol, chlorinated carbohydrogen, fat, insoluble in water.		

Chromatography	Source : Communication XVII DFG Farbstoff-Kommission
DC	Kieselgel
Carrier	Acetic acid ester 11 ml + Pyridine 5 ml + Water 4 ml

Spectral photometry	Source : Communication XVII DFG Farbstoff-Kommission
Solvent	Chloroform
Absorption maximum	404, 604, 641 nm

Main applications
Cosmetics — Oil products.

Toxicological and dermatological data		Source
LD50 tested on rats	> 3160 mg/kg	Kosmetische Färbemittel 3. ed., 1991
Skin compatibility tested on rabbits	non-irritant	
Mucous membrane compatibility tested on a rabbit eye	non-irritant	

Certification status

European Union	Approved for the coloration of cosmetics of group 1 (all cosmetic products).
Argentina	Approved for cosmetics for external applications, but not on mucous membranes.
Brazil	Approved for cosmetics for external applications, but not on mucous membranes.
Bulgaria	Approved for cosmetics, but not for application in the eye and lip area.
Hungary	Approved for the coloration of cosmetics of group 2 (not on eyes).
Japan	Approved for drugs, "quasi-drugs" and cosmetics for external applications.
Korea (South)	Approved for cosmetics.
Poland	Approved for cosmetics, but not for application in the eye and lip area.
South Africa	Approved for the coloration of cosmetics of group 1 (all cosmetic products).
Taiwan	Approved for cosmetics.
Thailand	Approved for cosmetics.
USA	Approved for drugs and cosmetics (also in the form of paint lacquer), but not for application on eyes and lips. Utilization requires FDA certificate.

For acceptance of this colorant in other countries, based on above mentioned approvals, see also 9.1.8.

C.I.61570

Name	EU-No.	C.I. No.	Class	Chemical name / formula
Alizarincyaningrün G D&C Green # 5 (CTFA adopted name) Green # 201 (Japan) CAS # 4403-90-1 EINECS # 224-546-6		61570	Anthra- quinone	1,4-Bis-(o-sulfo-o- toluidine)- anthraquinone, Sodium salt
Color	Green solution in water.			
Solubility	Soluble in water.			
Chromatography	No information available.			
Chromatography DC Carrier	Source : Communication XVII DFG Farbstoff-Kommission Kieselgel Acetic acid ester 11 ml + Pyridine 5 ml + Water 4 ml			
Spectral photometry Solvent Absorption maximum	Source : Communication XVII DFG Farbstoff-Kommission Water 404, 605, 640 nm (own assay: 414, 610, 644 nm)			
Main applications Cosmetics	- Shampoo, foam bath, shower gel. - Liquid soap, toilet soap.			

Toxicological and dermatological data		Source
LD50 tested on rats	> 10000 mg/kg	Kosmetische Färbemittel
Mucous membrane compatibility tested on a rabbit eye	non-irritant	3. ed., 1991

Certification status

European Union	Approved for the coloration of cosmetics of group 1 (all cosmetic products).
Argentina	Approved for cosmetics, but not on eyes.
Brazil	Approved for cosmetics, but not on eyes.
Bulgaria	Approved for cosmetics, but not on eyes.
Hungary	Approved for the coloration of cosmetics of group 2 (not on eyes).
Israel	Approved for drugs and cosmetics.
Japan	Approved for drugs, "quasi-drugs" and cosmetics for external applications, also in the form of aluminum-lakes.

Korea (South)	Approved for cosmetics.
Malaysia	EU- or US-approved colorants are accepted for cosmetics.
Philippines	Approved for cosmetics, but not for application on eyes.
Poland	Approved for cosmetics, but not for application in the eye area.
South Africa	Approved for the coloration of cosmetics of group 1 (all cosmetic products).
Taiwan	Approved for cosmetics, also in the form of Aluminum lake.
Thailand	Approved for cosmetics.
Turkey	Approved for the coloration of cosmetics of group 1 (all cosmetic products).
USA	Approved for drugs and cosmetics (also in the form of paint lacquer), but not for application in the eye area (CFR21, April 1, 1993). According to Federal Register Vol. 59, No. 153, August 10, 1994 will be approved in the future for application in the eye area. Utilization requires FDA certificate.
Venezuela	Approved for cosmetics, but not for application in the eye area.

For acceptance of this colorant in other countries, based on above mentioned approvals, see also 9.1.8.

C.I.61585

Name	EU-No.	C.I. No.	Class	Chemical name / formula
Sandolan Walkblau N-BL C.I. Acid Blue 80 CAS # 4474-24-2 EINECS # 224-748-4		61585	Anthraquinone	1,4-Bis (3-sulfo-2,4,6-trimethyl-aniline)-anthraquinone, Sodium salt
Color	Blue solution in water.			
Solubility	Soluble in water.			
Chromatography DC Carrier	Source : Communication XVII DFG Farbstoff-Kommission Kieselgel Acetic acid ester 11 ml + Pyridine 5 ml + Water 4 ml			
Spectral photometry Solvent Absorption maximum	Source : Communication XVII DFG Farbstoff-Kommission Water 470 nm			
Main applications Cosmetics	- Shampoo, foam bath. - Liquid soap, toilet soap.			

Toxicological and dermatological data		Source
LD50 tested on rats	> 15000 mg/kg	Kosmetische Färbemittel 3. ed., 1991
Skin compatibility tested on rabbits	minimal irritation	
Mucous membrane compatibility tested on a rabbit eye	minor irritation	

Certification status

European Union	Approved for the coloration of cosmetics of group 4 (only for a short residence time on skin).
Bulgaria	Not approved for cosmetics.
Hungary	Approved for the coloration of cosmetics of group 2 (not on eyes).
Japan	Not approved for food, drugs and cosmetics.
Poland	Not approved for cosmetics.
South Africa	Approved for the coloration of cosmetics of group 4 (only for a short residence time on skin).
Turkey	Approved for the coloration of cosmetics of group 4 (only for a short residence time on skin).
USA	Not approved for cosmetics.

For acceptance of this colorant in other countries, based on above mentioned approvals, see also 9.1.8.

C.I.62045

Name	EU-No.	C.I. No.	Class	Chemical name / formula
C.I. Acid Blue 62 CAS # 4368-56-3 EINECS # unknown		62045	Anthraquinone	1-Amino-2-sulfo-4-cyclohexyl-amino-anthraquinone, Sodium salt
Color	Blue solution in ethanol.			
Solubility	Soluble in water and ethanol.			
Chromatography	No information available.			
Spectral photometry	No information available.			
Main applications	No information available.			

Toxicological and dermatological data		Source
LD50 tested on rats	11750 mg/kg	Kosmetische Färbemittel 3. ed., 1991
Skin compatibility tested on rabbits	weak edema	
Mucous membrane compatibility tested on a rabbit eye	minor irritation	

Certification status	
European Union	Approved for the coloration of cosmetics of group 4 (only for a short residence time on skin).
Bulgaria	Not approved for cosmetics.
Hungary	Approved for the coloration of cosmetics of group 2 (not on eyes).
Japan	Not approved for food, drugs and cosmetics.
Poland	Not approved for cosmetics.
South Africa	Approved for the coloration of cosmetics of group 4 (only for a short residence time on skin).
Turkey	Approved for the coloration of cosmetics of group 4 (only for a short residence time on skin).
USA	Not approved for food, drugs and cosmetics.

For acceptance of this colorant in other countries, based on above mentioned approvals, see also 9.1.8.

C.I.69800

Name	EU-No.	C.I. No.	Class	Chemical name / formula
Indanthrenblau RS C.I. Food Blue 4 C.I. Vat Blue 4 C.I. Pigment Blue 60 CAS # 81-77-6 EINECS # 201-375-5		69800	Anthra-quinone	5,9,14,18-Tetraoxo-5,6,9,14,15,18-hexahydrodinaphthol/2,3-a:2',3'h/phenazin
Color	Blue pigment.			
Solubility	Soluble in dimethylformamide, insoluble in water, methanol, dichloromethane and oil. Available commercially in a water-dispersible form.			
Chromatography	Not applicable.			
Spectral photometry	of the pigment : Source : Communication XVII DFG Farbstoff-Kommission			
Solvent	Dimethylformamide			
Absorption maximum	625 nm			
Solvent	Water (own assay of the water-dispersible form)			
Absorption maximum	610 nm			

Data Sheets

Main applications

Cosmetics
- Shampoo, shower gel, liquid soap (water-dispersible form).
- Toothpaste (water-dispersible form).
- Toilet soap (pigment and water-dispersible form).

Toxicological and dermatological data		**Source**
LD50 tested on rats	> 5000 mg/kg	Kosmetische Färbemittel
Sensibility tested on guinea pig	non-sensitive	3. ed., 1991

Certification status

European Union	Approved for the coloration of cosmetics of group 1 (all cosmetic products).
Brazil	Not approved anymore for food.
Chile	Not approved any more for food.
Hungary	Approved for the coloration of cosmetics of group 2 (not on eyes).
Japan	Not approved for food, drugs and cosmetics.
Poland	Approved for cosmetics.
South Africa	Approved for the coloration of cosmetics of group 1 (all cosmetic products).
Thailand	Approved for cosmetics.
Turkey	Approved for the coloration of cosmetics of group 1 (all cosmetic products).
USA	Not approved for food, drugs and cosmetics.
Zambia	Approved for food.

For acceptance of this colorant in other countries, based on above mentioned approvals, see also 9.1.8.

C.I.69825

Name	EU-No.	C.I. No.	Class	Chemical name / formula
Indanthrenblau BC C.I. Pigment Blue 64 C.I. Vat Blue 6 D&C Blue # 9 (CTFA adopted name) Blue # 204 (Japan) CAS # 130-20-1 EINECS # unknown		69825	Anthra-quinone	7,16-Dichloroindanthrone
Color	Blue pigment.			

Solubility	Insoluble in all standard solvents.
Chromatography	Not applicable.
Spectral photometry	Not applicable.
Main applications	No information available.

Toxicological and dermatological data	Source
No analytical data are available. The assessment of this colorant is done on the basis of current general knowledge of the physico-chemical properties and toxicological experience (Kosmetische Färbemitel, 3. ed., 1991).	

Certification status

European Union	Approved for the coloration of cosmetics of group 1 (all cosmetic products).
Hungary	Approved for the coloration of cosmetics of group 2 (not on eyes).
Japan	Approved for drugs, "quasi-drugs" and cosmetics for external applications.
Korea (South)	Approved for cosmetics.
South Africa	Approved for the coloration of cosmetics of group 1 (all cosmetic products).
Taiwan	Approved for cosmetics.
Turkey	Approved for the coloration of cosmetic of group 1 (all cosmetic products).
USA	Not approved for food, drugs and cosmetics.

For acceptance of this colorant in other countries, based on above mentioned approvals, see also 9.1.8.

C.I.71105

Name	EU-No.	C.I. No.	Class	Chemical name / formula
Hostapermorange GR C.I. Pigment Orange 43 C.I. Vat Orange 7 CAS # 4424-06-0 EINECS # 224-597-4		71105	Anthraquinone	Bisbenzimidazo /2,1-b:2',1' i/benzo /lmn//3,8/phenanthrolin-8,17-dion
Color	Orange pigment.			
Solubility	Low solubility in pyridine, insoluble in water, ethanol and dichloromethane.			

Data Sheets

Chromatography	Not applicable.
Spectral photometry	Not applicable.

Main applications
Cosmetics — Toilet soap.

Toxicological and dermatological data		Source
LD50 tested on rats	> 10000 mg/kg	Kosmetische Färbemittel 3. ed., 1991
Skin compatibility tested on rabbits	minimal irritation	
Mucous membrane compatibility tested on a rabbit eye	non-irritant	

Certification status

European Union	Approved for the coloration of cosmetics of group 3 (not on mucous membranes).
Argentina	Approved only for soap.
Austria	Approved for defined food products.
Bulgaria	Not approved for cosmetics.
Hungary	Approved for the coloration of cosmetics of group 1 (all cosmetic products).
Japan	Not approved for food, drugs and cosmetics.
Poland	Not approved for cosmetics.
South Africa	Approved for the coloration of cosmetics of group 3 (not on mucous membranes).
Turkey	Approved for the coloration of cosmetics of group 3 (not on mucous membranes.
USA	Not approved for food, drugs and cosmetics.

For acceptance of this colorant in other countries, based on above mentioned approvals, see also 9.1.8.

C.I.73000

Name	EU-No.	C.I. No.	Class	Chemical name / formula
Indigo C.I. Vat Blue 1 C.I. Pigment Blue 66 Blue # 201 (Japan) CAS # 482-89-30 EINECS # unknown		73000	Indigoide	Indigo

Color	Blue pigment.

Solubility	Soluble in chloroform and dimethylamide, insoluble in water.

Chromatography	Source : Communication XVII DFG Farbstoff-Kommission
DC	Kieselgel
Carrier	Acetic acid ester 11 ml + Pyridine 5 ml + Water 4 ml

Spectral photometry	Source : Communication XVII DFG Farbstoff-Kommission
Solvent	Dimethylformamide
Absorption maximum	607 nm

Main applications	No information available.

Toxicological and dermatological data		Source
LD50 tested on rats	> 3160 mg/kg	Kosmetische Färbemittel 3. ed., 1991
Skin compatibility tested on rabbits	minor irritation	

Certification status

European Union	Approved for the coloration of cosmetics of group 1 (all cosmetic products). According to Kosmetische Färbemittel, 3. ed., 1991, not recommended for application in the eye area.
Argentina	Approved only for soap.
Hungary	Approved for the coloration of cosmetics of group 2 (not on eyes).
Japan	Approved for drugs, "quasi-drugs" and cosmetics for external applications.
Korea (South)	Approved for cosmetics.
Singapore	Approved for food.
South Africa	Approved for the coloration of cosmetics of group 1 (all cosmetic products).
Taiwan	Approved for cosmetics.
Thailand	Approved for cosmetics.
Turkey	Approved for the coloration of cosmetics of group 1 (all cosmetic products).
USA	Not approved for food, drugs and cosmetics.

For acceptance of this colorant in other countries, based on above mentioned approvals, see also 9.1.8.

Data Sheets   267

C.I.73015

Name	EU-No.	C.I. No.	Class	Chemical name / formula
Indigotin C.I. Food Blue 1 C.I. Acid Blue 74 FD&C Blue # 2 (CFR21) Blue # 2 (Japan) CAS # 860-22-00 EINECS # 212-728-8		73015	Indigoide	Indigo-disulfo acid, Sodium salt

Color	Sodium salt blue solution in water, Aluminum lake blue powder.
Solubility	Sodium salt soluble in water (at 20 °C about 10 g/l) and glycerine (ca. 5 g/l), low solubility in ethanol. Aluminum lake insoluble in water, soluble in acid.
Chromatography DC Carrier	Source : Communication XVII DFG Farbstoff-Kommission Kieselgel Acetic acid ester 5011 ml + Ammonia 25% 10 ml + Methanol 20 ml
Spectral photometry Solvent Absorption maximum	Source : Communication XVII DFG Farbstoff-Kommission Water 610 nm
Main applications Food Drugs Cosmetics	- Candies, artificial ice-cream, liquors. - Aluminum lake for the coloration of capsules. - Aluminum lake for eye make-up.

Toxicological and dermatological data		Source
LD50 tested on rats	> 2000 mg/kg non-sensitive non-irritant	Kosmetische Färbemittel 3. ed., 1991
Skin compatibility tested on guinea pigs Mucous membrane compatibility tested on a rabbit eye ADI-value (WHO 1974, SCF 1975) :	0-5 mg/kg	

Certification status	
Argentina	Approved for food and cosmetics, but not for application in the eye area.

Australia	Approved for defined food products.
Austria	Approved for defined food products.
Brazil	Approved for defined food products.
Canada	Approved for defined food products.
Chile	Approved for food.
Colombia	Approved for food.
Cyprus	Approved for defined food products.
Dominican Republic	Approved for food.
Egypt	Approved for food.
Finland	Approved for defined food products.
Hong Kong	Approved for food.
Hungary	Approved for defined food products. Approved for the coloration of cosmetics of group 2 (not on eyes).
India	Approved for food.
Indonesia	Approved for food. Not approved for cosmetics.
Iran	Approved for food.
Israel	Approved for food, drugs and cosmetics.
Japan	Approved for defined food products, also in the form of Aluminum lakes. Approved for drugs, "quasi-drugs" and cosmetics for external applications, also in the form of Aluminum lake.
Kenya	Approved for food.
Korea (South)	Approved for food and cosmetics.
Kuwait	Approved for food.
Malaysia	Approved for defined food products.
Mexico	Approved for defined food products.
New Zealand	Approved for defined food products. EU-approved colorants for cosmetics are accepted.
Peru	Approved for defined food products.
Philippines	Approved for food and cosmetics.
Poland	Approved for defined food products and cosmetics.
Saudi Arabia	Approved for food.
Singapore	Approved for food.
South Africa	Approved for defined food products. Approved for the coloration of cosmetics of group 1 (all cosmetic products).
Sweden	Approved for defined food products.
Switzerland	Approved for defined food products.
Syria	Approved for food.
Taiwan	Approved for defined food products. Approved for cosmetics, also in the form of Aluminum lake.
Thailand	Approved for food.
Turkey	Approved for the coloration of cosmetics of group 1 (all cosmetic products).
Uruguay	Approved for food.
United Arab Emirates	Approved for food.
USA	Approved for defined food products and orally applied drugs. Utilization requires FDA certificate. Not approved for cosmetics.

Venezuela	Approved for food.
Zambia	Approved for food.

For acceptance of this colorant in other countries, based on above mentioned approvals, see also 9.1.8.

C.I.73312

Name	EU-No.	C.I. No.	Class	Chemical name / formula
C.I. Pigment Red 88 CAS # 14295-43-3 EINECS # unknown		73312	Indigoide	Tetrachloro-thio-indigo

Color	Red pigment.
Solubility	No information available.
Chromatography	No information available.
Spectral photometry	No information available.
Main applications	No information available.

Toxicological and dermatological data	Source
No information available.	

Certification status

European Union	Not approved for cosmetics.
Japan	Not approved for food, drugs and cosmetics.
USA	Not approved for food, drugs and cosmetics.

For acceptance of this colorant in other countries, based on above mentioned approvals, see also 9.1.8.

C.I.73360

Name	EU-No.	C.I. No.	Class	Chemical name / formula
Indanthrenbrillantrosa B C.I. Vat Red 1 C.I. Pigment Red 181 D&C Red # 30 (CTFA adopted name)		73360	Indigoide	6,6'-Dichloro-4,4'-dimethyl-thio-indigo

Red # 226 (Japan)
CAS # 2379-74-0
EINECS # 219-163-6

Color	Red pigment.
Solubility	Low solubility in chloroform and dimethylformamide, insoluble in water.
Chromatography DC Carrier	Source : Communication XVII DFG Farbstoff-Kommission Kieselgel Petrol ether (40-60 °C) 40 ml + Acetic acid ester 60 ml + Methylethylketone 4 ml + Benzol 20 ml.
Spectral photometry Solvent Absorption maximum	Source : Communication XVII DFG Farbstoff-Kommission Dimethylformamide 535 nm
Solvent Absorption maximum	Chloroform (Source : Kosmetische Färbemittel 3. ed., 1991) 537 nm
Main applications Cosmetics	- Toothpaste. - Lipstick.

Toxicological and dermatological data		Source
LD50 tested on rats	> 3160 mg/kg	Kosmetische Färbemittel 3. ed., 1991
Skin compatibility tested on rabbits	non-irritant	
Mucous membrane compatibility tested on a rabbit eye	non-irritant	

Certification status	
European Union	Approved for the coloration of cosmetics of group 1 (all cosmetic products, max. level not more than 3% of total mass).
Argentina	Approved for cosmetics, but not for application in the eye area.
Brazil	Approved for cosmetics, but not for application in the eye area.
Hungary	Approved for the coloration of cosmetics of group 1 (all cosmetic products, max. level not more than 3% of total mass).
Israel	Approved for drugs and cosmetics.
Japan	Approved for drugs, "quasi-drugs" and cosmetics for external applications.
Korea (South)	Approved for cosmetics.
Philippines	Approved for cosmetics, but not for application in the eye area.
Poland	Approved for cosmetics.
South Africa	Approved for the coloration of cosmetics of group 1 (all cosmetic products).
Taiwan	Approved for cosmetics, also in the form of Aluminum and Barium lake.

Data Sheets 271

Thailand	Approved for cosmetics.
Turkey	Approved for the coloration of cosmetics of group 1 (all cosmetic products).
USA	Approved for drugs and cosmetics (also in the form of paint lacquer), but not for application on eyes and lips. Utilization requires FDA certificate.

For acceptance of this colorant in other countries, based on above mentioned approvals, see also 9.1.8.

C.I.73385

Name	EU-No.	C.I. No.	Class	Chemical name / formula
Indanthren-rotviolett RH C.I. Vat Violet 2 C.I. Pigment Violet 36 CAS # 5462-29-3 EINECS # unknown		73385	Indigoide	5,5'-Dichloro-7,7'-dimethyl-thio-indigo

Color	Red violet pigment.
Solubility	Low solubility in dimethylformamide, insoluble in water, methanol and dichloromethane.
Chromatography	Source : Communication XVII DFG Farbstoff-Kommission Chromatogram cannot be made due to low solubility of the pigment
Spectral photometry Solvent Absorption maximum	Source : Communication XVII DFG Farbstoff-Kommission Dimethylformamide 562 nm
Main applications	No information available.

Toxicological and dermatological data		Source
No information available		
LD50 tested on rats	> 10000 mg/kg	Kosmetische Färbemittel
Skin compatibility tested on rabbits	non-irritant	3. ed., 1991
Mucous membrane compatibility tested on a rabbit eye	non-irritant	

Certification status

European Union	Approved for the coloration of cosmetics of group 1 (all cosmetic products).
Hungary	Approved for the coloration of cosmetics of group 1 (all cosmetic products).
Japan	Not approved for food, drugs and cosmetics.
South Africa	Approved for the coloration of cosmetics of group 1 (all cosmetic products).
Turkey	Approved for the coloration of cosmetics of group 1 (all cosmetic products).
USA	Not approved for food, drugs and cosmetics.

For acceptance of this colorant in other countries, based on above mentioned approvals, see also 9.1.8.

C.I.73900

Name	EU-No.	C.I. No.	Class	Chemical name / formula
Hostapermviolett ER02 C.I. Pigment Violet 19 CAS # 1047-16-1 EINECS # unknown		73900	Indigoide	5,12-Dihydrochin /2,3-b/acridin-7,14-dion

Color	Violet pigment.
Solubility	Insoluble in all standard solvents.
Chromatography	Not applicable.
Spectral photometry	Not applicable.
Main applications	No information available.

Toxicological and dermatological data		Source
LD50 tested on rats	> 10000 mg/kg	Kosmetische Färbemittel 3. ed., 1991
Skin compatibility tested on rabbits	non-irritant	
Mucous membrane compatibility tested on a rabbit eye	non-irritant	

Certification status

European Union	Approved for the coloration of cosmetics of group 4 (only for a short residence time on skin).

Bulgaria	Not approved for cosmetics.
Hungary	Not approved for cosmetics.
Japan	Not approved for food, drugs and cosmetics.
Malta	Not approved for cosmetics.
Poland	Not approved for cosmetics.
South Africa	Approved for the coloration of cosmetics of group 4 (only for a short residence time on skin).
Turkey	Approved for the coloration of cosmetics of group 4 (only for a short residence time on skin).
USA	Not approved for food, drugs and cosmetics.

For acceptance of this colorant in other countries, based on above mentioned approvals, see also 9.1.8.

C.I.73905

Name	EU-No.	C.I. No.	Class	Chemical name / formula
Hostapermrot EG C.I. Pigment Red 209 CAS # 3089-17-6 EINECS # unknown		73905	Indigoide	3,110-Dichlorochin /2,3-b/acridin- 7,14/5h, 12h/dion
Color	Red pigment.			
Solubility	Soluble in dimethylformamide, insoluble in water.			
Chromatography	No information available.			
Spectral photometry Solvent Absorption maximum	Source : Communication XVII DFG Farbstoff-Kommission Dimethylformamide 482, 513 nm			
Main applications	No information available.			

Toxicological and dermatological data		Source
LD50 tested on rats	> 15 g/kg	Ringbook Kosmetische Färbemittel 3. ed., 1991
Skin compatibility tested on rabbits	no observation	
Mucous membrane compatibility tested on a rabbit eye	no observation	

Certification status	
European Union	Not approved for cosmetics.

Hungary   Not approved for cosmetics.
Japan   Not approved for cosmetics.
USA   Not approved for food, drugs and cosmetics.
For acceptance of this colorant in other countries, based on above mentioned approvals, see also 9.1.8.

C.I.73915

Name	EU-No.	C.I. No.	Class	Chemical name / formula
C.I. Pigment Red 122 CAS # 16043-40-6 EINECS # unknown		73915	Indigoide	3,10-Dimethylchin /2,3-b/acridin-7, 14/5h, 12h/dion

Color	Red pigment.
Solubility	Insoluble in common solvents.
Chromatography	Not applicable.
Spectral photometry	Not applicable.
Main applications	No information available.

Toxicological and dermatological data		Source
LD50 tested on rats	> 10000 mg/kg	Ringbook Kosmetische Färbemittel 3. ed., 1991
Skin compatibility tested on rabbits	slight irritation	
Mucous membrane compatibility tested on a rabbit eye	non-irritant	

Certification status	
European Union	Approved for the coloration of cosmetics of group 4 (only for a short residence time on skin).
Bulgaria	Not approved for cosmetics.
Hungary	Not approved for cosmetics.
Japan	Not approved for cosmetics.
Malta	Not approved for cosmetics.
Poland	Not approved for cosmetics.
South Africa	Approved for the coloration of cosmetics of group 4 (only for a short residence time on skin).

Turkey	Approved for the coloration of cosmetics of group 4 (only for a short residence time on skin).
USA	Not approved for food, drugs and cosmetics.

For acceptance of this colorant in other countries, based on above mentioned approvals, see also 9.1.8.

C.I.74100

Name	EU-No.	C.I. No.	Class	Chemical name / formula
Heliogenblau G C.I. Pigment Blue 16 CAS # 574-93-60 EINECS # unknown	C 13	74100	Phthalo-cyanine	Phthalocyanine

Color	Blue pigment.
Solubility	Insoluble in all standard solvents.
Chromatography	Not applicable.
Spectral photometry	Not applicable.
Main applications	No information available.

Toxicological and dermatological data		Source
LD50 tested on rats	> 6000 mg/kg	Kosmetische Färbemittel 3. ed., 1991
Skin compatibility tested on rabbits	non-irritant	
Mucous membrane compatibility tested on a rabbit eye	minimal irritation	

Certification status

European Union	Approved for the coloration of cosmetics of group 4 (only for a short residence time on skin).
Bulgaria	Not approved for cosmetics.
Hungary	Approved for the coloration of cosmetics of group 2 (not on eyes).
Japan	Not approved for food, drugs and cosmetics.
Malta	Not approved for cosmetics.
Poland	Not approved for cosmetics.
South Africa	Approved for the coloration of cosmetics of group 4 (only for a short residence time on skin).

Turkey	Approved for the coloration of cosmetics of group 4 (only for a short residence time on skin).
USA	Not approved for food, drugs and cosmetics.

For acceptance of this colorant in other countries, based on above mentioned approvals, see also 9.1.8.

C.I.74160

Name	EU-No.	C.I. No.	Class	Chemical name / formula
Heliogenblau B C.I. Pigment Blue 15 Blue # 404 (Japan) CAS # 147-14-8 EINECS # 205-685-1		74160	Phthalo-cyanine	Copper-phthalo-cyanine
Color	Blue pigment.			
Solubility	Insoluble in water, commercially available in water-dispersible form.			
Chromatography	Not applicable.			
Spectral photometry	No information available.			
Spectral photometry Solvent Absorption maximum	Source : own assay of the water-dispersible form Water 612, 685 nm			
Main applications Cosmetics	- Eye makeup (pigment). - Toilet soap (pigment and water-dispersible form). - Shampoo, shower gel, liquid soap (water-dispersible form).			

Toxicological and dermatological data		Source
LD50 tested on rats	> 10000 mg/kg	Kosmetische Färbemittel 3. ed., 1991
Skin compatibility tested on rabbits	non- to slightly irritating	
Mucous membrane compatibility tested on a rabbit eye	non- to slightly irritating	

Certification status

European Union	Approved for the coloration of cosmetics of group 1 (all cosmetic products).
Argentina	Approved only for soap.
Hungary	Approved for the coloration of cosmetics of group 2 (not on eyes).
Japan	Approved for drugs, "quasi-drugs" and cosmetics for external applications, also in the form of aluminum-lakes, but not on mucous membranes.
Korea (South)	Approved for cosmetics.
Malta	Not approved for cosmetics.
South Africa	Approved for the coloration of cosmetics of group 1 (all cosmetic products).
Taiwan	Approved for facial toning masks, not for cosmetics.
Turkey	Approved for the coloration of cosmetics of group 1 (all cosmetic products).
USA	Not approved for food, drugs and cosmetics.

For acceptance of this colorant in other countries, based on above mentioned approvals, see also 9.1.8.

C.I.74180

Name	EU-No.	C.I. No.	Class	Chemical name / formula
Siriuslicht türkisblau GL C.I. Direct Blue 86 CAS # 1330-38-7 EINECS # 215-537-8		74180	Phthalo-cyanine	Copper-phthalo-cyanine-trisulfo acid, Sodium salt
Color	Blue solution in water.			
Solubility	Soluble in water.			
Chromatography DC Carrier	Source : Communication XVII DFG Farbstoff-Kommission Kieselgel n-Propanol 60 ml + Acetic acid ester 10 ml + Water 30 ml			
Spectral photometry Solvent Absorption maximum	Source : Communication XVII DFG Farbstoff-Kommission Water 618, 685 nm (own assay : 618, 658 nm)			
Main applications Cosmetics	- Shampoo, shower gel. - Liquid soap.			

Toxicological and dermatological data		Source
LD50 tested on rats	> 5000 mg/kg	Kosmetische Färbemittel 3. ed., 1991
Skin compatibility tested on mice	non-irritant	
Mucous membrane compatibility tested on a rabbit eye	slight reddening of	

Certification status	
European Union	Approved for the coloration of cosmetics of group 4 (only for a short residence time on skin).
Bulgaria	Not approved for cosmetics.
Hungary	Not approved for cosmetics.
Poland	Not approved for cosmetics.
South Africa	Approved for the coloration of cosmetics of group 4 (only for a short residence time on skin).
Turkey	Approved for the coloration of cosmetics of group 4 (only for a short residence time on skin).
USA	Not approved for food, drugs and cosmetics.

For acceptance of this colorant in other countries, based on above mentioned approvals, see also 9.1.8.

C.I.74260

Name	EU-No.	C.I. No.	Class	Chemical name / formula
Heliogengrün G C.I. Pigment Green 7 CAS # 1328-53-6 EINECS # 215-524-7		74260	Phthalo-cyanine	Poly-chloro-copper-phthalocyanine
Color	Green pigment.			
Solubility	Insoluble in water, but commercially available as a water-dispersible preparation.			
Chromatography	Not applicable.			
Spectral photometry Solvent Absorption maximum	(Own assay of the water-dispersible preparation.) Water 368, 650, 728 nm			
Main applications Cosmetics	- Toilet soap (pigment and water-dispersible preparation). - Shampoo, foam bath, liquid soap (water-dispersible preparation).			

Data Sheets 279

Toxicological and dermatological data		Source
LD50 tested on rats	> 10000 mg/kg	Kosmetische Färbemittel
Skin compatibility tested on mice	non-irritant	3. ed., 1991
Mucous membrane compatibility tested on a rabbit eye	non-irritant	

Certification status

European Union	Approved for the coloration of cosmetics of group 2 (not on eyes).
Argentina	Approved only for soap.
Bulgaria	Approved for cosmetics, but not in the eye area.
Hungary	Approved for the coloration of cosmetics of group 2 (not on eyes).
Japan	Not approved for food, drugs and cosmetics.
Poland	Approved for cosmetics, but not in the eye area.
South Africa	Approved for the coloration of cosmetics of group 2 (not on eyes).
Taiwan	Approved for cosmetics.
Turkey	Approved for the coloration of cosmetics of group 4 (only for a short residence time on skin).
USA	Not approved for food, drugs and cosmetics.

For acceptance of this colorant in other countries, based on above mentioned approvals, see also 9.1.8.

C.I.75100

Name	EU-No.	C.I. No.	Class	Chemical name / formula
Crocetin C.I. Natural Yellow 6/19 C.I. Natural Red 1 Crocetine (Japan) CAS # 89382-88-7, # 27876-94-4 EINECS # unknown		75100	Carotinoide	Crocetine (Dicarbon acid of the carotenoide sequence)
Color	Yellow solution in water.			
Solubility	Soluble in water.			

Chromatography	No information available.
Spectral photometry	No information available.
Main applications	No information available.

Toxicological and dermatological data	Source
No information available.	

Certification status

European Union	Approved for the coloration of cosmetics of group 1 (all cosmetic products).
Hungary	Approved for the coloration of cosmetics of group 1 (all cosmetic products).
Japan	Not approved for food and drugs.
	Approved for cosmetics (CTFA-list of Japanese cosmetic ingredients).
Singapore	Approved for food.
South Africa	Approved for the coloration of cosmetics of group 1 (all cosmetic products).
Sweden	Approved for defined food products.
Thailand	Approved for cosmetics.
Turkey	Approved for the coloration of cosmetics of group 1 (all cosmetic products).
	Approved for the coloration of cosmetics of group 4 (only for a short residence time on skin).
United Arab Emirates	Approved for food.
USA	Not approved for food, drugs and cosmetics.

For acceptance of this colorant in other countries, based on above mentioned approvals, see also 9.1.8.

C.I.75120

Name	EU-No.	C.I. No.	Class	Chemical name / formula
Bixin, Orlean C.I. Natural Orange 4 Annatto (CTFA adopted name) Annatto (Japan) CAS # 6983-79-5, # 1393-63-1 EINECS # 230-248-7	E 160b	75120	Carotenoide	Bixin (major colorant component of the commercially available annatto extracts, content 1-30%)

Norbixin CAS # 542-40-5 EINECS # 208-810-8	E 160b	75120	Carotenoide	Norbixin (manufactured from Bixin by alkaline processing)	

Color	Yellow to orange color in diluted solutions.
Solubility	Bixin soluble in oil, insoluble in water; Norbixin soluble in water.
Chromatography DC Carrier	of Bixin : Source : Communication XVII DFG Farbstoff-Kommission Kieselgel Chloroform 50 ml + Acetone 50 ml + Acetic Acid ester 1 ml
Spectral photometry Solvent Absorption maximum	of Bixin : Source : Communication XVII DFG Farbstoff-Kommission Chloroform 440, 466, 498 nm
Solvent Absorption maximum	of Norbixin (Source : Kosmetische Färbemittel, 3. ed., 1991) 480 nm
Main applications Food Cosmetics	 - Oil, margarine, mayonnaise, cheese. - Oil products, creams.

Toxicological and dermatological data		Source
The biological and toxicological literature covers only annatto extracts. ADI-value (SCF value 1975)	0-1.5 mg/kg as the sum of Bixin and Norbixin	Ringbook Colorants for food 1978

Certification status

European Union	Approved for defined food products (see 2.4.1.) and for the coloration of drugs and cosmetic preparations of group 1 (all cosmetic products).
Argentina	Approved for food and cosmetics.
Australia	Approved for defined food products.
Austria	Approved for defined food products.
Brazil	Approved for defined food products. Approved for cosmetics.
Canada	Approved for defined food products.
Chile	Approved for food.
Colombia	Approved for food.

Costa Rica	Approved for food.
Cyprus	Approved for defined food products.
Egypt	Approved for food.
Finland	Approved for defined food products.
Hungary	Approved for defined food products.
	Approved for the coloration of cosmetics of group 1 (all cosmetic products).
India	Approved for food.
Indonesia	Approved for food.
Iran	Approved for food.
Israel	Approved for food, drugs and cosmetics.
Japan	Approved for defined food products.
	Approved for drugs, "quasi-drugs" and cosmetics.
Kenya	Approved for food.
Korea (South)	Approved for food.
Kuwait	Approved for food.
Malaysia	Approved for defined food products.
Malta	Approved for food.
New Zealand	Approved for defined food products.
Norway	Approved for defined food products.
Philippines	Approved for food and cosmetics.
Poland	Approved for food and cosmetics.
Saudi Arabia	Approved for food.
Singapore	Approved for food.
South Africa	Approved for defined food products.
	Approved for the coloration of cosmetics of group 1 (all cosmetic products).
	Approved for the coloration of cosmetics of group 4 (only for a short residence time on skin).
Sweden	Approved for defined food products.
Switzerland	Approved for defined food products.
Syria	Approved for food.
Taiwan	Approved for defined food products.
Thailand	Approved for food.
Turkey	Approved for defined food products.
	Approved for the coloration of cosmetics of group 1 (all cosmetic products).
United Arab Emirates	Approved for food.
USA	Approved for defined food products, drugs and cosmetics, also for application in the eye area.
	Utilization requires FDA certificate.
Venezuela	Approved for cosmetics.
Zambia	Approved for food.

For acceptance of this colorant in other countries, based on above mentioned approvals, see also 9.1.8.

C.I.75125

Name	EU-No.	C.I. No.	Class	Chemical name / formula
Lycopin C.I. Natural Yellow 27 CAS # 502-65-8 EINECS # 207-949-1	E 160d	75125	Carotenoide	Lycopine

Color	Yellow to orange color in hydrocarbons.
Solubility	Soluble in chloroform, cyclohexane and oil.
Chromatography DC Carrier	Source : Communication XVII DFG Farbstoff-Kommission Kieselgel Petrol ether (100-160 °C) 40 ml + Petrol ether (40-60 °C) 50 ml + Isopropanol 20 ml
Spectral photometry Solvent Absorption maximum	Source : Communication XVII DFG Farbstoff-Kommission Chloroform 453, 478, 512 nm
Main applications	Lycopine exists in tomatoes and many other fruits. The isolated colorant is not of technical importance. Tomato extracts are used for the coloration of mayonnaise and sauces.

Toxicological and dermatological data	Source
ADI-value not specified (EU document III/9280/90)	

Certification status	
European Union	Approved for defined food products (see 2.4.1.) and for the coloration of drugs and cosmetic preparations of group 1 (all cosmetic products).
Hungary	Approved for the coloration of cosmetics of group 1 (all cosmetic products).
Japan	Not approved for food, drugs and cosmetics.
Malta	Approved for food.
South Africa	Approved for the coloration of cosmetics of group 1 (all cosmetic products).
Thailand	Approved for cosmetics.
Turkey	Approved for the coloration of cosmetics of group 1 (all cosmetic products).
USA	Not approved for food, drugs and cosmetics.

For acceptance of this colorant in other countries, based on above mentioned approvals, see also 9.1.8.

C.I.75130

Name	EU-No.	C.I. No.	Class	Chemical name / formula
Carotene Provitamin A C.I. Natural Yellow 26 Carotene (CTFA adopted name) Carotene (Japan) CAS # 7235-40-8 EINECS # 230-636-6	E 160a	75130	Carotenoide	Naturally occuring blend of isomeres of alpha-, beta- and gamma-carotene, with beta-carotene being the major compound (see C.I.40800), which is also manufactured synthetically.
CAS # 7488-99-5 (alpha) EINECS # unknown				
CAS # 7235-40-7 (beta) EINECS # 230-636-6 CAS # 10593-83-6 (gamma) EINECS # unknown				

Color	Yellow-orange solution in organic solvents and fatty oils.
Solubility	Soluble in chloroform, cyclohexane and oil. Beta-carotene (see C.I.40800) is commercially available in the form of a water-dispersible preparation.
Chromatography DC Carrier	Source : Communication XVII DFG Farbstoff-Kommission Kieselgel Cyclohexane 100 ml + acetic acid ester 50 ml
Spectral photometry Solvent Absorption maximum	Source : Communication XVII DFG Farbstoff-Kommission Chloroform 454, 485 nm (alpha) 466, 497 nm (beta) 446, 475, 509 nm (gamma)
Main applications Food Drugs Cosmetics	 - Oils, fats, margarine, mayonnaise, waterdispersible preparation for beverages, candies, dessert products. - Universally applicable. - Creams.

Data Sheets 285

Toxicological and dermatological data	Source

No analytical results are available. The classification of this colorant is done on the basis of general knowledge of the physical-chemical properties and toxicological experiences (Kosmetische Färbemittel, 3. Ed., 1991).
Data for β-Carotene see C.I.40800.

Certification status

European Union	Approved for defined food products (see 2.4.1.) and for the coloration of drugs and cosmetic preparations of group 1 (all cosmetic products).
Argentina	Approved for food and cosmetics.
Australia	Approved for defined food products.
Austria	Approved for defined food products.
Brazil	Approved for defined food products.
	Approved for cosmetics, but not in the eye area and for products for nail care or painting.
Canada	Approved for defined food products.
Chile	Approved for food products.
Colombia	Approved for food products.
Costa Rica	Approved for food products.
Cyprus	Approved for defined food products.
Egypt	Approved for food products.
Finland	Approved for defined food products.
Guatemala	Approved for defined food products.
Hungary	Approved for defined food products.
	Approved for the coloration of cosmetics of group 1 (all cosmetic products).
India	Approved for food products.
Indonesia	Approved for food products.
Iran	Approved for food products.
Israel	Approved for food, drugs and cosmetics.
Japan	Approved for defined food products.
Kenya	Approved for food products.
Korea (South)	Approved for food products.
Kuwait	Approved for food products.
Malaysia	Approved for defined food products.
Malta	Approved for food.
New Zealand	Approved for defined food products.
Norway	Approved for defined food products.
Panama	US-approved colorants for cosmetics are accepted.
Peru	Approved for food products.
Philippines	Approved for food and cosmetics.
Poland	Approved for food and cosmetics.
Saudi Arabia	Approved for food products.
Singapore	Approved for food products.
South Africa	Approved for the coloration of cosmetics of group 1 (all cosmetic·products).
Sweden	Approved for defined food products.

Switzerland	Approved for defined food products and drugs.
Syria	Approved for food products.
Taiwan	Approved for defined food products.
Thailand	Approved for cosmetics.
Tunisia	Approved for defined food products.
Turkey	Approved for defined food products.
	Approved for the coloration of cosmetics of group 1 (all cosmetic products).
United Arab Emirates	Approved for food products.
Uruguay	Approved for food products.
USA	Approved for food, drugs and cosmetics, also for the eye area. FDA certificate not required.
Zambia	Approved for food products.

For acceptance of this colorant in other countries, based on above mentioned approvals, see also 9.1.8.

C.I.75135

Name	EU-No.	C.I. No.	Class	Chemical name / formula
Rubixanthin C.I. Natural Yellow 27 CAS # 3763-55-1 EINECS # unknown	E 161d	75135	Carotenoide (Xanthophyll)	Hydroxyl-derivate of carotene
Color	Orange solution in chloroform.			
Solubility	Soluble in chloroform, low solubility in alcohol and petrol ether.			
Chromatography	No information available.			
Spectral photometry Solvent Absorption maximum	Source : Kosmetische Färbemittel 1991 Chloroform 439, 474, 509 nm			
Main applications	No information available, this colorant is currently not of any technical importance.			

Toxicological and dermatological data	Source
Results are not available. The assessment of this colorant is done on the basis of general knowledge of the physico-chemical properties and toxicological experience (Kosmetische Färbemittel, 3. ed., 1991)	

Certification status
See Xanthophyll

C.I.75138

Name	EU-No.	C.I. No.	Class	Chemical name / formula
Violaxanthin C.I. Natural Yellow 27 CAS # 126-29-4 EINECS # unknown	E 161e	75138	Carotenoide	Keto-hydroxyl-derivate of carotene

Color	Yellow to orange solution in hydrocarbon.
Solubility	Soluble in chloroform and hydrocarbon.
Chromatography	No information available.
Spectral photometry Solvent Absorption maximum	Source : Kosmetische Färbemittel 1991 Chloroform 424, 452, 482 nm
Main applications	No information available; the isolated colorant is currently of no technical importance.

Toxicological and dermatological data	Source
Results are not available. The assessment of this colorant is done on the basis of general knowledge of the physico-chemical properties and toxicological experience (Kosmetische Färbemittel, 3. ed., 1991)	

Certification status	
See Xanthophyll	

C.I.75136

Name	EU-No.	C.I. No.	Class	Chemical name / formula
Lutein, Xanthophyll C.I. Natural Yellow 29 CAS # 127-40-2 EINECS # 204-840-0	E 161b	75136	Carotenoide (Xanthophyll)	Hydroxyl derivative of Carotene

Color	Yellow to orange color in hydrocarbons.

Solubility	Soluble in chloroform, hydrocarbons.
Chromatography	No information available.
Spectral photometry Solvent Absorption maximum	Source : Kosmetische Färbemittel, 3. ed., 1991 Chloroform 428, 456, 487 nm
Main applications	Lutein is not available commercially in its pure form, but occurs as a compound in vegetable extracts, and it blends with other carotenoides.

Toxicological and dermatological data	**Source**
Results are not available. The assessment of this colorant is done on the basis of general knowledge of the physico-chemical properties and toxicological experience (Kosmetische Färbemittel, 3. ed., 1991)	

Certification status

See Xanthophyll

C.I.75137

Name	EU-No.	C.I. No.	Class	Chemical name / formula
Zeaxanthin C.I. Natural Yellow 29 CAS # 144-68-3 EINECS # unknown		75137	Carotenoide (Xanthophyll)	Zeaxanthin
Color	Yellow to yellow-orange color in oils.			
Solubility	Soluble in oil and organic solvents.			
Chromatography	No information available.			
Spectral photometry Solvent Absorption maximum	Source : Ringbook Farbstoffe für Lebensmittel 1978 n-Hexane 450-452 nm			
Main applications	(Source: Ringbook Farbstoffe für Lebensmittel 1978) Fat-soluble commercial products for the coloration of fats, water-dispersible products for the coloration of hot and cold drinks, creams, puddings, feed additives for egg yolk and broiler pigmentation.			

Toxicological and dermatological data	Source
ADI-value (SCF 1975) Approved without specifically defined ADI-value (Ringbook Farbstoffe für Lebensmittel 1978)	

Certification status	
European Union	Not approved for food, drugs and cosmetics.
Japan	Not approved for food, drugs and cosmetics.
USA	Not approved for food, drugs and cosmetics.
For acceptance of this colorant in other countries, based on above mentioned approvals, see also 9.1.8.	

C.I.75138

Name	EU-No.	C.I. No.	Class	Chemical name / formula
Violaxanthin C.I. Natural Yellow 27 CAS # 126-29-4 EINECS # unknown	E 161e	75138	Carotenoide	Keto-hydroxyl-derivate of carotene
Color	Yellow to orange solution in hydrocarbon.			
Solubility	Soluble in chloroform and hydrocarbon.			
Chromatography	No information available.			
Spectral photometry Solvent Absorption maximum	Source : Kosmetische Färbemittel 1991 Chloroform 424, 452, 482 nm			
Main applications	No information available; the isolated colorant is currently of no technical importance.			

Toxicological and dermatological data	Source
Results are not available. The assessment of this colorant is done on the basis of general knowledge of the physico-chemical properties and toxicological experience (Kosmetische Färbemittel, 3. ed., 1991)	

Certification status

See Xanthophyll

C.I.75170

Name	EU-No.	C.I. No.	Class	Chemical name / formula
Guanin Fischsilber C.I. Natural White 1 Guanin (Japan) CAS # 73-40-5 EINECS # unknown		75170	Natural	2-Amino-6-hydroxy-purin

Color	White to yellow pearl pigment (brilliant).
Solubility	Insoluble in water, soluble in diluted acid and lye with salt formation.
Chromatography	Not applicable.
Spectral photometry	No information available.
Spectral photometry Solvent Absorption maximum	Source : Kosmetische Färbemittel, 3. ed., 1991 Water (pH 6.2) 246, 275 nm
Main applications Cosmetics	- Decorative cosmetics.

Toxicological and dermatological data	Source
Results are not available. The assessment of this colorant is done on the basis of general knowledge of the physico-chemical properties and toxicological experience (Kosmetische Färbemittel, 3. ed., 1991)	

Certification status

European Union	Approved for the coloration of cosmetics of group 1 (all cosmetic products).
Argentina	Approved for cosmetics.
Brazil	Approved for cosmetics.
Hungary	Approved for the coloration of cosmetics of group 1 (all cosmetic products).
Japan	Approved for drugs, "quasi-drugs" and cosmetics.
Philippines	Approved for cosmetics.
South Africa	Approved for the coloration of cosmetics of group 1 (all cosmetic products).
Turkey	Approved for the coloration of cosmetics of group 1 (all cosmetic products).

USA	Approved for drugs and cosmetics for external applications, also on eyes. Utilization requires FDA certificate.
Venezuela	Approved for cosmetics.

For acceptance of this colorant in other countries, based on above mentioned approvals, see also 9.1.8.

C.I.75300

Name	EU-No.	C.I. No.	Class	Chemical name / formula
Curcumin Turmeric C.I. Natural Yellow 3 Turmeric Turmeric oleoresin (CFR21) CAS # 458-37-7 EINECS # 207-280-5	E 100	75300	Dicinna- moyl- methane	1,7-Bis (4-hydroxy-3-methoxyphenyl)-1,6-heptadien-3,5-dion
Color	Yellow solution in ethanol.			
Solubility	Soluble in ethanol and ether, lower solubility in water.			
Chromatography DC Carrier	Source : Ringbook Colorant for food 1978 Kieselgel Chloroform 90 ml + Methanol 5 ml			
Spectral photometry Solvent Absorption maximum Solvent Absorption maximum	Source : Ringbook Kosmetische Färbemittel 1984 and Ringbook Colorant for food, 1978 Ethanol 426 nm Alkaline alcohol solution 482 nm			
Main applications Food	Usually extracts of the curcuma root are utilized, which contain curcumin and two other methoxy-derivatives of curcumin - mustard, sauces.			

Toxicological and dermatological data		Source
LD50 tested on rats	>10000 mg/kg	Kosmetische Färbemittel 3. ed., 1991
ADI-value (WHO 1986, JEFCA 1990)	0-0.1 mg/kg	

Certification status

European Union	Approved for defined food products (see 2.4.1.) and for the coloration of drugs and cosmetic preparations of group 1 (all cosmetic products).
Argentina	Approved for food.
Australia	Approved for defined food products.
Austria	Approved for defined food products.
Brazil	Approved for defined food products.
Canada	Approved for defined food products.
Chile	Approved for food.
Colombia	Approved for food.
Costa Rica	Approved for food.
Cyprus	Approved for defined food products.
Finland	Approved for food.
Hungary	Approved for defined food products. Approved for the coloration of cosmetics of group 1 (all cosmetic products).
India	Approved for food.
Indonesia	Approved for food.
Iran	Approved for food.
Israel	Approved for food, drugs and cosmetics.
Japan	Approval for food status unclear. Not approved for cosmetics.
Korea (South)	Approved for food.
Kuwait	Approved for food.
Malaysia	Approved for defined food products.
Malta	Approved for food.
New Zealand	Approved for defined food products.
Norway	Approved for defined food products.
Philippines	Approved for food.
Poland	Approved for defined food products and cosmetics.
Saudi Arabia	Approved for food.
Singapore	Approved for food.
South Africa	Approved for the coloration of cosmetics of group 1 (all cosmetic products).
Sweden	Approved for defined food products.
Switzerland	Approved for defined food products.
Thailand	Approved for food.
Turkey	Approved for defined food products. Approved for the coloration of cosmetics of group 1 (all cosmetic products).
United Arab Emirates	Approved for food.
USA	Approved for defined food products. Utilization does not require FDA certificate. Not approved for drugs and cosmetics.
Zambia	Approved for food.

For acceptance of this colorant in other countries, based on above mentioned approvals, see also 9.1.8.

C.I.75470

Name	EU-No.	C.I. No.	Class	Chemical name / formula
Cochenille, Karmin C.I. Natural Red 4 Cochenille extract, Carmine , (CTFA adopted name, CFR21) Carmine (Japan) CAS # 1390-65-4 EINECS # 215-724-4 (Carmines), # 215-680-6 (Cochineal)	E 120	75470	Anthra-quinone	Aluminum-Calcium lacquer of carmine acid
Carmine acid CAS # 1260-17-9 EINECS # 215-023-3	E 120	75470	Anthra-quinone	-, free acid

Color	Aluminum-Calcium lacquer red powder, carmine acid red solution in water.
Solubility	Aluminum-Calcium lacquer insoluble in water, low solubility inorganic solvents. Carmine acid soluble in water and ethanol.
Chromatography DC Carrier	of carmine acid : Source : Communication XVII DFG Farbstoff-Kommission Kieselgel Water 20 ml + Acetone 40 ml + Ammonia 25% 10 ml
Spectral photometry Solvent Absorption maximum	of carmine acid : Source : Communication XVII DFG Farbstoff-Kommission Water 525, 567 nm (subject to pH, blue-reddish in alkaline solution)
Main applications Food Drugs Cosmetics	Commercially available are dried cochenille, Aluminum-Calcium lacquer (Carmine-Naccarat) and pure carmine acid. - Beverages, candies. - Juice. - Make-up, lipstick.

Toxicological and dermatological data		Source
LD50 tested on rats	> 15000 mg/kg	Ringbook
Sensitivity (human)	Allergic reaction on persons with lip injuries... (...Calcium carmine) no value defined 0-0.05 mg/kg approved only for some alcoholic beverages 0-5 mg/kg	Kosmetische Färbemittel 1984
ADI-value (WHO 1974) (SCF 1975)		Kosmetische Färbemittel, 3. ed., 1991
(CIAA list Mouton)		

Certification status

European Union	Approved for defined food products (see 2.4.1.) and for the coloration of drugs and cosmetic preparations of group 1 (all cosmetic products).
Argentina	Approval for food and cosmetics.
Australia	Approved for defined food products.
Austria	Approved for defined food products and cosmetics.
Canada	Approved for defined food products.
Chile	Approved for food.
Colombia	Approved for food.
Costa Rica	Approved for food.
Cyprus	Approved for defined food products.
Egypt	Approved for food.
Hungary	Approved for defined food products. Approved for the coloration of cosmetics of group 1 (all cosmetic products).
Indonesia	Approved for food.
Iran	Approved for food.
Israel	Approved for food, drugs and cosmetics.
Japan	Approved for drugs, "quasi-drugs" and cosmetics.
Kenya	Approved for food.
Korea (South)	Approved for food.
Malaysia	Approved for defined food products.
Malta	Approved for food.
New Zealand	Approved for defined food products.
Peru	Approved for food.
Philippines	Approved for food and cosmetics.
Poland	Approved for cosmetics.
Singapore	Approved for food.
South Africa	Approved for defined food products. Approved for the coloration of cosmetics of group 1 (all cosmetic products).

Switzerland	Approved for defined food products and drugs.
Syria	Approved for food.
Taiwan	Approved for defined food products.
Thailand	Approved for food and cosmetics.
Tunisia	Approved for defined food products.
Turkey	Approved for defined food products.
	Approved for the coloration of cosmetics of group 1 (all cosmetic products).
Uruguay	Approved for food.
USA	Approved for defined food products.
	Approved for orally and externally applied drugs.
	Approved for cosmetics, also for application in the eye area. Utilization does not require FDA certificate.
Venezuela	Approved for food and cosmetics.
Zambia	Approved for food.

For acceptance of this colorant in other countries, based on above mentioned approvals, see also 9.1.8.

C.I.75480

Name	EU-No.	C.I. No.	Class	Chemical name / formula
Henna, Lawsone C.I. Natural Orange 6 Henna (CTFA adopted name) CAS # 83-72-7 EINECS # unknown		75480	Naphtho-quinone	1-Hydroxy-naphtho-quinone

Color	Henna-powder : greenish.
Solubility	Soluble in water.
Chromatography	No information available.
Spectral photometry	No information available.
Main applications	Hair dying.

Toxicological and dermatological data	Source
No information available.	

Certification status

European Union	Not considered a cosmetic colorant, is used for hair dying.
Japan	Not considered a cosmetic colorant.
USA	Approved for hair dying, but not in the eye area.
	Utilization does not require FDA certificate.

For acceptance of this colorant in other countries, based on above mentioned approvals, see also 9.1.8.

C.I.75660

Name	EU-No.	C.I. No.	Class	Chemical name / formula
Morin C.I. Natural Yellow 8,11 CAS # 480-16-0 EINECS # unknown		75660	Flavone	3,5,7,2',4'-Penta-hydroxy-flavone
Color	Yellow solution in water.			
Solubility	Soluble in hot water, alkali, ethanol and acetic acid, low solubility in cold water and ether.			
Chromatography DC Carrier	Source : Communication XVII DFG Farbstoff-Kommission Kieselgel tert. Sodium citrate solution 2.5% 80 ml + Ammonia 25% 20 ml + Methanol 12 ml			
Spectral photometry Solvent Absorption maximum	Source : Communication XVII DFG Farbstoff-Kommission Water 320 nm			
Solvent Absorption maximum	Methanol (own assay) 398 nm			
Main applications	No information available.			

Toxicological and dermatological data		Source
LD50 tested on rats	> 6.3 g/kg	Ringbook Kosmetische Färbemittel, 1984
Skin compatibility tested on humans and rabbits	no observation	
Mucous membrane compatibility tested on a rabbit eye	no observation	

Data Sheets

Certification status

European Union	Not approved for cosmetics.
Hungary	Not approved for cosmetics.
Japan	Not approved for food, drugs and cosmetics.
USA	Not approved for food, drugs and cosmetics.

There is no information available from other countries, i.e., this colorant is not included in other national positive lists.

C.I. 75810

Name	EU-No.	C.I. No.	Class	Chemical name / formula
Chlorophyll C.I. Natural Green 3 CAS # 1406-65-1 (Chlorophyll a/b) CAS # 479-61-8 (Chlorophyll a) EINECS # 207-536-6		75810	Porphyrin	Chlorophyll a/b (in green plants as a blend of isomeres)
CAS # 519-62-0 (Chlorophyll b) EINECS # 208-272-4				
Chlorophyll-copper complex C.I. Natural Green 3 Copper Chlorophyll (Japan)	E 141	75810	Porphyrin	Chlorophyll a/b Copper complex
CAS # 8049-84-1 (Chlorophyll a/b copper complex) EINECS # 232-471-5				
CAS # 15739-09-0 (Chlorophyll a copper complex) EINECS # 239-830-5				
CAS # 24111-17-9 (Chlorophyll b copper complex) EINECS # 246-020-5				
Color	Chlorophyll a/b gives a green solution in methanol with a red fluorescence. Chlorophyll copper complex gives a green solution in ethanol.			

Solubility	Chlorophyll a/b and Chlorophyll copper complex are soluble in ethanol, methanol, chloroform, ether, fats and oils. Insoluble in water.
Chromatography DC Carrier	Source : Communication XVII DFG Farbstoff-Kommission Cellulose Petrol ether (100-160 °C) 50 ml + Benzol 35 ml + Chloroform 10 ml + Acetone 0.5 ml + Isopropanol 0.2 ml
Spectral photometry 1) Chlorophyll a/b Solvent Absorption maximum	 (Source: Communication XVII DFG Farbstoff-Kommission) Methanol 402, 500, 625, 655 nm
2) Chlorophyll a Solvent Absorption maximum	(Source: Kosmet. Färbemittel, 3. ed., 1991) Ether 381, 409, 428, 496, 530, 576, 613, 660 nm
3) Chlorophyll b Solvent Absorption maximum	(Source: Kosmet. Färbemittel, 3. ed., 1991) Ether 381, 409, 428, 496, 530, 576, 613, 660 nm
Main applications Food: Drugs: Cosmetics:	 - Fats and oils. - Salves, suppositories. - Oils, creams, toilet soap.

Toxicological and dermatological data		Source
LD50 tested on mice	>10000 mg/kg	Kosmetische Färbemittel 3. ed., 1991
ADI-value of chlorophyll not limited ADI-value as the sum of chlorophyll in (C.I.75815) and Chlorophyll-copper-complex (SCF 1975)	 0-15 mg/kg	Ringbook Farbstoffe f. Lebensmittel 1978

Certification status

European Union	Approved for defined food products (see 2.4.1.) and for the coloration of drugs and cosmetic preparations of group 1 (all cosmetic products).
Argentina	Approved for food products. Approved for cosmetics, but only in perfumes on an alcohol basis.
Australia	Approved for defined food products.
Austria	Approved for defined food products.
Brazil	Approved for defined food products.
Canada	Approved for defined food products.
Chile	Approved for food products.
Colombia	Approved for food products.

Data Sheets

Costa Rica	Approved for food products.
Cyprus	Approved for defined food products.
Egypt	Approved for food products.
Finland	Approved for defined food products.
Hungary	Approved for defined food products.
	Approved for the coloration of cosmetics of group 2 (not on eyes).
India	Approved for food products.
Indonesia	Approved for food products.
Iran	Approved for food products.
Israel	Approved for food products.
Japan	Approved only in chewing gum.
	Not approved in cosmetics.
Kenia	Approved for food products.
Korea (South)	Approved for food products.
Kuwait	Approved for food products.
Malaysia	Approved for defined food products.
Malta	Approved for food products.
New Zealand	Approved for defined food products.
Norway	Approved for defined food products.
Peru	Approved for food products.
Poland	Approved for defined food products.
Saudi Arabia	Approved for food products.
Singapore	Approved for food products.
South Africa	Approved for defined food products.
	Approved for cosmetic preparations of group 1 (all cosmetic products).
Sudan	Approved for food products.
Sweden	Approved for defined food products.
Switzerland	Approved for defined food products.
Taiwan	Approved for defined food products.
Thailand	Approved for food products.
Turkey	Approved for cosmetic preparations of group 1 (all cosmetic products).
United Arab Emirates	Approved for food products.
USA	Not approved for food products, drugs and cosmetics.
Zambia	Approved for food products.

There is no information available from other countries, i.e., this colorant is not included in other national positive lists.

C.I.75815

Name	EU-No.	C.I. No.	Class	Chemical name / formula
Chlorophyllin	E 141	75815	Porphyrin	Chlorophyllin-

C.I. Natural Green 5　　　　　　　　　　　　　　　　　　copper-complex, So-
Sodium copper chloro-　　　　　　　　　　　　　　　　　dium salt
phyllin　(Japan)
CAS # 11006-34-1
EINECS # 234-242-6

Potassium sodium copper　E 141　　75815　　Porphyrin　Chlorophyllin-
chlorophyllin　　　　　　　　　　　　　　　　　　　　　copper-complex,
(CTFA adopted name,　　　　　　　　　　　　　　　　　Potassium-sodium
CFR21)　　　　　　　　　　　　　　　　　　　　　　　complex
CAS # 1337-20-8
EINECS # 215-652-3

Color	Green solution in water.
Solubility	Soluble in water (Sodium salt at 20 °C about 70 g/l), low solubility in ethanol, insoluble in vegetable oil.
Chromatography DC Carrier	Source : Communication XVII DFG Farbstoff-Kommission Cellulose Petrol ether (100-160 °C) 50 ml + Benzol 35 ml + Chloroform 10 ml + Acetone 0.5 ml + Isopropanol 0.2 ml
Spectral photometry Solvent Absorption maximum Solvent Absorption assay	of the Sodium salt Source : Kosmetische Färbemittel, 3. ed., 1991 Water (pH 7.5) 405 nm Water (own assay) 404, 500, 629, 660 nm
Main applications Food Drugs Cosmetics	 - Candies, jelly products, liquor. - General utilization. - Products for mouth- and tooth care.

Toxicological and dermatological data		Source
LD50 tested on rats (Na-K-Cu-Chlorophyllin-complex)	7000 mg/kg	Kosmetische Färbemittel 3. ed., 1991
ADI-value (SCF 19975) as the sum of chlorophyllin and chlorophyll- copper-complex	0-15 mg/kg	Ringbook Color- ants for food 1978

Certification status

European Union	Approved for defined food products (see 2.4.1.) and for the coloration of drugs and cosmetic preparations of group 1 (all cosmetic products).
Argentina	Approved for mouth and tooth care products with a maximum dosage of 0.1%.

Brazil	Approved for mouth- and tooth care products with a maximum dosage of 0.1%.
Canada	Approved for defined food products.
Chile	Approved for food.
Colombia	Approved for food.
Costa Rica	Approved for food products.
Cyprus	Approved for defined food products.
Finland	Approved for defined food products.
Guatemala	Approved for food.
Hungary	Approved for defined food products. Approved for the coloration of cosmetics of group 2 (not on eyes).
Iran	Approved for food.
Japan	Approved for defined food products. Approved for drugs, "quasi-drugs" and cosmetics.
Kenya	Approved for food.
Korea (South)	Approved for food.
Kuwait	Approved for food.
Malta	Approved for food.
New Zealand	Approved for defined food products.
Philippines	Approved for mouth- and tooth care products with a maximum dosage of 0.1%.
Poland	Approved for food and cosmetics.
Saudi Arabia	Approved for food.
Singapore	Approved for food.
South Africa	Approved for defined food products. Approved for the coloration of cosmetics of group 1 (all cosmetic products).
Sudan	Approved for food.
Sweden	Approved for defined food products.
Switzerland	Approved for defined food products and drugs.
Syria	Approved for food.
Taiwan	Approved for defined food products. Maximum levels must be respected (Sodium-copper-chlorophyllin). For defined food products also approved in the form of Sodium-iron-chlorophyllin.
Thailand	Approved for food and cosmetics.
Tunisia	Approved for defined food products.
Turkey	Approved for the coloration of cosmetics of group 1 (all cosmetic products).
Uruguay	Approved for food.
United Arab Emirates	Approved for food.
USA	Approved for drugs and cosmetics in the form of Potassium-Sodium-Chlorophyllin, maximum dosage 0.1%.
Venezuela	Approved for food. Approved for cosmetics (mouth- and tooth care products with a maximum dosage of 0.1%).
Zambia	Approved for food.

For acceptance of this colorant in other countries, based on above mentioned approvals, see also 9.1.8.

C.I.77000

Name	EU-No.	C.I. No.	Class	Chemical name / formula
Aluminum C.I. Pigment Metal 1 Aluminum powder (CTFA adopted name) Aluminum powder (Japan) CAS # 7429-90-5 EINECS # 231-073-3	E 173	77000	Inorganic Pigment	

Color	Shiny silver brilliant pigment.
Solubility	Soluble in diluted acids and lye with hydrogen generation.
Chromatography	Not applicable.
Spectral photometry	Not applicable.
Main applications	
Food	- Surface coloration of capsules, decoration and brilliant effects.
Drugs	- Capsule coloration.
Cosmetics	- Make-up.

Toxicological and dermatological data — **Source**

ADI-value not established (CIAA list Mouton).
Results are not available. The assessment of this colorant is done on the basis of general knowledge of the physico-chemical properties and toxicological experience (Kosmetische Färbemittel, 3. ed., 1991).

Certification status

European Union	Approved for defined food products (see 2.4.1.) and for the coloration of drugs and cosmetic preparations of group 1 (all cosmetic products).
Argentina	Approved for food and cosmetics.
Austria	Approved for surface coloration and decoration of food.
Brazil	Approved for surface coloration and decoration of food. Approved for cosmetics.
Canada	Approved for defined food products.
Colombia	Approved for food.
Cyprus	Approved for surface coloration and decoration of food.
Finland	Approved for surface coloration and decoration of food.

Hungary	Approved for defined food products.
	Approved for the coloration of cosmetics of group 1 (all cosmetic products).
Iran	Approved for surface coloration and decoration of food.
Israel	Approved for food.
Japan	Approved for drugs, "quasi-drugs" and cosmetics.
Kenya	Approved for food.
Kuwait	Approved for surface coloration and decoration of food.
Malaysia	Approved for surface coloration and decoration of food.
Malta	Approved for surface coloration and decoration of food.
New Zealand	Approved for defined food products.
Philippines	Approved for cosmetics.
Poland	Approved for cosmetics.
Saudi Arabia	Approved for food.
Singapore	Approved for surface coloration and decoration of food.
South Africa	Approved for surface coloration and decoration of food.
	Approved for the coloration of cosmetics of group 1 (all cosmetic products).
Sweden	Approved for defined food products.
Switzerland	Approved for surface coloration and decoration of food.
Thailand	Approved for cosmetics.
Turkey	Approved for defined food products.
	Approved for the coloration of cosmetics of group 1 (all cosmetic products).
Uruguay	Approved for food.
United Arab Emirates	Approved for food.
USA	Approved for externally applied drugs and cosmetics, also for application in the eye area (particle size > 200 mesh 100%, < 325 mesh 95%).
Venezuela	Approved for cosmetics.
Zambia	Approved for food.

For acceptance of this colorant in other countries, based on above mentioned approvals, see also 9.1.8.

C.I.77002

Name	EU-No.	C.I. No.	Class	Chemical name / formula
Aluminum hydroxide Aluminum oxide with water C.I. Pigment White 24 Alumina (CFR21) Aluminum hydroxide (Japan)		77002	Inorganic Pigment	$Al_2O_3 \times H_2O$

CAS # 21645-51-2
EINECS # unknown

Color	White pigment.
Solubility	Insoluble in water.
Chromatography	Not applicable.
Spectral photometry	Not applicable.
Main applications	No information available.

Toxicological and dermatological data	Source
Results are not available. The assessment of this colorant is done on the basis of general knowledge of the physico-chemical properties and toxicological experience (Kosmetische Färbemittel, 3. ed., 1991).	

Certification status

European Union	Approved for the coloration of cosmetics of group 1 (all cosmetic products).
Hungary	Approved for the coloration of cosmetics of group 1 (all cosmetic products).
Japan	Approved for cosmetics.
Kenya	Approved for food.
South Africa	Approved for the coloration of cosmetics of group 1 (all cosmetic products).
Thailand	Approved for cosmetics.
Turkey	Approved for the coloration of cosmetics of group 1 (all cosmetic products).
USA	Approved for drugs, is present in all aluminum paints due to manufacturing process.

For acceptance of this colorant in other countries, based on above mentioned approvals, see also 9.1.8.

C.I.77004

Name	EU-No.	C.I. No.	Class	Chemical name / formula
Kaolin C.I. Pigment White 19 Kaolin (CTFA adopted name)		77004	Inorganic Pigment	Aluminum silicate with moisture

Data Sheets   305

Kaolin (Japan)
CAS # 1332-58-7,
    # 1302-78-9,
    # 1327-36-2
EINECS # unknown

Color	White pigment.
Solubility	Insoluble in water and all other standard solvents.
Chromatography	Not applicable.
Spectral photometry	Not applicable.
Main applications	No information on utilization as paint lacquer.

Toxicological and dermatological data	Source

Results are not available. The assessment of this colorant is done on the basis of general knowledge of the physico-chemical properties and toxicological experience (Kosmetische Färbemittel, 3. ed., 1991).

Certification status

European Union	Approved for the coloration of cosmetics of group 1 (all cosmetic products).
Bulgaria	Not approved for cosmetics
Hungary	Approved for the coloration of cosmetics of group 1 (all cosmetic products).
Japan	Approved for drugs, "quasi-drugs" and cosmetics.
South Africa	Approved for the coloration of cosmetics of group 1 (all cosmetic products).
Turkey	Approved for the coloration of cosmetics of group 1 (all cosmetic products).
USA	Is not considered as a cosmetics colorant, but as a cosmetic base material.

For acceptance of this colorant in other countries, based on above mentioned approvals, see also 9.1.8.

C.I.77007

Name	EU-No.	C.I. No.	Class	Chemical name / formula
Ultramarine C.I. Pigment Blue 29	C 12	77007	Inorganic Pigment	Sulfur containing sodium-aluminum-

C.I. Pigment Green 16 silicate
Ultramarines
 (CTFA adopted name)
Ultramarine, -pink, -
violet (Japan)
CAS # 1317-97-1 (blue)
    # 57455-37-5 (blue)
EINECS # - (polymer :
listed in EINECS)

Color	Blue, violet, pink, red and green pigments.
Solubility	Insoluble in water, soluble in acids with development of hydrogen sulfur.
Chromatography	Not applicable.
Spectral photometry	Not applicable.
Main applications Cosmetics	- Make-up, lipstick, eye cosmetic. - Toilet soap.

Toxicological and dermatological data	Source
Results are not available. The assessment of this colorant is done on the basis of general knowledge of the physico-chemical properties and toxicological experience (Kosmetische Färbemittel, 3. ed., 1991).	

Certification status	
European Union	Approved for defined food products (see 2.4.1.) and for the coloration of drugs and cosmetic preparations of group 1 (all cosmetic products).
Argentina	Approved for cosmetics for external applications, including eye make-up.
Brazil	Approved for cosmetics for external applications, including eye make-up.
Hong Kong	Approved for food.
Hungary	Approved for defined food products. Approved for the coloration of cosmetics of group 2 (not on eyes).
Israel	Approved for cosmetics.
Japan	Approved for drugs, "quasi-drugs" and cosmetics.
Philippines	Approved for cosmetics for external applications, including eye make-up.
Poland	Approved for cosmetics.
Singapore	Approved for the coloration of capsules and for decoration of sugar icings.

Data Sheets

South Africa	Approved for the coloration of cosmetics of group 1 (all cosmetic products).
Turkey	Approved for the coloration of cosmetics of group 1 (all cosmetic products).
USA	Approved for externally applied cosmetics (including eye make-up), but not for mouth wash water, tooth paste and products for the lip area. Utilization does not require FDA certificate.
Venezuela	Approved for cosmetics for external application.

For acceptance of this colorant in other countries, based on above mentioned approvals, see also 9.1.8.

C.I.77013

Name	EU-No.	C.I. No.	Class	Chemical name / formula
C.I. Pigment Green 24 Ultramarines (CTFA adopted name) Ultramarine (Japan) CAS # 1317-97-1, # 1345-00-2, # 12769-96-9 EINECS # unknown		77013	Inorganic Pigment	Sulfur-containing aluminum-sodium silicate

Color	Green pigment.
Solubility	Insoluble in water.
Chromatography	Not applicable.
Spectral photometry	Not applicable.
Main applications Cosmetics	- Decorative cosmetics.

Toxicological and dermatological data	Source
No information available.	

Certification status

European Union	Not approved for food, drugs and cosmetics.
Hungary	Not approved for cosmetics.

Japan	Approved for cosmetics (group 1).
USA	Approved for cosmetics for external applications (including eye make-up), but not for the mouth and lip area.

For acceptance of this colorant in other countries, based on above mentioned approvals, see also 9.1.8.

C.I.77015

Name	EU-No.	C.I. No.	Class	Chemical name / formula
C.I. Pigment Red 101/102 CAS # 12141-46-2 EINECS # unknown		77015	Inorganic Pigment	Aluminum silicate with iron oxide
Color	Red pigment.			
Solubility	Soluble in water, low solubility in ethanol.			
Chromatography	Not applicable.			
Spectral photometry	Not applicable.			
Main applications	No information available.			

Toxicological and dermatological data		Source
Results are not available. The assessment of this colorant is done on the basis of general knowledge of the physico-chemical properties and toxicological experience (Kosmetische Färbemittel, 3. ed., 1991).		

Certification status

European Union	Approved for the coloration of cosmetics of group 1 (all cosmetic products).
Hungary	Approved for the coloration of cosmetics of group 2 (not on eyes).
Japan	Not approved for food, drugs and cosmetics.
South Africa	Approved for the coloration of cosmetics of group 1 (all cosmetic products).
Turkey	Approved for the coloration of cosmetics of group 1 (all cosmetic products).
USA	Not approved for food, drugs and cosmetics.

For acceptance of this colorant in other countries, based on above mentioned approvals, see also 9.1.8.

C.I.77019

Name	EU-No.	C.I. No.	Class	Chemical name / formula
Glimmer, Muscovit C.I. Pigment White 20, 26 Mica (CTFA adopted name) Mica (Japan) CAS # 12001-26-2 EINECS # unknown		77019	Inorganic Pigment	Potassium-Aluminum silicate

Color	White to opaque pigment.
Solubility	Insoluble in water and other common solvents.
Chromatography	Not applicable.
Spectral photometry	Not applicable.
Main applications Cosmetics	- Decorative cosmetics.

Toxicological and dermatological data	Source

No information available. This product is not listed in Kosmetische Färbemittel, 3. ed., 1991.

Certification status

European Union	Approved for the coloration of cosmetics of group 1 (all cosmetic products). Glimmer (Mica) is listed in the EU guideline 86/179/EWG and in the German cosmetic ordinance together with Titanium dioxide and Bismut oxychloride. C.I.77019 is not listed separately.
Argentina	Approved for cosmetics.
Brazil	Approved for cosmetics.
Hungary	Not approved for food, drugs and cosmetics.
Japan	Approved for all drugs, "quasi-drugs" and cosmetics.
Philippines	Approved for cosmetics.
USA	Not approved for food, drugs and cosmetics.
Venezuela	Approved for cosmetics.

For acceptance of this colorant in other countries, based on above mentioned approvals, see also 9.1.8.

C.I.77120

Name	EU-No.	C.I. No.	Class	Chemical name / formula
Schwerspat Blanc fixe Barium sulfate (CTFA adopted name) Barium sulfate (Japan) CAS # 7727-43-7 EINECS # unknown		77120	Inorganic Pigment	Barium sulfate

Color	White pigment.
Solubility	Insoluble in water and all other common solvents.
Chromatography	Not applicable.
Spectral photometry	Not applicable.
Main applications	Not known as a colorant.

Toxicological and dermatological data	Source

Results are not available. The assessment of this colorant is done on the basis of general knowledge of the physico-chemical properties and toxicological experience (Kosmetische Färbemittel, 3. ed., 1991).

Certification status

European Union	Approved for the coloration of cosmetics of group 1 (all cosmetic products).
Hungary	Approved for the coloration of cosmetics of group 2 (not on eyes).
Japan	Not considered as a cosmetic colorant, but as a base cosmetic ingredient.
South Africa	Approved for the coloration of cosmetics of group 1 (all cosmetic products).
Thailand	Approved for cosmetics.
Turkey	Approved for the coloration of cosmetic of group 1 (all cosmetic products).
USA	Not considered as a cosmetic colorant, but as a base cosmetic ingredient.

For acceptance of this colorant in other countries, based on above mentioned approvals, see also 9.1.8.

C.I.77163

Name	EU-No.	C.I. No.	Class	Chemical name / formula
Perlweiss C.I. Pigment White 14/31 Bismut oxychloride (CTFA adopted name) Bismut oxychloride (Japan) CAS # 7787-59-9, EINECS # unknown		77163	Inorganic Pigment	Bismut oxychloride
Color	White pearl pigment.			
Solubility	Insoluble in water, soluble in mineral acids.			
Chromatography	Not applicable.			
Spectral photometry	Not applicable.			

Main applications
Cosmetics — Decorative cosmetics.

Toxicological and dermatological data		Source
LD50 tested on rats	> 5.0 mg/kg	Ringbook Kosmetische Färbemittel 1984
Skin compatibility tested on guinea pig	no observation	
Mucous membrane compatibility tested on a rabbit eye	no observation	

Certification status

European Union	Approved for the coloration of cosmetics of group 1 (all cosmetic products).
Argentina	Approved for cosmetics.
Brazil	Approved for cosmetics.
Bulgaria	Approved for cosmetics, but not for the lip area.
Hungary	Approved for the coloration of cosmetics of group 1 (all cosmetic products).
Japan	Approved for drugs, "quasi-drugs" and cosmetics.
Philippines	Approved for cosmetics.
Poland	Approved for cosmetics, but not for application in the lip area.
South Africa	Approved for the coloration of cosmetics of group 1 (all cosmetic products).
Thailand	Approved for cosmetics.

Turkey	Approved for the coloration of cosmetic of group 1 (all cosmetic products).
USA	Approved for externally applied drugs and cosmetics, also for application in the eye area. Utilization requires FDA certificate.
Venezuela	Approved for cosmetics.

For acceptance of this colorant in other countries, based on above mentioned approvals, see also 9.1.8.

C.I.77220

Name	EU-No.	C.I. No.	Class	Chemical name / formula
Calcium carbonate Kreide C.I. Pigment White 18 Calcium carbonate (CTFA adopted name) precipitated calcium carbonate, heavy calcium carbonate (Japan) CAS # 471-34-1 EINECS # 207-439-9	E 170	77220	Inorganic Pigment	Calcium carbonate $CaCO_3$
Color	White pigment.			
Solubility	Low solubility in water, soluble in diluted acids.			
Chromatography	Not applicable.			
Spectral photometry	Not applicable.			
Main applications Food	- Surface coloration of capsules and decoration of food.			

Toxicological and dermatological data	Source
Results are not available. The assessment of this colorant is done on the basis of general knowledge of the physico-chemical properties and toxicological experience (Kosmetische Färbemittel, 3. ed., 1991).	

Certification status

| European Union | Approved for defined food products (see 2.4.1.) and for the coloration of drugs and cosmetic preparations of group 1 (all cosmetic products). |

Argentina	Approved for food.
Finland	Approved for defined food products.
Hungary	Approved for defined food products. Approved for the coloration of cosmetics of group 1 (all cosmetic products).
Iran	Approved for surface coloration and decoration of food.
Japan	Approved for drugs, "quasi-drugs" and cosmetics.
Norway	Approved for cosmetics.
South Africa	Approved for defined food products. Approved for the coloration of cosmetics of group 1 (all cosmetic products).
Sweden	Approved for defined food products.
Switzerland	Approved for surface coloration and decoration of food
Thailand	Approved for cosmetics.
Turkey	Approved for the coloration of cosmetics of group 1 (all cosmetic products).
USA	Not considered as a cosmetic colorant, is considered a cosmetic base material.

For acceptance of this colorant in other countries, based on above mentioned approvals, see also 9.1.8.

C.I.77231

Name	EU-No.	C.I. No.	Class	Chemical name / formula

Gips
C.I. Pigment White 25
Calcium sulfate
  (CTFA adopted name)
Calcium sulfate (Japan)
CAS # 1010-41-4,
    # 7778-18-9
EINECS # unknown
		77231	Inorganic Pigment	Calcium sulfate

Color	White pigment.			
Solubility	Low solubility in water (at 20 °C about 2 g/l).			
Chromatography	Not applicable.			
Spectral photometry	Not applicable.			
Main applications	Not known as a colorant.			

Toxicological and dermatological data	Source

Results are not available. The assessment of this colorant is done on the basis of general knowledge of the physico-chemical properties and toxicological experience (Kosmetische Färbemittel, 3. ed., 1991).

Certification status

European Union	Approved for the coloration of cosmetics of group 1 (all cosmetic products).
Hungary	Approved for the coloration of cosmetics of group 1 (all cosmetic products).
Japan	Not considered a cosmetic colorant, is considered a cosmetic base material.
South Africa	Approved for the coloration of cosmetics of group 1 (all cosmetic products).
Thailand	Approved for cosmetics.
Turkey	Approved for the coloration of cosmetics of group 1 (all cosmetic products).
USA	Not considered a cosmetic colorant, is considered a cosmetic base material.

For acceptance of this colorant in other countries, based on above mentioned approvals, see also 9.1.8.

C.I.77266

Name	EU-No.	C.I. No.	Class	Chemical name / formula
Rußschwarz C.I. Pigment Black 6,7 Carbon black (Japan) CAS # 7440-44-0, # 1333-86-4 EINECS # 231-153-3		77266	Inorganic Pigment	Carbon, manufactured from hydrocarbon
Color	Black pigment.			
Solubility	Insoluble in water, fat and oils.			
Chromatography	Not applicable.			
Spectral photometry	Not applicable.			
Main applications Cosmetics	- Decorative cosmetics.			

Data Sheets

Toxicological and dermatological data	Source
Results are not available. The assessment of this colorant is done on the basis of general knowledge of the physico-chemical properties and toxicological experience (Kosmetische Färbemittel, 3. ed., 1991).	

Certification status

European Union	Approved for the coloration of cosmetics of group 1 (all cosmetic products).
Hungary	Approved for the coloration of cosmetics of group 1 (all cosmetic products).
Japan	Approved for drugs, "quasi-drugs" and cosmetics.
South Africa	Approved for the coloration of cosmetics of group 1 (all cosmetic products).
Thailand	Approved for cosmetics.
Turkey	Approved for the coloration of cosmetics of group 1 (all cosmetic products).
USA	Not approved for food, drugs and cosmetics.

For acceptance of this colorant in other countries, based on above mentioned approvals, see also 9.1.8.

C.I.77267

Name	EU-No.	C.I. No.	Class	Chemical name / formula
Knochenkohle C.I. Pigment Black 9 CAS # 8021-99-6 EINECS # unknown		77267	Inorganic Pigment	Blend of Carbon (10%), Calcium phosphate (78%), Calcium carbonate (8%) and other inorganic salts.
Color	Black pigment.			
Solubility	No information available.			
Chromatography	Not applicable.			
Spectral photometry	Not applicable.			
Main applications	No information available.			

Toxicological and dermatological data	Source

Results are not available. The assessment of this colorant is done on the basis of general knowledge of the physico-chemical properties and toxicological experience (Kosmetische Färbemittel, 3. ed., 1991).

Certification status

European Union	Approved for the coloration of cosmetics of group 1 (all cosmetic products).
Hungary	Approved for the coloration of cosmetics of group 1 (all cosmetic products).
Japan	Not approved for food, drugs and cosmetics.
South Africa	Approved for the coloration of cosmetics of group 1 (all cosmetic products).
Turkey	Approved for the coloration of cosmetics of group 1 (all cosmetic products).
USA	Not approved for food, drugs and cosmetics.

For acceptance of this colorant in other countries, based on above mentioned approvals, see also 9.1.8.

C.I.77268

Name	EU-No.	C.I. No.	Class	Chemical name / formula
Kohleschwarz Carbo medicinalis vegetabilis (Vegetable coal) C.I. Food Black 3 C.I. Pigment Black 8 CAS # 1339-82-8 EINECS # 215-669-6	E 153	77268:1	Inorganic Pigment	Carbon (vegetable carbon with the properties of medical carbon/coal)
Color	Black pigment.			
Solubility	Insoluble in water and organic solvents.			
Chromatography	Not applicable.			
Spectral photometry	Not applicable.			
Main applications Food Cosmetics	 - Capsules, cheese coatings. - Mascara.			

Data Sheets

Toxicological and dermatological data	Source

Results are not available. The assessment of this colorant is done on the basis of general knowledge of the physico-chemical properties and toxicological experience (Kosmetische Färbemittel, 3. ed., 1991).

Certification status

European Union	Approved for the coloration of cosmetics of group 1 (all cosmetic products).
Austria	Approved for defined food products.
Bulgaria	Not approved for cosmetics.
Canada	Approved for defined food products.
Chile	Approved for food products.
Colombia	Approved for food products.
Costa Rica	Approved for food products.
Finland	Approved for defined food products.
Hungary	Approved for the coloration of cosmetics of group 1 (all cosmetic products).
Iran	Approved for food products.
Japan	Not approved for food, drugs and cosmetics.
Kenya	Approved for food products.
Malaysia	Approved for defined food products.
Malta	Approved for defined food products. Not approved for cosmetics.
Norway	Approved for defined food products.
Peru	Approved for food products.
Poland	Not approved for cosmetics.
Singapore	Approved for the coloration of capsules and for the decoration of sugar-based coatings.
South Africa	Approved for the coloration of cosmetics of group 1 (all cosmetic products).
Thailand	Approved for food products.
Turkey	Approved for the coloration of cosmetics of group 1 (all cosmetic products).
USA	Not approved for food, drugs and cosmetics.
Zambia	Approved for food products.

For acceptance of this colorant in other countries, based on above mentioned approvals, see also 9.1.8.

C.I.77288

Name	EU-No.	C.I. No.	Class	Chemical name / formula
Chromoxidgrün C.I. Pigment Green 17 Chromium oxide green (CTFA adopted name)		77288	Inorganic Pigment	Chrome-(III)-oxide

Chromium oxide green
(Japan)
CAS # 1308-38-9,
EINECS # 215-160-9

Color	Green pigment.
Solubility	Insoluble in water, low solubility in acid and lye.
Chromatography	Not applicable.
Spectral photometry	Not applicable.
Main applications Cosmetics	- Make-up. - Toilet soap.

Toxicological and dermatological data		Source
LD50 tested on rats	> 5 g/kg	Ringbook Kosmetische Färbemittel, 1984
Skin compatibility tested on rabbits	no observation	
Mucous membrane compatibility tested on a rabbit eye	slight reddening, disappears after 48 h	

Certification status	
European Union	Approved for the coloration of cosmetics of group 1 (all cosmetic products).
Argentina	Approved for externally applied cosmetics including eye make-up.
Brazil	Approved for externally applied cosmetics including eye make-up.
Bulgaria	Approved for cosmetics, but not in the lip area.
Hungary	Approved for the coloration of cosmetics of group 1 (all cosmetic products).
Japan	Approved for cosmetics, but not for the mouth and lip area.
Philippines	Approved for externally applied cosmetics including eye make-up.
Poland	Approved for cosmetics, but not for the mouth and lip area.
South Africa	Approved for the coloration of cosmetics of group 1 (all cosmetic products).
Thailand	Approved for cosmetics.
Turkey	Approved for the coloration of cosmetics of group 1 (all cosmetic products).
USA	Approved for externally applied drugs and cosmetics (also in the eye area, but not for mouth wash water, tooth paste and

	products for the lip area.)
	Utilization does not require FDA certificate.
Venezuela	Approved for cosmetics for external application including eye make-up.

For acceptance of this colorant in other countries, based on above mentioned approvals, see also 9.1.8.

C.I.77289

Name	EU-No.	C.I. No.	Class	Chemical name / formula
Chrome oxide with water Chromium hydrogen oxide (CTFA adopted name) Hydrated chromium oxide (Japan) CAS # 12001-99-9 EINECS # unknown		77289	Inorganic Pigment	Chromium-(III)-oxide-hydrate

Color	Green pigment.
Solubility	Insoluble in water.
Chromatography	Not applicable.
Spectral photometry	Not applicable.
Main applications Cosmetics	- Make-up. - Toilet soap.

Toxicological and dermatological data	Source

Results are not available. The assessment of this colorant is done on the basis of general knowledge of the physico-chemical properties and toxicological experience (Kosmetische Färbemittel, 3. ed., 1991).

Certification status

European Union	Approved for the coloration of cosmetics of group 1 (all cosmetic products). According to Ringbook Kosmetische Färbemittel, 1984, not recommended for the mouth and lip area.

Argentina	Approved for externally applied cosmetics, including eye make-up.
Brazil	Approved for externally applied cosmetics, including eye make-up.
Bulgaria	Approved for externally applied cosmetics, including eye make-up.
Hungary	Approved for the coloration of cosmetics of group 1 (all cosmetic products).
Japan	Approved for externally applied cosmetics, including eye make-up, but not for the mouth and lip area.
Philippines	Approved for externally applied cosmetics, including eye make-up.
Poland	Approved for externally applied cosmetics, including eye make-up.
South Africa	Approved for the coloration of cosmetics of group 1 (all cosmetic products).
Turkey	Approved for the coloration of cosmetics of group 1 (all cosmetic products).
USA	Approved for externally applied cosmetics, including eye make-up, but not for mouth wash water, tooth paste and products for the lip area.

For acceptance of this colorant in other countries, based on above mentioned approvals, see also 9.1.8.

C.I.77400

Name	EU-No.	C.I. No.	Class	Chemical name / formula
Copper C.I. Pigment Metal 2 Copper powder (CTFA adopted name) CAS # 7440-50-8 EINECS # unknown		77400	Inorganic Pigment	Cu
Bronze powder (CTFA adopted name) CAS # unknown EINECS # unknown		77400	Inorganic Pigment	Cu with traces of Zn, Al and Sn.
Color	Copper-colored pigments.			
Solubility	Insoluble in water and organic solvents.			
Chromatography	Not applicable.			

Data Sheets

Spectral photometry   Not applicable.

Main applications
Cosmetics   - Decorative cosmetics.

Toxicological and dermatological data	Source

Results are not available. The assessment of this colorant is done on the basis of general knowledge of the physico-chemical properties and toxicological experience (Kosmetische Färbemittel, 3. ed., 1991).

Certification status of copper

European Union	Approved for the coloration of cosmetics of group 1 (all cosmetic products).
Argentina	Approval for cosmetics.
Hungary	Approved for the coloration of cosmetics of group 1 (all cosmetic products).
Japan	Not approved for food, drugs and cosmetics.
Philippines	Approved for cosmetics.
South Africa	Approved for the coloration of cosmetics of group 1 (all cosmetic products).
Turkey	Approved for the coloration of cosmetics of group 1 (all cosmetic products).
USA	Approved for drugs and cosmetics for external applications, also for the eye area. Utilization does not require FDA certificate.

For acceptance of this colorant in other countries, based on above mentioned approvals, see also 9.1.8.

Certification status of bronze

European Union	Not approved for food, drugs and cosmetics.
Japan	Not approved for food, drugs and cosmetics.
USA	Approved for drugs and cosmetics for external applications, also for the eye area. Utilization does not require FDA certificate.

For acceptance of this colorant in other countries, based on above mentioned approvals, see also 9.1.8.

C.I.77480

Name	EU-No.	C.I. No.	Class	Chemical name / formula
Gold C.I. Pigment Metal 3	E 175	77480	Inorganic Pigment	Au

Gold leaf (Japan)
CAS # 7440-57-5,
EINECS # 231-165-9

Color	Gold-colored pigment.
Solubility	Insoluble in water and solvents.
Chromatography	Not applicable.
Spectral photometry	Not applicable.

Main applications
Food   - Used for candy and beverage manufacturing in the form of powder or gold leaf for decoration and other external effects.
Drugs   - Capsules.

Toxicological and dermatological data	Source

Results are not available. The assessment of this colorant is done on the basis of general knowledge of the physico-chemical properties and toxicological experience (Kosmetische Färbemittel, 3. ed., 1991).

Certification status

European Union	Approved for defined food products (see 2.4.1.) and for the coloration of drugs and cosmetic preparations of group 1 (all cosmetic products).
Argentina	Approved for food.
Brazil	Approved for defined food products.
Colombia	Approved for food.
Cyprus	Approved for defined food products.
Finland	Approved for defined food products.
Hungary	Approved for the coloration of cosmetics of group 1 (all cosmetic products).
Japan	Not approved for food. Approval status for cosmetics unclear.
Kuwait	Approved for food.
Malaysia	Approved for defined food products.
Malta	Approved for food.
New Zealand	Approved for defined food products.
Poland	Approved for defined food products.
Saudi Arabia	Approved for food.
South Africa	Approved for defined food products. Approved for the coloration of cosmetics of group 1 (all cosmetic products).
Sweden	Approved for defined food products.
Switzerland	Approved for defined food products.

Thailand	Approved for cosmetics.
Turkey	Approved for the coloration of cosmetics of group 1 (all cosmetic products).
Uruguay	Approved for food.
United Arab Emirates	Approved for food.
USA	Not approved for food, drugs and cosmetics.

For acceptance of this colorant in other countries, based on above mentioned approvals, see also 9.1.8.

C.I.77489

Name	EU-No.	C.I. No.	Class	Chemical name / formula
Iron oxide Iron oxide (CTFA adopted name) CAS # 1345-25-1 EINECS # unknown	E 172	77489	Inorganic Pigment	Iron-(II)-oxide, FeO

According to Color Index FeO (black), in many laws C.I.77489 is used as a collective number for yellow, brown and black iron oxides and iron hydroxides (see also C.I.77491, 77492, 77499).

Color	Black pigment.
Solubility	Insoluble in water and alkali, soluble in acids.
Chromatography	Not applicable.
Spectral photometry	Not applicable.
Main applications	No information available.

Toxicological and dermatological data	Source

Results are not available. The assessment of this colorant is done on the basis of general knowledge of the physico-chemical properties and toxicological experience (Kosmetische Färbemittel, 3. ed., 1991).

Certification status

European Union	Approved for defined food products (see 2.4.1.) and for the coloration of drugs and cosmetic preparations of group 1 (all cosmetic products).
Hungary	Approved for the coloration of cosmetics of group 1 (all cosmetic products).

Japan	Not approved for food, drugs and cosmetics.
Poland	Approved for defined food products.
Singapore	Approved for the coloration of capsules and decorations for sugar icings.
South Africa	Approved for the coloration of cosmetics of group 1 (all cosmetic products).
Tunisia	Approved for defined food products.
Turkey	Approved for the coloration of cosmetics of group 1 (all cosmetic products).
United Arab Emirates	Approved for food.
USA	Approved for cosmetics for external applications including eye make-up. Utilization does not require FDA certificate.

For acceptance of this colorant in other countries, based on above mentioned approvals, see also 9.1.8.

C.I.77491

Name	EU-No.	C.I. No.	Class	Chemical name / formula
Iron oxide red C.I. Pigment Red 101,102 Synthetic iron oxide (CFR21) Iron oxides (CFR21, CTFA adopted name) Red oxide of iron (Japan) CAS # 61309-37-1 EINECS # 215-168-2	E 172	77491	Inorganic Pigment	Iron-(III)-oxide
Color	Red-brown pigment.			
Solubility	Insoluble in water, soluble in acid.			
Chromatography	Not applicable.			
Spectral photometry	Not applicable.			
Main applications Food Drugs Cosmetics	 - Candies, capsules. - Capsules. - Cream, make-up, lipstick, powder. - Toilet soap.			

Toxicological and dermatological data	Source

Results are not available. The assessment of this colorant is done on the basis of general knowledge of the physico-chemical properties and toxicological experience (Kosmetische Färbemittel, 3. ed., 1991).

Certification status

European Union	Approved for defined food products (see 2.4.1.) and for the coloration of drugs and cosmetic preparations of group 1 (all cosmetic products).
Argentina	Approved for food and cosmetics.
Australia	Approved for defined food products.
Austria	Approved for defined food products.
Brazil	Approved for defined food products.
Canada	Approved for defined food products.
Cyprus	Approved for defined food products.
Finland	Approved for defined food products.
Hungary	Approved for defined food products.
	Approved for the coloration of cosmetics of group 1 (all cosmetic products).
Iran	Approved for food.
Israel	Approved for food, drugs and cosmetics.
Japan	Approved for defined food products.
	Approved for drugs, "quasi-drugs" and cosmetics.
Kenya	Approved for food.
Kuwait	Approved for food.
Malaysia	Approved for defined food products.
Malta	Approved for food.
New Zealand	Approved for defined food products.
Philippines	Approved for food and cosmetics.
Poland	Approved for defined food products and cosmetics.
Saudi Arabia	Approved for food.
Singapore	Approved for the coloration of capsules and decorations for sugar icings.
South Africa	Approved for defined food products.
	Approved for the coloration of cosmetics of group 1 (all cosmetic products).
Sweden	Approved for defined food products.
Switzerland	Approved for defined food products and drugs.
Taiwan	Approved for defined food products.
Thailand	Approved for cosmetics.
Tunisia	Approved for defined food products.
Turkey	Approved for the coloration of cosmetics of group 1 (all cosmetic products).
Uruguay	Approved for food.
United Arab Emirates	Approved for food.
USA	Not approved for food.
	Approved for pet food with a maximum dosage of 0.25%.

USA (continued) Approved for drugs with restrictions (CFR 21,§73.1200)
  Approved for cosmetics, also for the eye area.
  Utilization does not require FDA certificate.
Venezuela Approved for cosmetics.
For acceptance of this colorant in other countries, based on above mentioned approvals, see also 9.1.8.

C.I.77492

Name	EU-No.	C.I. No.	Class	Chemical name / formula
Ironoxide yellow C.I. Pigment Yellow 42,43 Synthetic iron oxide (CFR21) Iron oxides (CFR21/CTFA adopted name) Yellow oxide of iron (Japan) CAS # 51274-00-1 EINECS # 257-098-5	E 172	77492	Inorganic Pigment	Iron-oxide-hydrate
Color	Yellow pigment.			
Solubility	Insoluble in water, soluble in acids.			
Chromatography	Not applicable.			
Spectral photometry	Not applicable.			
Main applications	No information available.			
Main applications Food Drugs Cosmetics	- Candies, capsules. - Capsules - Creams, make-up-lipstick, powder. - Toilet soap.			
Toxicological and dermatological data				**Source**

Results are not available. The assessment of this colorant is done on the basis of general knowledge of the physico-chemical properties and toxicological experience (Kosmetische Färbemittel, 3. ed., 1991).

Data Sheets

Certification status

European Union	Approved for defined food products (see 2.4.1.) and for the coloration of drugs and cosmetic preparations of group 1 (all cosmetic products).
Argentina	Approved for food and cosmetics.
Australia	Approved for defined food products.
Austria	Approved for defined food products.
Brazil	Approved for defined food products.
Canada	Approved for defined food products.
Finland	Approved for defined food products.
Hungary	Approved for defined food products. Approved for the coloration of cosmetics of group 1 (all cosmetic products).
Iran	Approved for food.
Israel	Approved for food. Approved for drugs, "quasi-drugs" and cosmetics.
Kenya	Approved for food.
Kuwait	Approved for food.
Malaysia	Approved for defined food products.
Malta	Approved for food.
New Zealand	Approved for defined food products.
Philippines	Approved for food and cosmetics.
Poland	Approved for defined food products and cosmetics.
Saudi Arabia	Approved for food.
Singapore	Approved for the coloration of capsules and decorations for sugar icings.
South Africa	Approved for defined food products. Approved for the coloration of cosmetics of group 1 (all cosmetic products).
Sweden	Approved for defined food products.
Switzerland	Approved for defined food products and drugs.
Taiwan	Approved for cosmetics.
Thailand	Approved for cosmetics.
Turkey	Approved for the coloration of cosmetics of group 1 (all cosmetic products).
Uruguay	Approved for food.
United Arab Emirates	Approved for food.
USA	Not approved for food. Approved for pet food with a maximum dosage of 0.25%. Approved for drugs with restrictions (CFR 21,§73.1200) Approved for cosmetics, also for the eye area. Utilization does not require FDA certificate.
Venezuela	Approved for food.
Zambia	Approved for food.

For acceptance of this colorant in other countries, based on above mentioned approvals, see also 9.1.8.

C.I.77499

Name	EU-No.	C.I. No.	Class	Chemical name / formula

Iron oxide black
C.I. Pigment Black 11
Synthetic iron oxide (CFR21)
Iron oxides (CFR21 / CTFA adopted name)
Black oxide of iron (Japan)
CAS # 12227-89-3,
    # 1309-37-1 (Fe_2O_3)
    # 1317-61-9 (Fe_3O_4)
EINECS # 257-098-5
    # 215-277-5
	E 172	77499	Inorganic Pigment	Iron-(II)-oxide + Iron-(III)-oxide

Color	Black pigment.
Solubility	Insoluble in water, soluble in acid.
Chromatography	Not applicable.
Spectral photometry	Not applicable.
Main applications Food Drugs Cosmetics	 - Candies, capsules. - Capsules. - Cream, make-up, lipstick, powder. - Toilet soap.

Toxicological and dermatological data   **Source**

Results are not available. The assessment of this colorant is done on the basis of general knowledge of the physico-chemical properties and toxicological experience (Kosmetische Färbemittel, 3. ed., 1991).

Certification status

European Union	Approved for defined food products (see 2.4.1.) and for the coloration of drugs and cosmetic preparations of group 1 (all cosmetic products).
Argentina	Approved for food and cosmetics.
Australia	Approved for defined food products.
Austria	Approved for defined food products.
Brazil	Approved for defined food products.

Data Sheets

Canada	Approved for defined food products.
Cyprus	Approved for defined food products.
Finland	Approved for defined food products.
Hungary	Approved for defined food products. Approved for the coloration of cosmetics of group 1 (all cosmetic products).
Iran	Approved for food.
Israel	Approved for food, drugs and cosmetics.
Japan	Not approved for food, drugs and cosmetics.
Kenya	Approved for food.
Kuwait	Approved for food.
Malaysia	Approved for defined food products.
Malta	Approved for food.
New Zealand	Approved for defined food products.
Philippines	Approved for food and cosmetics.
Poland	Approved for defined food products and cosmetics.
Saudi Arabia	Approved for food.
Singapore	Approved for the coloration of capsules and decorations for sugar icings.
South Africa	Approved for the coloration of cosmetics of group 1 (all cosmetic products).
Sweden	Approved for defined food products.
Switzerland	Approved for defined food products and drugs.
Taiwan	Approved for defined food products.
Thailand	Approved for cosmetics.
Tunisia	Approved for defined food products.
Turkey	Approved for the coloration of cosmetics of group 1 (all cosmetic products).
Uruguay	Approved for food.
United Arab Emirates	Approved for food.
USA	Not approved for food. Approved for pet food with a maximum dosage of 0.25%. Approved for drugs with restrictions (CFR 21,§73.1200) Approved for cosmetics, also for the eye area. Utilization does not require FDA certificate.
Venezuela	Approved for cosmetics
Zambia	Approved for food.

For acceptance of this colorant in other countries, based on above mentioned approvals, see also 9.1.8.

C.I.77510

Name	EU-No.	C.I. No.	Class	Chemical name / formula
Prussian Blue C.I. Pigment Blue 27 Ferric ferrocyanide (CTFA adopted name)		77510	Inorganic Pigment	Iron (III)-hexa-ferrocyanide

Ferric ferrocyanide (Japan)
CAS # 14038-43-8
EINECS # unknown

Color	Blue pigment.
Solubility	Insoluble in water, diluted acid and organic solvents.
Chromatography	Not applicable.
Spectral photometry	Not applicable.

Main applications
Cosmetics — Decorative cosmetics.

Toxicological and dermatological data		Source
LD50 tested on rats	> 8 g/kg	Ringbook Kosmetische Färbemittel, 1984
Skin compatibility tested on rabbits	no observation	
Mucous membrane compatibility tested on a rabbit eye	no observation	

Certification status

European Union	Approved for the coloration of cosmetics of group 1 (all cosmetic products). According to Ringbook Kosmetische Färbemittel, 1984, not recommended for application in the mouth and lip area.
Argentina	Approved for cosmetics for external applications including eye make-up, but not on eyes and lips.
Brazil	Approved for cosmetics for external applications including eye make-up, but not on eyes and lips.
Hungary	Approved for the coloration of cosmetics of group 1 (all cosmetic products).
Japan	Approved for drugs, "quasi-drugs" and cosmetics.
Poland	Approved for cosmetics.
South Africa	Approved for the coloration of cosmetics of group 1 (all cosmetic products).
Thailand	Approved for cosmetics.
Turkey	Approved for the coloration of cosmetic of group 1 (all cosmetic products).
USA	Approved for externally applied drugs and cosmetics (also for the eye area), but not for mouth wash water, tooth paste and products for the lip area.
Venezuela	Approved for cosmetics for external applications including eye make-up, but not on eyes and lips

For acceptance of this colorant in other countries, based on above mentioned approvals, see also 9.1.8.

Data Sheets

C.I.77520

Name	EU-No.	C.I. No.	Class	Chemical name / formula
C.I. Pigment Blue 27 Ferric ammonia-ferro-cyanide (CTFA adopted name) Ferric Ammonium Ferrocyanide (Japan) CAS # 25869-00-5 EINECS # unknown		77520	Inorganic Pigment	Ferric ammonia-ferrocyanide

Color	Blue pigment.
Solubility	Insoluble in water.
Chromatography	Not applicable.
Spectral photometry	Not applicable.
Main applications Cosmetics	- Decorative cosmetics.

Toxicological and dermatological data	Source
Results are not available. The assessment of this colorant is done on the basis of general knowledge of the physico-chemical properties and toxicological experience (Kosmetische Färbemittel, 3. ed., 1991).	

Certification status

European Union	Not approved for food, drugs and cosmetics
Japan	Approved for drugs, "quasi-drugs" and cosmetics.
USA	Approved for drugs and cosmetics (also for the eye area), but not for mouth wash water, tooth paste and products for the lip area.

For acceptance of this colorant in other countries, based on above mentioned approvals, see also 9.1.8.

C.I.77711

Name	EU-No.	C.I. No.	Class	Chemical name / formula
Magnesium oxide C.I. (no generic name)		77711	Inorganic Pigment	MgO

Magnesium oxide
(CTFA adopted name)
Magnesium oxide (Japan)
CAS # 1309-48-4,
EINECS # unknown

Color	White pigment.
Solubility	Insoluble in water.
Chromatography	Not applicable.
Spectral photometry	Not applicable.
Main applications	No information available.

Toxicological and dermatological data   Source

No information available.

Certification status

European Union	Not considered as a cosmetic colorant.
Japan	Approved for cosmetics.
USA	Not considered a cosmetic colorant, is considered a cosmetic base material.

For acceptance of this colorant in other countries, based on above mentioned approvals, see also 9.1.8.

C.I.77713

Name	EU-No.	C.I. No.	Class	Chemical name / formula
Magnesium carbonate C.I. Pigment White 18 Magnesium carbonate (CTFA adopted name) Magnesium carbonate, light & heavy (Japan) CAS # 546-93-0, EINECS # unknown		77713	Inorganic Pigment	Magnesium carbonate
Color		White pigment.		

Solubility	Insoluble in water and alkali, soluble in mineral acids.
Chromatography	Not applicable.
Spectral photometry	Not applicable.
Main applications Cosmetics:	- Powder.

Toxicological and dermatological data	Source
Results are not available. The assessment of this colorant is done on the basis of general knowledge of the physico-chemical properties and toxicological experience (Kosmetische Färbemittel, 3. ed., 1991).	

Certification status

European Union	Approved for the coloration of cosmetics of group 1 (all cosmetic products).
Hungary	Approved for the coloration of cosmetics of group 1 (all cosmetic products).
Japan	Approved for drugs, "quasi-drugs" and cosmetics.
South Africa	Approved for the coloration of cosmetics of group 1 (all cosmetic products).
Thailand	Approved for cosmetics.
Turkey	Approved for the coloration of cosmetics of group 1 (all cosmetic products).
USA	Not considered a cosmetic colorant, is considered a cosmetic base material.

For acceptance of this colorant in other countries, based on above mentioned approvals, see also 9.1.8.

C.I.77718

Name	EU-No.	C.I. No.	Class	Chemical name / formula
Magnesium silicate Talc, Talcum C.I. Pigment White 26 Talc (CTFA adopted name) Magnesium silicate (Japan) Talc (Japan) CAS # 14807-96-6 EINECS # unknown		77718	Inorganic Pigment	Magnesium silicate

Color	White pigment.
Solubility	Insoluble in water.
Chromatography	Not applicable.
Spectral photometry	Not applicable.
Main applications Drugs Cosmetics	Not used as a colorant but as a basic ingredient. - Powder. - Powder.

Toxicological and dermatological data	Source
No information available.	

Certification status

European Union	Not considered as a cosmetic colorant. Is used as a basic ingredient for drugs and cosmetics.
Japan	Talc and Magnesium silicate are mentioned separately in the Japanese cosmetic colorant list. Both are approved for cosmetics.
USA	Approved for drugs. Not considered a cosmetic colorant, is considered a cosmetic base material.

For acceptance of this colorant in other countries, based on above mentioned approvals, see also 9.1.8.

C.I.77742

Name	EU-No.	C.I. No.	Class	Chemical name / formula
Manganese violet C.I. Pigment Violet 1 Manganese violet (CTFA adopted name) Ammonium manganese pyrophosphate, Manganese Violet (Japan) CAS # 10101-66-3 EINECS # unknown		77742	Inorganic Pigment	Ammonium-manganese-pyrophosphate
Color		Violet pigment.		

Solubility	Insoluble in water.
Chromatography	Not applicable.
Spectral photometry	Not applicable.
Main applications Cosmetics	- Decorative cosmetics.
Toxicological and dermatological data	**Source**

Results are not available. The assessment of this colorant is done on the basis of general knowledge of the physico-chemical properties and toxicological experience (Kosmetische Färbemittel, 3. ed., 1991).

Certification status

European Union	Approved for the coloration of cosmetics of group 1 (all cosmetic products). According to Ringbook Kosmetische Färbemittel 1984 not recommended for the mouth and lip area.
Argentina	Approved for cosmetics.
Brazil	Approved for externally applied cosmetics including eye make-up, but not for application in the mouth and lip area.
Hungary	Approved for the coloration of cosmetics of group 1 (all cosmetic products).
Japan	Approved for externally applied cosmetics including eye make-up, but not for application in the mouth and lip area.
Philippines	Approved for cosmetics.
South Africa	Approved for the coloration of cosmetics of group 1 (all cosmetic products).
Thailand	Approved for cosmetics.
Turkey	Approved for the coloration of cosmetic of group 1 (all cosmetic products).
USA	Approved for cosmetics, also in the eye area. Utilization does not require FDA certificate.

For acceptance of this colorant in other countries, based on above mentioned approvals, see also 9.1.8.

C.I.77745

Name	EU-No.	C.I. No.	Class	Chemical name / formula
Manganese phosphate C.I. (no generic name) CAS # 10236-39-2 EINECS # unknown		77745	Inorganic Pigment	Manganese-(II)-phosphate, heptahydrate

Color	Red pigment.
Solubility	Insoluble in water.
Chromatography	Not applicable.
Spectral photometry	Not applicable.
Main applications	No information available.
Toxicological and dermatological data	Source

No information available.

Certification status

European Union	Approved for the coloration of cosmetics of group 1 (all cosmetic products).
Hungary	Approved for the coloration of cosmetics of group 1 (all cosmetic products).
Japan	Not approved for food, drugs and cosmetics.
South Africa	Approved for the coloration of cosmetics of group 1 (all cosmetic products).
Thailand	Approved for cosmetics.
Turkey	Approved for the coloration of cosmetics of group 1 (all cosmetic products).
USA	Not approved for food, drugs and cosmetics.

For acceptance of this colorant in other countries, based on above mentioned approvals, see also 9.1.8.

C.I.77820

Name	EU-No.	C.I. No.	Class	Chemical name / formula
Silver Silver (CTFA adopted name) CAS # 7440-22-4, EINECS # unknown	E 174	77820	Inorganic Pigment	Ag

Color	Silver colored pigment.
Solubility	Insoluble in water.
Chromatography	Not applicable.

| Spectral photometry | Not applicable. |

Main applications	
Food	- Capsules, decorations and for shiny effects.

Toxicological and dermatological data	Source

Results are not available. The assessment of this colorant is done on the basis of general knowledge of the physico-chemical properties and toxicological experience (Kosmetische Färbemittel, 3. ed., 1991).

Certification status

European Union	Approved for defined food products (see 2.4.1.) and for the coloration of drugs and cosmetic preparations of group 1 (all cosmetic products).
Argentina	Approval for food and cosmetics.
Brazil	Approved for surface coloration and decoration of food.
Canada	Approved for defined food products.
Colombia	Approved for food.
Finland	Approved for surface coloration and decoration of food.
Hungary	Approved for the coloration of cosmetics of group 1 (all cosmetic products).
Iran	Approved for food.
Israel	Approved for food.
Japan	Not approved for food, drugs and cosmetics.
Kenya	Approved for food.
Malaysia	Approved for surface coloration and decoration of food.
Malta	Approved for food.
New Zealand	Approved for defined food products.
Saudi Arabia	Approved for food.
Singapore	Approved for surface coloration and decoration of sugar icings.
South Africa	Approved for surface coloration and decoration of food. Approved for the coloration of cosmetics of group 1 (all cosmetic products).
Thailand	Approved for cosmetics.
Turkey	Approved for the coloration of cosmetics of group 1 (all cosmetic products).
Uruguay	Approved for food.
United Arab Emirates	Approved for food.
USA	Approved for the coloration of products for the nail area (maximum dosage 1%). Utilization does not require FDA certificate.

For acceptance of this colorant in other countries, based on above mentioned approvals, see also 9.1.8.

C.I.77891

Name	EU-No.	C.I. No.	Class	Chemical name / formula
Titanium dioxide C.I. Pigment White 6 Titanium dioxide (CTFA adopted name) Titanium dioxide (Japan) CAS # 13463-67-7 EINECS # 236-675-5	E 171	77891	Inorganic Pigment	TiO_2
CAS # 1317-80-2 (Rutil) EINECS # unknown				
CAS # 1317-70-0 (RAnatas) EINECS # 215-280-1				

Color	White pigment.
Solubility	Insoluble in water and organic solvents.
Chromatography	Not applicable.
Spectral photometry	Not applicable.
Main applications	No information available.
Main applications Food Drugs Cosmetics	 - Capsules, candies, chewing gum. - Capsules. - Cream, make-up, lipstick, powder. - Toilet soap (in a blend with titanium dioxide, the light stability of organic solvents can change).

Toxicological and dermatological data		Source
LD50 tested on rats	> 10000 mg/kg	Kosmetische Färbemittel 3. ed., 1991
Skin compatibility tested on rabbits	small erythremes	
Mucous membrane compatibility tested on a rabbit eye	minor, temporary reddening	

Certification status	
European Union	Approved for defined food products (see 2.4.1.) and for the coloration of drugs and cosmetic preparations of group 1 (all cosmetic products). See also C.I. 77019.

Data Sheets

Argentina	Approved for food and cosmetics.
Australia	Approved for defined food products.
Austria	Approved for defined food products.
Brazil	Approved for defined food products and cosmetics.
Canada	Approved for defined food products.
Chile	Approved for food.
Colombia	Approved for food.
Costa Rica	Approved for food products.
Cyprus	Approved for defined food products.
Egypt	Approved for food.
Finland	Approved for defined food products and drugs.
Guatemala	Approved for food.
Hungary	Approved for defined food products.
	Approved for the coloration of cosmetics of group 1 (all cosmetic products).
India	Approved for food.
Indonesia	Approved for food.
Iran	Approved for food.
Israel	Approved for food, drugs and cosmetics.
Japan	Approved for defined food products.
	Approved for drugs, "quasi-drugs" and cosmetics.
Kenya	Approved for food.
Kuwait	Approved for food.
Malaysia	Approved for defined food products.
Malta	Approved for food.
New Zealand	Approved for defined food products.
Norway	Approved for defined food products.
Philippines	Approved for food and cosmetics.
Poland	Approved for cosmetics.
Saudi Arabia	Approved for food.
Singapore	Approved for the coloration of capsules and decoration of sugar icings.
South Africa	Approved for defined food products.
	Approved for the coloration of cosmetics of group 1 (all cosmetic products).
Sweden	Approved for defined food products and drugs.
Switzerland	Approved for defined food products and drugs.
Taiwan	Approved for defined food products.
Thailand	Approved for food and cosmetics.
Tunisia	Approved for defined food products.
Turkey	Approved for defined food products.
	Approved for the coloration of cosmetics of group 1 (all cosmetic products).
Uruguay	Approved for food.
United Arab Emirates	Approved for food.
USA	Approved for defined food products, drugs and cosmetics, also for application in the eye area.
	Utilization does not require FDA certificate.
Venezuela	Approved for cosmetics.
Zambia	Approved for food.

For acceptance of this colorant in other countries, based on above mentioned approvals, see also 9.1.8.

C.I.77947

Name	EU-No.	C.I. No.	Class	Chemical name / formula
Zinc white C.I. Pigment White 4 Zinc oxide (CTFA adopted name) Zinc oxide, low temperature burned zinc oxide (Japan) CAS # 1314-13-2, EINECS # unknown	E 172	77947	Inorganic Pigment	Zinc oxide
Color	White or yellow-white pigment.			
Solubility	Insoluble in water, soluble in diluted acids and ammonia.			
Chromatography	Not applicable.			
Spectral photometry	Not applicable.			
Main applications	Not used as a colorant in pharmaceutical products, is used as a functional ingredient (zinc salve).			

Toxicological and dermatological data	Source
Results are not available. The assessment of this colorant is done on the basis of general knowledge of the physico-chemical properties and toxicological experience (Kosmetische Färbemittel, 3. ed., 1991).	

Certification status

European Union	Approved for the coloration of cosmetics of group 1 (all cosmetic products).
Argentina	Approval for cosmetics.
Hungary	Approved for the coloration of cosmetics of group 1 (all cosmetic products).
Japan	Approved for drugs, "quasi-drugs" and cosmetics.
Philippines	Approved for cosmetics.
South Africa	Approved for the coloration of cosmetics of group 1 (all cosmetic products).
Thailand	Approved for cosmetics.
Turkey	Approved for the coloration of cosmetics of group 1 (all cosmetic products).

USA	Approved for externally applied drugs and cosmetics, also for application in the eye area. Utilization does not require FDA certificate.
Venezuela	Approved for cosmetics.

For acceptance of this colorant in other countries, based on above mentioned approvals, see also 9.1.8.

C.I.77990

Name	EU-No.	C.I. No.	Class	Chemical name / formula
Zirconium oxide C.I. Pigment White 12 Zirconium dioxide (CTFA adopted name) Zirconium dioxide (Japan)	E 172	77990	Inorganic Pigment	ZrO_2

Color	White pigment.
Solubility	Insoluble in water.
Chromatography	Not applicable.
Spectral photometry	Not applicable.
Main applications	No information available.

Toxicological and dermatological data	Source
No information available.	

Certification status

European Union	Not approved for food, drugs and cosmetics.
Japan	Approved for cosmetics.
USA	Not considered a cosmetic colorant, is considered a cosmetic base material.

For acceptance of this colorant in other countries, based on above mentioned approvals, see also 9.1.8.

Aluminum, Zinc, Magnesium and Calcium Stearate

Name	EU-No.	C.I. No.	Class	Chemical name / formula
Aluminum, Zinc, Magnesium and Calcium stearate Aluminum stearate (CTFA adopted name) Aluminum stearate (Japan) CAS # 637-12-7 EINECS # unknown			Stearate	
Zinc stearate (CTFA adopted name) Zinc stearate (Japan) CAS # 557-05-1 EINECS # unknown			Stearate	
Magnesium stearate (CTFA adopted name) Magnesium stearate (Japan) CAS # 557-04-0 EINECS # unknown			Stearate	
Calcium stearate (CTFA adopted name) Calcium stearate (Japan) CAS # 1592-23-0 EINECS # unknown			Stearate	
Color	White powder.			
Solubility	Soluble in oil, insoluble in water.			
Chromatography	Not applicable.			
Spectral photometry	Not applicable.			
Main applications	Not known as a colorant.			
Toxicological and dermatological data				**Source**
No information available.				

Data Sheets

Certification status

European Union	Approved for the coloration of cosmetics of group 1 (all cosmetic products).
Japan	Approved for cosmetics.
South Africa	Approved for the coloration of cosmetics of group 1 (all cosmetic products).
Turkey	Approved for the coloration of cosmetic of group 1 (all cosmetic products).
USA	Above mentioned stearates are not considered a cosmetic colorant, are considered a cosmetic base material.

For acceptance of this colorant in other countries, based on above mentioned approvals, see also 9.1.8.

Anthocyan

Name	EU-No.	C.I. No.	Class	Chemical name / formula
Anthocyan Grape skin extract (enoncianina) (CFR21)	E 163		Benzo-pyrylium salt	Colorant from cherries, various berries, red cabbage
Red grape extract (Enocyanine) CAS # 84929-27-1 EINECS # 284-511-6				
CAS # 134-04-3 EINECS # 205-127-7	(Pelargonidine : in red grapes, strawberries, mulberry)			
CAS # 528-58-5 EINECS # 208-438-6	(Cyanidine : in red grapes, cherries, raspberries, blackberries)			
CAS # 134-01-0 EINECS # 205-125-6	(Peonidine : in red grapes)			
CAS # 528-53-0 EINECS # 208-437-0	(Delphinidine : in red grapes, blueberries)			
CAS # 1429-30-7 EINECS # unknown	(Petunidine : in red grapes, mooseberries)			
CAS # 643-84-5 EINECS # 211-403-8	(Malvidine : in red grapes)			

Color	Red to blue-red solution.
Solubility	Soluble in water.
Chromatography DC Carrier	Source : own assay Schleicher & Schüll 2043 b Mgl Acetic acid ester 11 ml + Pyridine 5 ml + Water 4 ml
Spectral photometry	Source : Ringbook Kosmetische Färbemittel 1984. The absorption maxima of anthocyanes are subject to pH, and are in the range of 520-546 nm
Main applications	Above mentioned isolated colorant have no technical importance for the time being. Extracts from the red grape skins are used, sometimes also in the form of spray-dried products.
Food	- Candies, beverages.

Toxicological and dermatological data		Source
ADI-value (JEFCA) for anthocyanes from grape skin	0-2.5 mg/kg	

Certification status

European Union	Approved for defined food products (see 2.4.1.) and for the coloration of drugs and cosmetic preparations of group 1 (all cosmetic products).
Australia	Approved for defined food products.
Canada	Approved for defined food products.
Chile	Approved for food.
Colombia	Approved for food.
Cyprus	Approved for defined food products.
Finland	Approved for defined food products.
Iran	Approved for food.
Israel	Approved for food.
Japan	Approved for defined food products. Not approved for cosmetics.
Korea (South)	Approved for food.
Malta	Approved for food.
New Zealand	Approved for defined food products.
Norway	Approved for defined food products.
Peru	Approved for food.
Saudi Arabia	Approved for food.
South Africa	Approved for defined food products. Approved for the coloration of cosmetics of group 1 (all cosmetic products).
Sweden	Approved for defined food products.
Switzerland	Approved for defined food products.

Thailand	Approved for cosmetics.
Turkey	Approved for the coloration of cosmetic of group 1 (all cosmetic products).
United Arab Emirates	Approved for food.
USA	Approved for defined food products. Utilization does not require FDA certificate. Not approved for drugs and cosmetics.

For acceptance of this colorant in other countries, based on above mentioned approvals, see also 9.1.8.

Astaxanthin

Name	EU-No.	C.I. No.	Class	Chemical name / formula
Astaxanthin CAS # 472-61-7 EINECS # unknown			Carotenoide (Xanthophyll)	Astaxanthin

Color	Orange-red in oil.
Solubility	Soluble in oil and organic solvents.
Chromatography	No information available.
Spectral photometry	No information available.
Main applications	Feed additive for egg yolk, broiler and fish pigmentation.

Toxicological and dermatological data	Source
No information available.	

Certification status

European Union	Not approved for food, drugs and cosmetics.
Japan	Not approved for food, drugs and cosmetics.
USA	Not approved for food, drugs and cosmetics.

There is no information available from other countries, i.e., this colorant is not included in other national positive lists.

Betaine

Name	EU-No.	C.I. No.	Class	Chemical name / formula
Betaine, Beet root CAS # 7659-95-2 EINECS # 231-628-5	E 162		Betaine	Betaine, colorant red beet
Red beet extract CAS # 89957-90-4 EINECS # 289-611-3				

Color	Red solution in water.
Solubility	Soluble in water.
Chromatography DC Carrier	Source : Communication XVII DFG Farbstoff-Kommission Cellulose n-Propanol 60 ml + Glacial acetic acid 10 ml + Water 30 ml
Spectral photometry Solvent Absorption maximum	Source : Communication XVII DFG Farbstoff-Kommission Water 478, 526 nm
Main applications Food	The isolated colorant Betaine has no technical importance. It is used mainly in juice concentrates or spray-dried products for the coloration of fruit yogurt, soups, sauces, chewing gum, dessert products and ice-cream.

Toxicological and dermatological data	Source
Acute toxicity tested on rats : no mortality even at high dosage levels	Kosmetische Färbemittel 3. ed., 1991

Certification status

European Union	a) Red beet concentrate are not legally considered a food colorant, but are seen as food with coloring properties. b) Betaine : Approved for defined food products (see 2.4.1.) and for the coloration of drugs and cosmetic preparations of group 1 (all cosmetic products).
Australia	Approved for defined food products.
Austria	Approved for defined food products.
Brazil	Approved for defined food products.
Canada	Approved for defined food products.

Data Sheets

Chile	Approved for food.
Colombia	Approved for food.
Cyprus	Approved for defined food products.
Finland	Approved for defined food products.
Japan	Approved for defined food products. Not approved for cosmetics.
Kenya	Approved for food.
Korea (South)	Approved for food.
Kuwait	Approved for food.
Malta	Approved for food.
New Zealand	Approved for defined food products.
Peru	Approved for food.
Philippines	Approved for food.
Saudi Arabia	Approved for food.
Singapore	Approved for food.
South Africa	Approved for defined food products. Approved for the coloration of cosmetics of group 1 (all cosmetic products).
Sweden	Approved for defined food products.
Switzerland	Approved for defined food products.
Thailand	Approved for cosmetics.
Turkey	Approved for defined food products. Approved for the coloration of cosmetics of group 1 (all cosmetic products).
United Arab Emirates	Approved for food.
USA	Approved for defined food products. Utilization does not require FDA certificate. Not approved for drugs and cosmetics.
Zambia	Approved for food.

For acceptance of this colorant in other countries, based on above mentioned approvals, see also 9.1.8.

Betonite

Name	EU-No.	C.I. No.	Class	Chemical name / formula
Bentonite (CTFA adopted name) Bentonite (Japan) CAS # 1302-78-9 EINECS # unknown			Inorganic pigment	$Al_2/Si_4O_{10}(OH)_2$
Color		White pigment.		

Solubility	Insoluble.
Chromatography	Not applicable.
Spectral photometry	Not applicable.
Main applications	No information available.

Toxicological and dermatological data	Source
No information available.	

Certification status

European Union	Not considered a cosmetic colorant, is considered a base cosmetic material.
Japan	Not considered a cosmetic colorant, is considered a base cosmetic material.
USA	Not considered a cosmetic colorant, is considered a base cosmetic material.

There is no information available from other countries, i.e., this colorant is not included in other national positive lists.

Bismuth Citrate

Name	EU-No.	C.I. No.	Class	Chemical name / formula
Bismuth citrate (CTFA adopted name) CAS # 813-93-45, EINECS # unknown				Bismuth salt of citric acid
Color	No information available.			
Solubility	No information available.			
Chromatography	No information available.			
Spectral photometry	No information available.			
Main applications	Hair dying.			

Data Sheets

Toxicological and dermatological data	Source

No information available.

Certification status

European Union	Not considered a cosmetic colorant, but a functional cosmetic or pharmaceutical ingredient.
Japan	Not considered a cosmetic colorant, but a functional cosmetic or pharmaceutical ingredient.
USA	Not considered a cosmetic colorant, but a functional cosmetic or pharmaceutical ingredient.

For acceptance of this colorant in other countries, based on above mentioned approvals, see also 9.1.8.

Bromo Cresol Green

Name	EU-No.	C.I. No.	Class	Chemical name / formula
Bromo cresol green CAS # 641-19-0 (Ringbook Kosmet. Färbemittel 1984) CAS # 76-60-8 (Kosmet. Färbemittel 1991) EINECS # unknown			Triarylmethane	3',3'',5',5''-Tetrabromo-m-cresol-sulfophthalein
Color	Yellow solution in ethanol.			
Solubility	Soluble in ethanol and dichloromethane, low solubility in water.			
Chromatography DC Carrier	Source : Communication XVII DFG Farbstoff-Kommission Kieselgel tert. Sodium citrate solution 2.5% 80 ml + Ammonia 25% 20 ml			
Spectral photometry Solvent Absorption maximum	Source : Communication XVII DFG Farbstoff-Kommission Ethanol 423 nm			
Main applications Cosmetics	- Shampoo, shower gel. - Liquid soap.			

Toxicological and dermatological data		Source
LD50 tested on rats	> 17900 mg/kg	Kosmetische Färbemittel
Skin compatibility tested on humans	non-irritant	3. ed. 1991
Mucous membrane compatibility tested on a rabbit eye	non-irritant	

Certification status	
European Union	Approved for the coloration of cosmetics of group 4 (only for a short residence time on skin).
Japan	Not approved for food, drugs and cosmetics.
South Africa	Approved for the coloration of cosmetics of group 4 (only for a short residence time on skin).
Turkey	Approved for the coloration of cosmetics of group 4 (only for a short residence time on skin).
USA	Not approved for food, drugs and cosmetics.

For acceptance of this colorant in other countries, based on above mentioned approvals, see also 9.1.8.

Bromthymol Blue

Name	EU-No.	C.I. No.	Class	Chemical name / formula
Bromthymol blue CAS # 76-59-5 EINECS # unknown			Triaryl- methane	3',3''-Dibromo- thymolsulfo- naphthalein

Color	Yellow solution in ethanol.
Solubility	Soluble in ethanol, dichloromethane and in aqueous alkaline solutions, low solubility in water.
Chromatography DC Carrier	Source : Communication XVII DFG Farbstoff-Kommission Kieselgel Acetic acid ester 11 ml + Pyridine 5 ml + Water 4 ml
Spectral photometry Solvent Absorption maximum	Source : Communication XVII DFG Farbstoff-Kommission Ethanol 420 nm
Main applications	No information available, color change from yellow to blue at pH 6.0-7.6.

Toxicological and dermatological data

		Source
LD50 tested on rats	> 19900 mg/kg	Kosmetische Färbemittel 3. ed., 1991
Skin compatibility tested on humans	non-irritant	
Mucous membrane compatibility tested on a rabbit eye	after 5 hours minor reddening of mucous membrane, reversible after 24 hours	

Certification status

European Union	Approved for the coloration of cosmetics of group 4 (only for a short residence time on skin).
Japan	Not approved for food, drugs and cosmetics.
South Africa	Approved for the coloration of cosmetics of group 4 (only for a short residence time on skin).
Turkey	Approved for the coloration of cosmetics of group 4 (only for a short residence time on skin)
USA	Not approved for food, drugs and cosmetics.

For acceptance of this colorant in other countries, based on above mentioned approvals, see also 9.1.8.

Brown FK

Name	EU-No.	C.I. No.	Class	Chemical name / formula
Brown FK C.I. Food Brown 1 CAS # 8062-14-4 EINECS # unknown	E 154		Azo	Blend of 6 azo colorants (I) 4-(2,4 Diaminophenylazo)-benzoyl sulfonic acid, sodium salt (II) 4-(4,6-Diamino-m-toluylazo)-benzoyl sulfonic acid, sodium salt

Brown FK (continued)

(III) 4,4'-(4,6-Diamino-1,3-phenylene-bisazo)-dibenzoyl sulfonic acid, sodium salt
(IV) 4,4'-(2,4-Diamino-5-methyl-1,3-phenylene-bisazo)-dibenzoyl sulfonic acid, sodium salt
(V) 4,4'-(2,4-Diamino-5-methyl-1,3-phenylene-bisazo)-dibenzoyl sulfonic acid, sodium salt
(VI) 4,4',4''-(2,4-Diaminobenzoyl-1,3,5-trisazo)-tribenzoyl sulfonic acid, sodium salt

Color	Brown solution in water.
Solubility	Soluble in water.
Chromatography	No information available.
Spectral photometry Solvent Absorption maximum	Source : Farbstoffe für Lebensmittel, 2. ed., 1988) Water 420-460 nm (wide range)
Main applications Food	- Used traditionally in UK in coloring smoked herring.

Toxicological and dermatological data		Source
LD50 tested on rats	> 8000 mg/kg	Farbstoffe f. Lebensmittel, 2. ed., 1988
ADI-value (SCF 1984, WHO 1985)	0-0.15 mg/kg	

Certification status

European Union	Approved for defined food products (see 2.4.1). Not approved for drugs and cosmetics.
Japan	Not approved for food, drugs and cosmetics.
USA	Not approved for food, drugs and cosmetics.

For acceptance of this colorant in other countries, based on above mentioned approvals, see also 9.1.8.

Calamine

Name	EU-No.	C.I. No	Class	Chemical name / formula
Calamine Hemimorphit Calamine (CTFA adopted name) Calamine (Japan) CAS # 8011-96-6, EINECS # unknown				$Zn_4/Si_2O_7(OH)_2/:H_2O$

Color	Exists in minerals in different forms : colorless, white, light green, brown with a distinct glassy appearance.
Solubility	Insoluble in water.
Chromatography	Not applicable.
Spectral photometry	Not applicable.
Main applications	No information available.

Toxicological and dermatological data	Source
No information available.	

Certification status

European Union	Not considered a cosmetic colorant, but a functional cosmetic or pharmaceutical ingredient.
Japan	Not considered a cosmetic colorant, but a functional cosmetic or pharmaceutical ingredient.
USA	Not considered a cosmetic colorant, but a functional cosmetic or pharmaceutical ingredient.

There is no information available from other countries, i.e., this colorant is not included in other national positive lists.

Capsanthine, Capsorubin

Name	EU-No.	C.I. No.	Class	Chemical name / formula
Capsanthine CAS # 456-42-9 EINECS # 207-364-1	E 160c		Carote- noide	Colorant from red bell pepper
Capsorubin CAS # 470-38-2 EINECS # 207-425-2				
Bell pepper extract Paprika, Paprika oleoresin (CFR21)				

Color	Orange solution in oil.
Solubility	The isolated colorants are of no technical importance. Oil-soluble paprika extracts and water-dispersible products are commercially available.
Chromatography DC Carrier	Source : Communication XVII DFG Farbstoff-Kommission Kieselgel Cyclohexane 40 ml + Acetic acid ester 10 ml
Spectral photometry Solvent Absorption maximum	Source : Communication XVII DFG Farbstoff-Kommission Methanol 446, 465 nm
Main applications Food	- Soups, sauces, convenience food, mayonnaise, sometimes also in candies.

Toxicological and dermatological data		Source
ADI-value (CIAA Liste Mouton)	0-5 mg/kg	

Certification status

European Union	a) Paprika extracts, where the colorant has not been enriched selectively, are considered food with coloring properties. b) Selectively enriched extracts and colorants : Approved for the coloration of defined food products (see 2.4.1.), of drugs and cosmetics of group 1 (all cosmetic products).

Austria	Approved for defined food products.
Finland	Approved for food.
Japan	Not approved for food, drugs and cosmetics.
South Africa	Approved for the coloration of cosmetics of group 1 (all cosmetic products).
Turkey	Approved for the coloration of cosmetics of group 1 (all cosmetic products).
United Arab Emirates	Approved for food.
USA	Paprika (CFR 21, 73.340) and paprika oleoresin (CFR 21, 73.345) are approved for defined food products. Utilization does not require FDA certificate. Not approved for drugs and cosmetics.

For acceptance of this colorant in other countries, based on above mentioned approvals, see also 9.1.8.

Caramel

Name	EU-No.	C.I. No.	Class	Chemical name / formula
Caramel	E 150a E 150b E 150c E 150d			standard caramel sulfite lye caramel Ammonia caramel Ammonia sulfite caramel
Caramel (CFR21) Caramel (Japan) CAS # 8028-89-5 (for all caramel types) EINECS # 232-435-9 (for all caramel types)				
Color	Brown solution in water.			
Solubility	Soluble in water.			
Chromatography	No information available.			
Spectral photometry	absorption curves are non-specific, cannot be used for analytical purposes.			

Main applications
Food :
a) standard (caustic) caramel
  alcohol stable, used for spirits and sweet wines

b) sulfite lye caramel
   alcohol stable, for spirits
c) ammonia caramel
   beer, soups and sauces
d) Ammonia sulfite caramel
   acid stable, for alcoholic and carbonated beverages

Toxicological and dermatological data		Source
LD50 tested on rats	> 20400 mg/kg for ammonia caramel	Kosmetische Färbemittel 3. ed., 1991
ADI-value (SCF 1987)	0-200 mg/kg for ammonia and ammonia sulfite caramel	

Certification status

European Union	Approved for defined food products (see 2.4.1.) and for the coloration of drugs and cosmetic preparations of group 1 (all cosmetic products).
Argentina	Approved for food and cosmetics.
Australia	Approved for defined food products.
Austria	Approved for defined food products.
Brazil	Approved for defined food products and cosmetics.
Canada	Approved for defined food products.
Chile	Approved for food.
Colombia	Approved for food.
Costa Rica	Approved for food products.
Cyprus	Approved for defined food products.
Egypt	Approved for food.
Finland	Approved for defined food products.
Hungary	Approved for defined food products. EU-approved colorants for cosmetics are accepted.
India	Approved for food.
Indonesia	Approved for food.
Iran	Approved for food.
Israel	Approved for food, drugs and cosmetics.
Japan	Approved for defined food products. Approved for cosmetics.
Kenya	Approved for food.
Korea (South)	Approved for food.
Kuwait	Approved for food.
Malaysia	Approved for defined food products.
Malta	Approved for food.
New Zealand	Approved for defined food products.
Norway	Approved for defined food products.
Peru	Approved for food.
Philippines	Approved for food.

Poland	Approved for food and cosmetics.
Saudi Arabia	Approved for food.
Singapore	Approved for food.
South Africa	Approved for defined food products.
	Approved for the coloration of cosmetics of group 1 (all cosmetic products).
Sweden	Approved for defined food products.
Switzerland	Approved for defined food products and drugs.
Syria	Approved for food.
Tunisia	Approved for defined food products.
Turkey	Approved for defined food products.
	Approved for the coloration of cosmetics of group 1 (all cosmetic products).
Uruguay	Approved for food.
United Arab Emirates	Approved for food, but only E 150a and E 150d.
USA	Approved for defined food products, drugs and cosmetics, also for application in the eye area.
	Utilization does not require FDA certificate.
Venezuela	Approved for food and cosmetics.
Zambia	Approved for food.

For acceptance of this colorant in other countries, based on above mentioned approvals, see also 9.1.8.

Citranaxanthine

Name	EU-No.	C.I. No.	Class	Chemical name / formula
Citranaxanthine CAS # 3604-90-8, EINECS # unknown			Carotenoide (Xanthophyll)	Citranaxanthine
Color	Orange to red-brown solution.			
Solubility	Soluble in oil and organic solvents.			
Chromatography DC Carrier	Source : Communication XVII DFG Farbstoff-Kommission Kieselgel Cyclohexane 40 ml + Acetic acid ester 10 ml			
Spectral photometry Solvent Absorption maximum	Source : Ringbook Kosmetische Färbemittel 1984 Chloroform 590 nm			

Main applications	Source : Ringbook Kosmetische Färbemittel 1984 Water-dispersible commercial products are used as feed additives for egg yolk pigmentation.

Toxicological and dermatological data		Source
LD50 tested on rats	6400 mg/kg	Kosmetische Färbemittel 3. ed., 1991
Skin compatibility tested on rabbits	non-irritant	
Mucous membrane compatibility tested on a rabbit eye	non-irritant	
ADI-value (SCF 1977) must be included in the ADI of 0.5 mg/kg for all carotenoides with provitamin A activity	0-0.4 mg/kg	

Certification status

European Union	Not approved for food, drugs and cosmetics.
Japan	Not approved for food, drugs and cosmetics.
USA	Not approved for food, drugs and cosmetics.

There is no information available from other countries, i.e., this colorant is not included in other national positive lists.

Dihydroxyacetone

Name	EU-No.	C.I. No.	Class	Chemical name / formula
Dihydroxyacetone Aluminum powder (CTFA adopted name) Dihydroxyacetone (Japan) CAS # 96-26-4 EINECS # unknown			Ketone	1,3-Dihydroxy-2-propanone

Color	Colorless crystal.
Solubility	Soluble in water.
Chromatography	No information available.
Spectral photometry	No information available.
Main applications	Used in cosmetic products which cause a browning of the skin without being exposed to UV-rays (auto-browning).

Data Sheets 359

Toxicological and dermatological data	Source
No information available.	

Certification status

European Union	Is not considered a cosmetic colorant. Used as a cosmetic functional ingredient in auto-browning products.
Japan	Approved for cosmetics, but not for products for the eye, lip and mouth area.
USA	Approved for drugs and cosmetics for browning of the skin, but not for mouth wash water, tooth paste and products for the lip and mouth area. Utilization does not require FDA certificate.

For acceptance of this colorant in other countries, based on above mentioned approvals, see also 9.1.8.

Disodium EDTA-Copper

Name	EU-No.	C.I. No.	Class	Chemical name / formula
Disodium EDTA-copper (CTFA adopted name) CAS # 14025-15-1 EINECS # unknown				

Color	Blue-green solution in water.
Solubility	Soluble in water.
Chromatography	No information available.
Spectral photometry	No information available.
Main applications	For complex formation.

Toxicological and dermatological data	Source
No information available.	

Certification status

European Union	Not considered a cosmetic colorant, is considered a base cosmetic material.

Japan	Not considered a cosmetic colorant, is considered a base cosmetic material.
USA	Approved only for cosmetic shampoos, not for drugs. Utilization does not require FDA certificate.

There is no information available from other countries, i.e., this colorant is not included in other national positive lists.

Ferrous Gluconate

Name	EU-No.	C.I. No.	Class	Chemical name / formula
Ferrous gluconate (CFR21)	(579)		Gluconate	Iron salt of gluconic acid
Color	No information available.			
Solubility	No information available.			
Chromatography	No information available.			
Spectral photometry	No information available.			
Main applications	Used for the blackening of olives.			

Toxicological and dermatological data				Source
No information available.				

Certification status

European Union	Not considered a food colorant, is used in the blackening of olives (maximum dosage 320 ppm).
Japan	Approval status unknown.
USA	Approved for the coloration of olives.

There is no information available from other countries, i.e., this colorant is not included in other national positive lists.

Guaiazulene

Name	EU-No.	C.I. No.	Class	Chemical name / formula
Guaiazulene (CTFA adopted name) Guaiazulne (Japan) CAS # 489-84-9 EINECS # 207-701-2				1,4-Dimethyl-7-isopropyl-azulene

Color	Blue solution in methanol.
Solubility	Soluble in methanol and parafin oil.
Chromatography	No information available.
Spectral photometry Solvent Absorption maximum	Source : own assay Methanol 600 nm
Main applications	Used in pharmaceutical products (due to its anti-infection properties) and in cosmetics (care products). Note : Azulene diffuses into plastic and discolors the packing material.

Toxicological and dermatological data		Source
LD50 tested on rats	> 1450 mg/kg	Safety data sheet Azulen / DRAGOCO
mice	> 1550 mg/kg	
Skin compatibility tested on humans	non-irritant	
Mucous membrane compatibility tested on a:		
rabbit eye	slight irritation	
guinea pig eye	no observation	

Certification status

European Union	Not considered a cosmetic colorant, but a function cosmetic or pharmaceutical ingredient.
Japan	Approved for drugs, "quasi-drugs" and cosmetics.
USA	Approved for cosmetics but not for mouth wash water, tooth pate and products for the eye and lip area. Utilization does not require FDA certificate.

For acceptance of this colorant in other countries, based on above mentioned approvals, see also 9.1.8.

Pyrophyllite

Name	EU-No.	C.I. No.	Class	Chemical name / formula
Pyrophyllite, Aluminum silicate Pyrophyllite (CTFA adopted name) Aluminum silicate (Japan) CAS # 12269-78-2 # 1327-36-2 EINECS # unknown				

Color	White pigment.
Solubility	Insoluble.
Chromatography	Not applicable.
Spectral photometry	Not applicable.
Main applications	No information available.

Toxicological and dermatological data	Source
No information available.	

Certification status

European Union	Not considered a cosmetic colorant, but a functional cosmetic or pharmaceutical ingredient.
Japan	Approved for drugs, "quasi-drugs" and cosmetics.
USA	Approved for externally applied drugs and cosmetics. Utilization does not require FDA certificate.

For acceptance of this colorant in other countries, based on above mentioned approvals, see also 9.1.8.

Riboflavin, Riboflavin-5'-Phosphate

Name	EU-No.	C.I. No.	Class	Chemical name / formula
Riboflavin, Lactoflavin Vitamin B2 Riboflavin (CFR21) Riboflavin (Japan) CAS # 83-88-5 EINECS # 201-507-1	E 101		Isoall-oxazine	6,7-Dimethyl-9-(1'-D-ribityl)-iso-alloxazine
Riboflavin-5'-phosphate CAS # 146-17-8 EINECS # 204-988-6	E 101 previously E 101a		Isoall-oxazine	-, Phosphate
Color	Yellow sollution in water.			
Solubility	Riboflavin : Low solubility in water (about 70 g/l) and ethanol, insoluble in ether and chloroform, is decomposed by alkali			
Chromatography DC Carrier	of Riboflavin : Source : Communication XVII DFG Farbstoff-Kommission Kieselgel Acetic acid ester 11 ml + Ammonia 25% 10 ml + Methanol 20 ml			
Spectral photometry Solvent Absorption maximum	of Riboflavin : Source : Ringbook Kosmetische Färbemittel 1984 Water 445 nm			
Main applications Food	Mayonnaise, soup, dessert products, candies, can be used for vitamin fortification. If approved, Riboflavin-5'-phosphate is preferred due to its better solubility.			

Toxicological and dermatological data		Source
LD50 tested on rats	> 10000 mg/kg	Kosmetische Färbemittel 3. ed., 1991

ADI-values :
Riboflavin (WHO 1969) 0-0.5 mg/kg Ringbook Color-
Riboflavin-5'-phosphate no ADI value ants for food 1978
  specified (EU-
  document
  III/9280/90)

Certification status	
European Union	Riboflavin/riboflavin-5'-phosphate Approved for defined food products (see 2.4.1.) and for the coloration of drugs and cosmetic preparations of group 1 (all cosmetic products).
Argentina	Approved for food.
Australia	Approved for defined food products.
Austria	Riboflavin/riboflavin-5'-phosphate. Approved for defined food products.
Brazil	Approved for defined food products.
Canada	Approved for defined food products.
Chile	Approved for food.
Colombia	Riboflavin/riboflavin-5'-phosphate. Approved for food.
Cyprus	Approved for defined food products.
Finland	Approved for defined food products.
India	Approved for food.
Indonesia	Approved for food.
Iran	Approved for food.
Israel	Approved for food.
Japan	Approved for defined food products. Approved for cosmetics (CTFA list of Japanese Cosmetic Ingredients).
Kenya	Approved for food.
Korea (South)	Approved for food.
Kuwait	Approved for food.
Malta	Approved for food.
New Zealand	Approved for defined food products.
Norway	Approved for defined food products.
Philippines	Riboflavin/riboflavin-5'-phosphate. Approved for food.
Poland	Approved for cosmetics.
Saudi Arabia	Approved for food.
Singapore	Approved for food.
South Africa	Approved for defined food products. Approved for the coloration of cosmetics of group 1 (all cosmetic products).
Sweden	Approved for defined food products.
Switzerland	Approved for defined food products and drugs.
Syria	Approved for food.
Taiwan	Riboflavin/riboflavin-5'-phosphate. Approved for defined food products. Maximum levels must be respected.

Thailand	Approved for food.
Tunisia	Approved for defined food products.
Turkey	Approved for defined food products.
	Approved for the coloration of cosmetics of group 1 (all cosmetic products).
Uruguay	Approved for food.
United Arab Emirates	Approved for food.
USA	Approved for defined food products.
	Utilization does not require FDA certificate.
	Not approved for drugs and cosmetics.
Zambia	Approved for food.

For acceptance of this colorant in other countries, based on above mentioned approvals, see also 9.1.8.

Sudan Blue B

Name	EU-No.	C.I. No.	Class	Chemical name / formula
Sudan blue B Sudan blue 672 C.I. Solvent Blue 79 Blue # 403 (Japan) (?) CAS # 64553-79-5 (?) EINECS # unknown			Anthra- quinone	unknown
Color	Blue solution in organic solvents.			
Solubility	Soluble in organic solvents.			
Chromatography	No information available.			
Spectral photometry	No information available.			
Main applications	No information available.			

Toxicological and dermatological data	Source
No information available.	

Certification status

European Union	Not approved for food, drugs and cosmetics.
Japan	Approval status unclear.
USA	Not approved for food, drugs and cosmetics.

For acceptance of this colorant in other countries, based on above mentioned approvals, see also 9.1.8.

Vitrolan Rosa BE

Name	EU-No.	C.I. No.	Class	Chemical name / formula
Vitrolan Rosa BE C.I. Acid Red 195 CAS # 12220-24-5 EINECS # unknown			Monoazo	4-(2'-Oxo-4'-sulfo-naphthylazo)-1-phenyl-3-methyl-5-oxo-pyrazol, Sodium salt, Chromium complex

Color	Red solution in water. Sodium salt red solution in water, Aluminum lake red powder.
Solubility	Soluble in water (at 20 °C about 30 g/l).
Chromatography	No information available.
Spectral photometry	No information available.
Main applications	No information available.

Toxicological and dermatological data		Source
LD50 tested on rats	> 7000 mg/kg	Kosmetische Färbemittel 3. ed., 1991
Skin compatibility tested on rabbits	non-irritant	
Mucous membrane compatibility tested on a rabbit eye	non-irritant	

Certification status

European Union	Approved for the coloration of cosmetics of group 3 (not on mucous membranes).
Japan	Not approved for food, drugs and cosmetics.
South Africa	Approved for the coloration of cosmetics of group 3 (not on mucous membranes).
Turkey	Approved for the coloration of cosmetics of group 3 (not on mucous membranes.
USA	Not approved for food, drugs and cosmetics.

For acceptance of this colorant in other countries, based on above mentioned approvals, see also 9.1.8.

Xanthophyll

Name	EU-No.	C.I. No.	Class	Chemical name / formula
Xanthophyll CAS # 6983-79-5, EINECS # 230-248-7	E 161		Carote- noide	Keto- and/or Hy- droxyl derivate of carotene
Lutein Xanthophyll	E 161b	see C.I. 75136		
Kryptoxanthin CAS # 472-70-8 EINECS # unknown	E 161c			
Rubixanthin	E 161d	see C.I. 75135		
Violaxanthin	E 161e	see C.I. 75138		
Rhodoxanthin CAS # 116-30-3 EINECS # unknown	E 161f			
Canthaxanthin	E 161g	see C.I. 40850		
Astaxanthin		see Asta- xanthin		
Citranaxanthin		see Citrana- xanthin		
Zeaxanthin		see Zea- xanthin		
Color	Yellow to orange solution in hydrocarbons.			
Solubility	Soluble in chloroform and hydrocarbons.			
Chromatography	No information available.			
Spectral photometry Solvent	Chloroform			

Absorption maximum	a) Flavoxanthin	430, 459 nm
	b) Lutein	428, 456, 487 nm
	c) Kryptoxanthin	433, 463, 497 nm
	d) Rubixanthin	439, 474, 509 nm
	e) Violaxanthin	424, 452, 482 nm
	f) Rhodoxanthin	482, 510, 546 nm
	g) Canthaxanthin	485 nm
Main applications	These colorants (with the exception of lutein (xanthophyll) and canthaxanthin) is not of technical importance. For application see each colorant.	

Toxicological and dermatological data	Source
Results are not available. The assessment of this colorant is done on the basis of general knowledge of the physico-chemical properties and toxicological experience (Kosmetische Färbemittel, 3 ed., 1991).	

Certification status

European Union	Approved for defined food products (see 2.4.1.) and for the coloration of drugs and cosmetic preparations of group 1 (all cosmetic products). In the EU Colorant Guideline 94/36/EU on food colorants, only lutein (E 161b) and canthaxanthin (E 161g) are mentioned.
Australia	Approved for defined food products.
Brazil	Approved for defined food products.
Canada	Approved for defined food products.
Cyprus	Approved for defined food products.
Hungary	C.I.75135 E 161d Approved for the coloration of cosmetics of group 1 (all cosmetic products).
Israel	Approved for food.
Japan	Approved for defined food products. Not approved for cosmetics.
Kenya	Approved for food.
New Zealand	Approved for defined food products.
South Africa	Approved for defined food products. C.I.75135 E 161d: Approved for the coloration of cosmetic of group 1 (all cosmetic products).
Switzerland	Approved for defined food products.
Thailand	Approved for food.
Turkey	Approved for the coloration of cosmetics of group 1 (all cosmetic products).
USA	Not approved for food, drugs and cosmetics.

For acceptance of this colorant in other countries, based on above mentioned approvals, see also 9.1.8.

10 Literature

10.1. General information

- Color Index : Third edition, Vol. 1-4 (1971), Revised Third Edition, Vol. 5 - 6 (1975); The Society of Dyers and Colourists, P.O.Box 244, Perkin House 82, Grattan Road, Bradford West, Yorkshire BD1 2JB / England and the American Association of Textile Chemists and Colorists, P.O.Box 12215, Research Triangle Park, North Carolina 27709, USA.

- Deutsche Forschungsgemeinschaft (DFG), Ergenisse einer Tagung westeuropäischer Wissenschaftler zur Prophylaxe des Krebses, Bad Godesberg, 1954.

- DIN 55994 Farbmittel, Einteilung nach koloristischen und chemischen Gesichtspunkten, April 1990.

- Uwe Claussen, Angewandte Fluoreszenz: Weisstöner; Chemie in unserer Zeit, Heft 5/1973, 141.

- Johann Wolfgang von Goethe, Zur Farbenlehrel Die bibliophilem Taschenbücher Nr. 75, 2.Auflage 1982, Harenberg Kommunikation, Dotmund, 1979.

- Goethes Farbenlehre, ausgewählt und erläutert von RUPRECHT MATTAI; Otto Maier Verlag Verlag Ravensburg, 1971.

- Claudia Gottmann, Das Portrait: Michel Eugene Chevreul (1986-1891!); Chemie in unserer Zeit, Heft 6/1979, 176.

- Hans Kittel (Herausgeber), Lehrbuch der Lacke und Beschichtungen, Band II - Pigmente, Füllstoffe, Farbstoffe - Verlag W.A.Colomb in der Heenemann GmbH, Berlin Oberschwandorf, 1974.

- Martin Klessinger, Konstituttion und Lichtabsorption organischer Farbstoffe; Chemie in unserer Zeit Heft 1/1978, 1.

- Otto Krätz, Das Portrait: Peter Griess (1829–1888), Chemie in unserer Zeit, Heft 2/1976, 525.

- Otto Krätz, Zur Geschichte der Farbenchemie, Chemie für Labor und Betrieb, Heft 12/1979, 525.

- Edgar Lüscher (Herausgeber), Physik - Gestern, heute, morgen -; Moos Verlag München 1971.

- Max Lüscher, Farben - visualisierte Gefühle, DRAGOCO Report 4/5 -1981.

- Daniel M. Marmion, Handbook of U.S. Colorants for Foods, Drugs, and Cosmetics, Second Edition 1984, ISBN 0-471-09312-2.

- Alfred von Nagel, Fuchsin Alizarin Indigo - Der Beginn eines Weltunternehmens; Schriftenreihe des Frimenarchives der Badischen Anilinund Soda-Fabrik AG, 1.

- Otto-Albrecht Neumüller, Römpps-Chemie-Lexikon, 8. neubearbeitet und erweiterte Auflage; Franck;sche Verlagshandlung Stuttgart, 1979.

- Willibald Pschyrembel, Klinisches Wörterbuch mit klinischen Syndromen, 252. Auflage; Walter de Gruyter, Berlin - New York 1975.

- Gustav Schultz, Farbstofftabellen, 7. Auflage, neu bearbeitet und herausgegeben von DR. LUDWIG LEHMANN; Akademische Verlagsgesellschaft m.b.H. Leipzig 1931.

- Ullmanns Enzyklopädie der technischen Chemie, 3. Auflage; Urban und Schwarzenberg, München/Berlin 1953.

- Georg Wittke, Farbstoffchemie, Studienbücher Chemie, Verlag Morits Diesterweg/Otto Salle, Frankfurt a.M. 1979.

10.2. Food

- DFG-Farbstoff-Komission, Mitteilung 6: Toxikologische Daten von Farbstoffen und ihre Zulassung für Lebensmittel in verschiedenen Ländern; Franz Steiner Verlag GmbH, Wiesbaden, 2.Auflage 1957.

- DFG-Farbstoff-Kommission, Mitteilung 9 (gleichzeitig Zusammenfassung der Mitteilungen 1, 2, 4, 5 und 7), 20.12.1956; Franz Steiner Verlag GmbH, Wiesbaden.

- DFG-Farbstoff-Kommission, Farbstoffe für Lebensmittel, 1978, Harald Bold Verlag KG Boppard.

- E.E.C. Colours Group, Newsletter Dec. 5th, 1983, Increase of ADI-values.

- Grosse Anfrage der Fraktion Die Grünen "Nutzen und Risiken des Einsatzes synthetischer Lebensmittelfarbstoffe"; Deutscher Bundestag 10. Wahlperiode, Drucksache 10/3182, 16.4.1985, Sachgebiet 2125.

- Antwort der Bundesregierung auf die Grosse Anfrage der Fraktion Die Grünen - Drucksache 10/3182 -"Nutzen und Risiken des Einsatzes synthetischer Lebensmittelfarbstoffe", Deutscher Bundestag 10.Wahlperiode, Drucksache 10/5275, 1.4.1986, Sachgebiet 2125.

Literature

- Zusatzstoffe, Ihre Wirkung und Anwendung in Lebensmitteln (Herausgeber Fachgruppe "Lebensmittelchemie und gerichtliche Chemie" in der Gesellschaft Deutscher Chemiker); Behr's Verlag Hamburg, 1986.

- Zusatzstoffe in Lebensmitteln - Eine Information; Bund für Lebensmittelrecht und Lebensmittelkunde e.V.; Godesberger Allee 157, 53000 Bonn 2 (1987).

- Barbara Bertram, Farbstoffe: Wie gefährlich sind sie wirklich? Eine Übersicht über Stoffe zur Lebensmittel- und Arnzneimittelfärbung; Deutsche Apotherkerzeitung. 127. Jahrgang Nr. 10 (1987), 499.

- Barbara Bertram Farbstoffe in Lebensmitteln und Arzneimitteln. Eine Farbstoffübersicht mit toxikologischer Bewertung. Wissenschaftliche Verlagsgesellschaft mbH, Stuttgart 1989.

- Käte K. Glandorf, Peter Kuhnert, Handbuch Lebensmittelzusatz- stoffe, Behr's Verlag Hamburg 1991.

- Heinrich Kläui, Otto Isler. Warum und womit färbt man Lebensmittel?; Chemie in unserer Zeit, Heft 1/1981.

- Susanne Langguth, Food und Fakten—Wie sicher sind unsere Lebensmittel; Edition Interfromm, Osnabrück; Fromm (1986).

- Erich Lück, Chemie im Kochtopf—Chemische Vorgäne beim Herstellen von Speisen; Chemie in unserer Zeit, Heft 5/1985, 156.

- Erich Lück, Gert-Wolfhard von Rymon Lipinski, Lebens- mittelzusatzstoffe—Eine zeitgerechte Darstellung und Beurteilung; Deutsche Lebensmittelrundschau, 76. Jahrgang Oktober 1980, Heft 10, 339.

- Klaus Stüven, Grundsätzliches über Farbstoffe für Lebensmittel Lebens- mitteltechnik 6/80, 25.

- G.Vettorazzi, Advances in the safety evaluation of food additives, Food Additives and Contaminants, 1987, Vol.4, No.4, 331-356.

10.3. Drugs

- Pharmazeutika, Bestimmungsliste, 4. Überarbeitete Auflage 1985; IMP Kom- munikationsgesellschaft, Neu-Isenburg.

- Rote Liste 1982, Verzeichnis von Fertigarzneimitteln der Mitglieder des Bundesverbandes der Pharmazeutischen Industrie e.V. (Herausgeber).

- List of drugs dyes, Position as per December 1982l Capsugel - communication

- Peter Aeckerli, Zulässigkeit der Farbmittel in der Pharmazeutischen Industrie, Pharmazeutische Industrie 32, 160-168 (1970).

- Michel Und Wattenwyl, Farbstoffe in der Arzneimittelindustrie; Problematik und Möglichkeiten; Mitteilungsblatt der Capsugel-AG 1979.

10.4. Cosmetics

- DFG-Farbstoff-Kommission, Mitteilung 3 (Kosmetische Färbemittel) 2.Aufl. 21.11.1959; Franz Steiner Verlag GmbH, Wiesbaden.

- DFG-Farbstoff-Kommission, Kosmetische Färbemittel (Rotes Ringbuch) 1977; Harald Boldt Verlag, Boppard.

- DFG-Farbstoff-Kommission, Kosmetische Färbemittel (Rotes Ringbuch) 1984; Verlag Chemie GmbH, Weinheim.

- DFG-Farbstoff-Kommission, Kosmetische Färbemittel, 3. völlig überarbeitete Auflage 1991, VCH Weinheim.

- Wolfgang Bruhn, Sonnenstrahlung, Sonnenschutz und die Bräunung der menschlichen Haut (1); DRAGOCO-Report 2/1978.

- Dietmar Bücher, Färbemittel für Kosmetika, Seifen und Waschmittel; Seifen-Öle-Fette-Wachse, Nr.8/1980, 207.

- G. Möschl, F. Soehngen, M. Kieser, Perlglanzpigmente für Kosmetika; Seifen-Öle-Fette-Wachse, Nr.4/1980, 93-98 and Nr. 20/1985, 643-645.

- G.A. Nowak, Die kosmetischen Präparate, 3. verbesserte und erweiterte Auflage, Band 2, Rezeptur-Rohstoffe-wissenschaftlichen Grundlagen; Verlag für chemische Industrie H.Ziolkowsky KG, Augsburg 1984.

- Rolf Ohrmann, Duft und Farbe als Kommunikationselement in Badepräparaten; DRAGOCO-Report 6/1985.

- Susan Rush, Stability properties of colors used in Cosmetics and toiletries; Cosmetics and Toiletries, 1989, Vol 104, 47-53.

- Peter Tetweiler und J. Stephan Jellinek, Farbe in Mundwässern; DRAGOCO-Report 4/5-1982.

10.5. Analysis and color determination

- Specifications for identity and purity of food additives, Vol.II Food Colours, Food and Agriculture Organization of the United Nations, Rome, 1963.

- Specifications for the identity and purity of food additives and their toxicological evaluation; food colours, antimicrobials an antioxidants; Eighth

Literature

- report of the Joint FAO/WHO Expert Committee on the Food Additives, Rome 1965.

- Specifications for the identity and purity of food colours, FAO Food and Nutrition paper 31/1, Food and Agriculture Organization of the United Nations, Rome 1984.

- DFG-Farbstoff-Kommission, Mitteilung 8: Vegleichsmuster der vorgeschlagenen synthetischen Lebensmittelfarbstoffe, 23.Nov. 1956.

- DFG-Farbstoff-Kommission, Mitteilung 12 vom Juni 1964, Ausgabedatum Januar 1965: Untersuchungsmethoden zur Prüfung der Reinheit von Lebensmittelfarbstoffen; Franz Steiner Verlag GmbH, Wiesbaden.

- DG-Farbstoff-Kommission, Untersuchungsmethoden zur Prüfung der Reinheit von Lebensmittelfarbstoffen, 1980; Harald Boldt Verlag, Boppard.

- DFG-Farbstoff-Kommission, Mitteilung XIV: Anleitung zur Abtrennung und Identifizierung von Farbstoffen in gefärbten Lebensmittelnn, 1980; Harald Boldt Verlag KG, Boppard.

- DFG-Farbstoff-Kommission, Mitteilung XVII: Identifizierung von Farbstoffen in Kosmetika, Hrsg. Günter Lehmann mit Unterstützung von Barbara Binkle, 1986; VCH Verlagsgesellschaft, Weinheim.

- Lehrgang "Einführung in die Farbmessung" Auflage 1978; Bundesanstalt für Materialprüfung, Fachgruppe 5.4 Farbmetrik, Berlin Dahlem.

- Bedienungsanleitung des Farbmessgerätes LF90 für Farbmessung und Remissionsmessung and Oberflächen und Pulvern, Dr. Bruno Lange, Berlin.

- Exakte Farbkommunikation - Vom Farbgefühl bis zur objektiven Messung -: Minolta 1987.

- Die kleine Farbmessatfel nach Wilhelm Ostwal, Ausgabe A: Verlag Musterschmidt, Göttingen o.J.

- DIN-Farbkarte DIN 6164; Beuth Verlag GmbH, Berlin 1984.

- RAL - Farben und ihre Verwendung; RAL -F4, 7.Ausgabe.

- DIN 54004 - Bestimmung der Lichtechtheit von Färbungen und Drucken mit Künstlichem Tageslicht; Beuth Verlag.

- Anni Berger, Andreas Brockes, Farbmessung in der Textilindustrie; Bayer - Farben Revue, Sonderheft 3/1, Leverkusen 1971.

- Bisalski, Pflanzenfarben-Atlas mit Farbzeichen nach DIN 6164; Musterschmiedt-Verlag, Göttingen - Berlin - Frankfurt 1957.

- F. Brücker, Farbmessung als Massnahme der Qualitätssicherung; Elektro-Anzeiger Nr. 9/1979, Verlag W.Girardet, Essen.

- A. Kornerup und J.H. Wanscher, Taschenlexikon der Farben (1440 Farbnuancen und 600 Farbnamen); Musterschmiedt-Verlag, Zürich - Göttingen 1963.

- Müllers Mobiler Farbkörper 743/1093, Chromos-Verlag, Winterthur (1968).

- Grete Ostwald, In Farbe setzen; Technik für alle, Heft 9/1939, Franck'sche Verlagshandlung, Stuttgart.

- Paul Rabe, Zur Frage der Bestimmung der Lichtechtheit, Sonderdruck aus "Rayon, Zellwolle und andere Chemiefasern", Heft 12, Dezember 1957.

- Eugen Ristenpart, Die Ostwaldsche Farblehre und ihre Nutzen; Technischer Verlag Herbert Cram, Berlin 1948.

- Thaler und Sommer, Die papierchromatographische Trennung wasserlöslicher Teerfarbstoffe; Zeitschrift für Lebensmitteluntersuchung und Forschung, 97. Baand, Heft 5, 345.

10.6. Food legislation

Apart from the sources mentioned under 10.6.1 to 10.6.3. all information regarding the legal status of colorants in different countries are based on information (food laws, ordinances) archived at DRAGOCO Holzminden, and on internal communication of DRAGOCO overseas subsidiaries and representatives as well as customers in Europe, Asia, Africa, America and Australia as well as information from the Bundesstelle für Aussenhandelsinformation, Agrippastrasse 87-93, 50676 Köln, Tel. 0221-20570.

10.6.1. Food

- Richtlinie des Rates vom 23. Oktober 1962 : Festlegung der Farbstoffe für Lebensmittel und der Reinheitskriterien.

- Richtlinie des Rates vom 24. Oktober 1967 : Zufügung von Erythrosin und Brillantsäuregrün.

- Lebensmitel- und Bedarfsgegenstände-Gesetz vom 15.8.1974, BGBl. Teil 1, S.1945.

- Verordnung über das Inverkehrbringen von Zusatzstoffen und einzelnen wie Zusatzstoffe verwendete Lebensmittel (Zusatzstoffverkehrsverordnung) vom 22.12.1977, BGBl. 1977, Teil I, Nr. 88, 2653.

Literature 375

- Verordnung über die Zulassung von Zusatzstoffen zu Lebensmitteln (Zusatzstoffzulassungs-Verordung) vom 20.12.1977, BGBl 1977, Teil I, Nr. 88, 2711.

- Verordnung zur Neuordnung lebensmittelrechtlicher Kennzeichnungsvorschriften, BGBl. 1981, Teil I, Nr. 60, 1625, insbesondere Artikel 1 : Lebensmittelkennzeichnungsverodnung und Artikel 2: Zusatzstoff-Zulassungsverordnung.

- Bekanntmachung der Liste der zugelassenen Lebensmittelzusatzstoffe (Fundstellenliste) und des Verzeichnisses der EWG-Nummern vom 1. September 1982; Bundesanzeiger 48/62.

- Verordnung über das Inverkehrbringen von zusatzstoffen und einzelnen wie Zusatzstoffe verwendeten Stoffen (Zusatzstoff-Verkehrsverordnung) vom 10.7.1984, BGBl. 1984, Teil I, Nr. 30 (enthält bei Azorubin E 122 einen Druckfehler : Nebenfarbstoffe irrtümlich 0.1% statt 1%).

- Verordnung zur Änderung der Zusatstoff-Zulassungsverordnung vom 13.Juni 1990, BGBl. 1990, Teil I, Nr. 27, 1053.

- Overseas Food Legislation, Second edition, June 1984.

- Information from Leatherhead Food R.A., The British Food Manufacturing Industries research Association, Randalls Road, Leatherhead, Surrey, KT 22 7RY.

- Code of Federal Regulations 21, (1993), source see 2.4.3.

10.6.2. Cosmetics

- CTFA International Color Handbook (Editor Linda C. Packenham, Emalee G. Murphy, esq.), published by the Cosmetic, Toiletry and Fragrance Association Inc. 1110 Vermont Avenue, N.W., Suite 800, Washington, D.C. 20005, Telex 892673 CTFA WSH.

- CTFA International Color Handbook Second Edition, (Editor J. M. Rempe, L. Santucci, Esq.), published by the Cosmetic, Toiletry and Fragrance Association Inc. 1101 17th Street, Suite 300, Washington, D.C. 20005, Phone 2022-31-1770, Fax 202-331-1969.

- Code of Federal Regulations 21, (1993), Source see 2.4.3.

- Principles of cosmetic licensing in Japan, 2nd. edition; Yakuji Nippi Ltd. 1 Kanda Izumicho, Chiyoda-Ku, Tokyo, 101 Japan.

- Richtlinie des Rates vom 27.Juli 1976 zur Angleichung der Rechtsvorschriften der Mitgliedstaaten über kosmetische Mittel (76/768/EWG).

- Siebente Richtlinie der Kommission vom 28. Februar 1986 zur Anpassung der Anhänge II, III, IV und V der Richtkinie 76/768/EWG des Rates zur Angleichung der Rechtsvorschrfiten der Mitgliedstaaten über kosmetische Mittel an den technischen Fortschritt (86/179/EWG).

- richtlinie 93/35/EWG des Rates vom 14. Juli 1993 zur sechsten Änderung der Richtlinie 76/768/EWG zur Angleichung der Rechtsvorschriften der Mitgliedstaaten über kosmetische Mittel.

- Verordnung über kosmetische Mittel (Kosmetik-Verordnung) vom 16.Dezember 1977, BGBl. 1977, Teil I, Nr. 86, 2589.

- Bekanntmachung der Neufassung der Kosmetik-Verordnung vom 19. Juni 1985, BGBl. 1985, Teil I, Nr. 32, 1083.

- Zuletzt geändert durch die 22. Verordnung zur Änderung der Kosmetik-Verordnung vom 24.März 1994, BGBl. 1994, Teil I, Nr. 20, 674.

- Birgit Hofmann, Gesetzliche Grundlagen der Färbemittel in der Bundesrepublik Deutschlad, der EG, in Japan und in den Vereinigten Staaten; Seife - Fette - Öle - Wachse - 116.Jahrgang, Nr. 8/1990, 299-306.

- E. Pfrommer, Rechtliche Bestimungen für Eisenoxide; Parfümerie und Kosmetik, 75. Jahrg., Nr. 2/94, 74-79.

Index

Additive colorant blending, 3, 4
ADI (acceptable daily intake) value, 63, 92
Alizarin, 9
Aluminum lakes of water-soluble colorants, 85
Aluminum stearate (data sheet), 342–343
American Association of Textile Chemists and Colorists, 11
Analysis, 47–89
    identification of colorants, 80–89
        aluminum lakes, 85
        isolation of coloring agent in the finished product and its identification, 88–89
        oil-soluble food and cosmetic colorants, 84–85
        pigments, 85–87
        water-soluble food and cosmetic colorants, 80–83
    literature on analysis and color determination, 372–374
    purity requirements, 77–80
        colorants for cosmetic products, 80
        colorants for food and drugs, 77–80
Anthocyan (natural food colorant), 13
    data sheet, 343–345
Antiauxochrome groups, 8
ß-Apo-5'-carotenal (natural food colorant), 13
Argentina, control of cosmetic product coloration in, 45
Astaxathin (data sheet), 345
Australia:
    certification status of colorants in, 93
    control of cosmetic product coloration in, 45
Austria, certification status of colorants in, 95
Auxochrome groups, 8
Azo compounds, 8, 10

Barium sulfate (data sheet), 310
Bathing products, colorants for, 6
Bathing salts, 55
Bathing tablets, 55
Berries, natural colorant for, 13
Betaine (data sheet), 346–347
Betanin (natual food colorant), 13
Betonite (data sheet), 347–348
Bismuth citrate (data sheet), 348–349
Black pigments, 86
Blue pigments, 86
    calculation example for, 70, 73
Brazil, control of cosmetic product coloration in, 45
British Society of Dyers and Colourists, 11
Bromo cresol green (data sheet), 349–350
Bromthymol blue (data sheet), 350–351
Brown FK (data sheet), 351–352
Brown pigments, 86

Cadmium levels in cereal samples, 77
Calamine (data sheet), 353
Calcium stearate (data sheet), 342–343
Canada, certification status of colorants in, 94
Capsanthine (data sheet), 354–355
Capsorubin (data sheet), 354–355
Caramel (data sheet), 355–357
Carriers for food colorants (EU guidelines), 20, 31
Carotene (natural food colorant), 13
Carrot extract (pro-vitamin A), 53
Carrots, natural colorant for, 13
CAS (Chemical Abstract System) number, 31
Central American countries, control of cosmetic product coloration in, 45
Cereal, cadmium levels in samples of, 77
Certification status of colorants (data sheet information), 93–95
Chile, certification status or colorants in, 93
China (PRC), certification status of colorants in, 93
Chlorophyll, 13
Chromatographic analysis in identification of colorants, 80–83
    paper chromatography for water-soluble colorants, 81–82
    thin-layer chromatography for oil-soluble colorants, 84
Chromium hydrogen oxide (data sheet), 319–320
Chromophores, 8
CIE (Commission International de l'Eclairage)-Lab color system, 7, 68, 70, 72
Citranaxathine (data sheet), 357–358
Citrus fruit, natural colorant for, 13
Colombia, certification status of colorants in, 94

Colorant blending, additive and subtractive, 3, 4
Colorants (definition), 7–10
Color determination, literature on, 372–374
Colorimetry, 64–67
Color Index (C.I.), 11–12
[*Color Index (C.I.) colorant data sheets follow*]:
C.I. Acid Black 1, 178–179
C.I. Acid Black 2, 245–246
C.I. Acid Blue 1, 200–201
C.I. Acid Blue 5, 201–202
C.I. Acid Blue 7, 204–205
C.I. Acid Blue 9, 206–208
C.I. Acid Blue 62, 261–262
C.I. Acid Blue 74, 267–269
C.I. Acid Blue 80, 260–261
C.I. Acid Blue 104, 216–217
C.I. Acid Dye (2-amino-3,5-xylolsulfoacid), 132–133
C.I. Acid Dye (2,3,4-trimethylaniline), 155–156
C.I. Acid Green 1, 97–98
C.I. Acid Green 3, 205
C.I. Acid Green 5, 208–209
C.I. Acid Green 9, 209–210
C.I. Acid Green 16, 217–218
C.I. Acid Green 22, 210–211
C.I. Acid Green 50, 220–221
C.I. Acid Orange 7, 133–134
C.I. Acid Orange 10, 158–159
C.I. Acid Orange 11, 228–229
C.I. Acid Orange 20, 128–129
C.I. Acid Orange 137, 175–176
C.I. Acid Orange (sulfanil acid), 177–178
C.I. Acid Red 1, 164–165
C.I. Acid Red 13, 153–154
C.I. Acid Red 14, 130–132
C.I. Acid Red 18, 159–161
C.I. Acid Red 26, 154–155
C.I. Acid Red 27, 156–158, 215
C.I. Acid Red 33, 162–164
C.I. Acid Red 41, 161–162
C.I. Acid Red 50, 225–226
C.I. Acid Red 51, 237–239
C.I. Acid Red 52, 221–222
C.I. Acid Red 73, 189
C.I. Acid Red 87, 229–231
C.I. Acid Red 88, 138–139
C.I. Acid Red 92, 233–235
C.I. Acid Red 94, 239–240
C.I. Acid Red 95, 235–236
C.I. Acid Red 99, 232–233
C.I. Acid Red 155, 165–166
C.I. Acid Red 163, 185–186
C.I. Acid Red 180, 167–168
C.I. Acid Violet 9, 224–225
C.I. Acid Violet 43, 254–255
C.I. Acid Violet 50, 244–245
C.I. Acid Yellow 1, 98–99
C.I. Acid Yellow 3, 243–244
C.I. Acid Yellow 11, 168–169
C.I. Acid Yellow 13, 172
C.I. Acid Yellow 17, 171–172
C.I. Acid Yellow 23, 173–175
C.I. Acid Yellow 36, 126–127
C.I. Acid Yellow 40, 170
C.I. Acid Yellow 73, 226–228
C.I. Acid Yellow 121, 166–167
C.I. Basic Blue 11, 218–219
C.I. Basic Blue 26, 219–220
C.I. Basic Blue 99, 247–248
C.I. Basic Brown 16, 115–116
C.I. Basic Brown 17, 116–117
C.I. Basic Red 76, 114–115
C.I. Basic Violet 1, 214
C.I. Basic Violet 2, 213
C.I. Basic Violet 10, 222–223
C.I. Basic Violet 14, 212
C.I. Basic Yellow 76, 123–124
C.I. Basic Yellow 86, 227–228
C.I. Direct Orange 34/39, 192–193
C.I. Disperse Violet 27, 251–252
C.I. Food Black 1, 191–192
C.I. Food Black 2, 190
C.I. Food Black 3, 316–317
C.I. Food Blue 1, 267–269
C.I. Food Blue 2, 206–208
C.I. Food Blue 3, 200–201
C.I. Food Blue 4, 262–263
C.I. Food Green 1, 205
C.I. Food Green 2, 208–209
C.I. Food Green 3, 202–203
C.I. Food Green 4, 220–221
C.I. Food Orange 2, 148–149
C.I. Food Orange 4, 158–159
C.I. Food Orange 5, 193–194
C.I. Food Orange 6, 194–196
C.I. Food Orange 7, 196–198, 198–200
C.I. Food Red 1, 129–130
C.I. Food Red 3, 130–132
C.I. Food Red 4, 153–154
C.I. Food Red 5, 154–155

Index

C.I. Food Red 6, 156–158, 215
C.I. Food Red 7, 159–161
C.I. Food Red 8, 161–162
C.I. Food Red 10, 164–165
C.I. Food Red 12, 162–164
C.I. Food Red 14, 237–239
C.I. Food Red 17, 152–153
C.I. Food Yellow 2, 124–125
C.I. Food Yellow 3, 149–151
C.I. Food Yellow 4, 173–175
C.I. Food Yellow 5, 171–172
C.I. Food Yellow 8, 127–128
C.I. Food Yellow 13, 241–244
C.I. Mordant Red 11, 249–250
C.I. Natural Green 3, 297–299
C.I. Natural Green 5, 299–301
C.I. Natural Orange 4, 280–282
C.I. Natural Orange 6, 295–296
C.I. Natural Red 4, 293–295
C.I. Natural White 1, 290–291
C.I. Natural Yellow 3, 291–292
C.I. Natural Yellow 6/19, 279–280
C.I. Natural Yellow 8/11, 296–297
C.I. Natural Yellow 26, 284–286
C.I. Natural Yellow 27 (lycopine), 283
C.I. Natural Yellow 27 (hydroxyl-derivative of carotene), 286, 289
C.I. Natural Yellow 27 (keto-hydroxyl derivative of carotene), 287
C.I. Natural Yellow 29 (hydroxyl-derivative of carotene), 287–288
C.I. Natural Yellow 29 (zeaxanthin), 288–289
C.I. Pigment Black 6/7, 314–315
C.I. Pigment Black 9, 315–316
C.I. Pigment Black 11, 328–329
C.I. Pigment Black 15, 275–277
C.I. Pigment Blue 16, 275–276
C.I. Pigment Blue 27 (ferric ammonium ferrocyanide), 331
C.I. Pigment Blue 27 (Prussian blue), 329–330
C.I. Pigment Blue 29, 305–307
C.I. Pigment Blue 60, 262–263
C.I. Pigment Blue 64, 263–264
C.I. Pigment Blue 66, 265–266
C.I. Pigment Brown 1, 120
C.I. Pigment Green 7, 278–279
C.I. Pigment Green 8, 96–97
C.I. Pigment Green 17, 317–319
C.I. Pigment Green 24, 307–308
C.I. Pigment Metal 1, 302–303
C.I. Pigment Metal 2, 320–321
C.I. Pigment Metal 3, 321–323
C.I. Pigment Orange 1, 104
C.I. Pigment Orange 5, 107
C.I. Pigment Orange 13, 182–183
C.I. Pigment Orange 34, 183–184
C.I. Pigment Orange 43, 264–265
C.I. Pigment Red 3, 110–111
C.I. Pigment Red 4, 108–109
C.I. Pigment Red 5, 121–122
C.I. Pigment Red 7, 119
C.I. Pigment Red 22, 117
C.I. Pigment Red 48, 145–146
C.I. Pigment Red 49, 139–141
C.I. Pigment Red 51, 136
C.I. Pigment Red 53, 136–138
C.I. Pigment Red 57, 143–145
C.I. Pigment Red 63, 146–148
C.I. Pigment Red 64, 141–143
C.I. Pigment Red 68, 135
C.I. Pigment Red 83, 249–250
C.I. Pigment Red 88, 269
C.I. Pigment Red 100, 125–126
C.I. Pigment Red 101/102 (aluminum silicate with iron oxide), 308
C.I. Pigment Red 101/102 (iron-III-oxide), 324–326
C.I. Pigment Red 112, 118
C.I. Pigment Red 122, 274–275
C.I. Pigment Red 172, 237–239
C.I. Pigment Red 181, 268–271
C.I. Pigment Red 191, 235–236
C.I. Pigment Red 209, 273–274
C.I. Pigment Violet 1, 334–335
C.I. Pigment Violet 19, 272–273
C.I. Pigment Violet 23, 246–247
C.I. Pigment Violet 36, 271–272
C.I. Pigment White 4, 340–341
C.I. Pigment White 6, 338–339
C.I. Pigment White 12, 341
C.I. Pigment White 14/31, 311–312
C.I. Pigment White 18 (calcium carbonate), 312–313
C.I. Pigment White 18 (magnesium carbonate), 332–333
C.I. Pigment White 19, 304–305
C.I. Pigment White 20, 309
C.I. Pigment White 24, 303–304
C.I. Pigment White 25, 313–314
C.I. Pigment White 26, 333–334

C.I. Pigment Yellow 1, 101–102
C.I. Pigment Yellow 3, 102–103
C.I. Pigment Yellow 12, 180
C.I. Pigment Yellow 13, 180–181
C.I. Pigment Yellow 16, 176–177
C.I. Pigment Yellow 42/43, 326–327
C.I. Pigment Yellow 83, 181–182
C.I. Pigment Yellow 100, 173–175
C.I. Pigment Yellow 104, 149–151
C.I. Pigment Yellow 115, 242–244
C.I. Solvent Blue 35, 256–257
C.I. Solvent Blue 63, 255–256
C.I. Solvent Green 7, 250–251
C.I. Solvent Orange 2, 109–110
C.I. Solvent Orange 3, 105
C.I. Solvent Orange 7, 111–112
C.I. Solvent Orange 16, 231–232
C.I. Solvent Red 1, 112–113
C.I. Solvent Red 3, 106
C.I. Solvent Red 23, 186–187
C.I. Solvent Red 24, 188
C.I. Solvent Red 48, 233–235
C.I. Solvent Red 73, 235–236
C.I. Solvent Red 80, 113–114
C.I. Solvent Red 140, 237–239
C.I. Solvent Violet, 13, 252–254
C.I. Solvent Yellow 6 (aniline), 100
C.I. Solvent Yellow 6 (α-toluidin), 100–101
C.I. Solvent Yellow 16, 122–123
C.I. Solvent Yellow 21, 166–167
C.I. Solvent Yellow 29, 184–185
C.I. Solvent Yellow 33, 240–241
C.I. Solvent Yellow 94, 226–228
C.I. Solvent Yellow 98, 248
C.I. Vat Blue 1, 265–266
C.I. Vat Blue 4, 262–263
C.I. Vat Blue 6, 263–264
C.I. Vat Orange 7, 264–265
C.I. Vat Red 1, 269–271
C.I. Vat Violet 2, 271–272
Coloring agents, 7–10
Color systems, 6–7
Cosmetic products, coloration of, 39–46
    importance of color in cosmetic products, 39
    isolation of coloring agent in the finished product, 88–89
    legal requirements, 39–46
        countries outside the EU, 45–46
        European Union/Federal Republic of Germany, 39–45

[Cosmetic products, coloration of]
    light interference in, 2
    literature on, 372
        legal status of colorants, 375–376
    product development, 54–58
        bathing salts, bathing tablets, 55
        eye makeup, 57
        hair dyeing and coloration products, 58
        lipstick, 57
        mouth and tooth care products, 57–58
        nail polish, 58
        oil and cream baths, 55
        oil-in-water emulsion, 56
        shading cream, makeup, 57
        shampoo, foam bath, shower gel, liquid soap, 54–55
        soap, 55–56
        water-in-oil emulsion 56
    purity standards for, 80
    technological possibilities, 39
    See also data sheets of colorants with Color Index (C.I.) numbers and without C.I. numbers
Costa Rica, certification status of colorants in, 94
Cream baths, 55
Curcuma spice, natural colorant for, 13

D&C Green #5 (data sheet), 259–260
D&C Green #6 (data sheet), 257–258
Data sheets of colorants for food, drugs, and cosmetics, 91–368
    Color Index (C.I.) generic name of the colorant, 96–341
    colorants without C.I. numbers, 342–368
    explanation of, 91–95
        certification status, 93–95
        chemical name, 92
        chromatography, 92
        color and solubility, 92
        major applications, 92
        names, 91
        spectral photometry, 92
        toxicological and dermatological information, 92
Definitions (basic), 1–12
    additive and subtractive colorant blending, 3, 4
    color and seeing colors, 1–3
        fluorescence and optical whiteners, 2–3
    coloring agents, colorants and pigments, 7–10

Index

[Definitions (basic)]
    colors and perceptions, 4–6
    color systems, 6–7
    interference, 3
    systematic of colorants, 11–12
        Color Index, 11–12
        EU number, 12
Dermatology, 63
Determination of color, 68–69
Determination of remission, 64
Dihydroxyacetone (data sheet), 358–359
DIN-Farbenkarte (DIN color chart), 6
Disodium EDTA-copper (data sheet), 359–360
Droplet reaction in concentrated sulfuric acid for identification of water-soluble colorants, 82, 83
Drug coloration, 37–38
    identification of colorants, 80–89
    importance of, 37
    isolation of coloring agent in the finished product, 88–89
    legal requirements, 37–38
        countries outside the EU, 38
        European Union/Federal Republic of Germany, 37–38
    literature on, 371–372
    product development, 53–54
    purity standards for, 77–80
    See also data sheets of colorants with Color Index (C.I.) numbers and without C.I. numbers
Dual-beam spectral photometer, 65
Dyer's woad, 9
Dyes, 10

Ecuador, certification status of colorants in, 94
Eggs, natural colorant for, 13
EINECS (European inventory of existing commerical chemical substances) number, 91
EL Salvador, certification status of colorants in, 94
European Union (EU):
    certification status of colorants in, 93
    food additive guidelines for, 12
    food products that can be colored, 19, 22–30
        approved colorants in foods (restricted use), 29–30

[European Union (EU)]
    colorants used only for defined purposes, 27–28
    foods not permitted to contain colorant additives, 22–23
    guidelines for solvents/carriers, 20, 31
    legal basis for food colorants in, 15–31
        colorants for declaration, stamping and egg colorants, 20
        demarcation of food colorants, 17
        food colorants approved by the EU, 17–18, 21–22
        food colorants not approved in all EU member states, 18
        food colorants not mentioned in new EU guidelines, 18
        food colorants permitted for limited use in Germany, 18
        food products, 19, 22–30
        maximum levels, 19–20
        new EU guidelines, 16
        past history, 15–16
        solvent/carriers, 20, 31
        special notes, 20
        transition period, 21
    legal requirements for cosmetic product coloration in, 39–45
    legal requirements for drug coloration in, 37–38
    purity standards for food colorants in, 77
European Union number (EU number), 12
Eye makeup, 57
    colorants for, 39

"Farbengesetz" (Germany's law on colorants), 39–40
Farbstoff-Kommission of the Deutsche Forschungs Gemeinschaft, 53
Fat pigments, special preparation for, 52
Ferrous gluconate (data sheet), 360
Finland, certification status of colorants in, 94
Fluorescence, 2–3
Foam bath, 54–55
    colorants for, 39
    formula for, 49
Food additive guidelines for the EU, 12
Food and Drug Administration (FDA):
    colorants requiring FDA certification, 32–33

[Food and Drug Administration (FDA)]
  colorants requiring no FDA certification 34–35
Food coloration, 13–35
  coloring ingredients, 14–15
  identification of, 80–89
  isolation of coloring agent in the finished product, 88–89
  legal basis, 15–35
    countries outside the EU, 31
    European Union, 15–31
    the U.S., 31–35
  literature on, 370–371
    legal status of colorants, 374–375
  need for coloration, 13–14
  product development, 52–53
  purity standards for, 77–80
  technical possibilities, 14
  See also data sheets of colorants with Color Index (C.I.) numbers and without C.I. numbers
Food products that can be colored (EU guidelines), 19, 22–30
  approved colorants in foods (restricted use), 29–30
  colorants used only for defined purposes, 27–28
  foods not permitted to contain colorant additives, 22–23
Fruits, citrus, natural colorant for, 13

Germany, Federal Republic of:
  legal requirements for cosmetic product coloration in, 39–45
  legal requirements for drug coloration in, 37–38
  Ostwald color system in, 6
  RAL color register in, 6
Glycerin-based soap, 56
Green pigments, 86
  calculation example for, 70, 74
Guaiazulene (data sheet), 361
Guatemala, certification status of colorants in, 94

Hair dyeing and coloration products, 58
Honduras, certification status of colorants in, 94
Hong Kong, certification status of colorants in, 94
Hungary, certification status of colorants in, 95

Identification of colorants, 80–89
  aluminum lakes, 85
  isolation of coloring agent in the finished product and its identification, 88–89
  oil-soluble food and cosmetic colorants, 84–85
  pigments, 85–87
  water-soluble food and cosmetic colorants, 80–83
INCI (International Cosmetic Ingredient Dictionary) names 91
Indigo plant, 9
Ingredients for coloring, 14–15
Inorganic colorants, 7
Inorganic pigments, identification of, 86
Interference, 3
International Commission on Lighting. See CIE-Lab color system
Iraq, certification status of colorants in, 94
Iron oxide (data sheet), 323–324
Isolation of coloring agents in the finished product, 88–89

Jamaica, certification status of colorants in, 94
Japan:
  certification status of colorants in, 94
  control of cosmetic product coloration in, 45

Lacquers:
  paint, 7
  processing of, 51–52
Lakes:
  aluminum, 85
  isolation in finished product, 89
Lambert-Beer law, 65–66
Legal basis for food coloration, 15–35
  countries outside the EU, 31
  European Union, 15–31
    colorants for declaration, stamping and egg colorants, 20
    demarcation of food colorants, 17
    food colorants approved by the EU, 17–18, 21–22
    food colorants not approved in all EU member states, 18
    food colorants not mentioned in new EU guidelines, 18
    food colorants permitted for limited use in Germany, 18
    food products, 19, 22–30
    maximum levels, 19–20

[Legal basis for food coloration]
    new EU guidelines, 16
    past history, 15–16
    solvent/carriers, 20, 31
    special notes, 20
    transition period, 21
    literature on legal status of colorants, 374–375
    United States, 31–35
        colorants for food, drugs and/or cosmetics, 32–35
Legal requirements for cosmetic product colorants, 39–46
    countries outside the EU, 45–46
    European Union/Federal Republic of Germany, 39–45
        declaration of colorants in cosmetic products, 41–45
    literature on legal status of colorants, 375–376
Legal requirements for drug coloration, 37–38
    countries outside the EU, 38
    European Union/Federal Republic of Germany, 37–38
Light absorption, correlation between wavelength, observed color and, 1, 2
Light interference, 3
Light stability test, 59–60
Lipstick, 57
    colorants for, 39
Liquid soap, 54–55
Literature, 369–376
    analysis and color determination, 372–374
    cosmetics, 372
    drugs, 371–372
    food, 370–371
    general information, 369–370
    legislation, 374–376
        cosmetics, 375–376
        food, 374–375
Lycopene (natural food colorant), 13

Magnesium oxide (data sheet), 331–332
Magnesium phosphate (data sheet), 335–336
Magnesium stearate (data sheet), 342–343
Makeup, 57
Malaysia, certification status of colorants in, 94
Measuring color, 68–75
    basics, 68
    calculation and evaluation, 70–75

[Measuring color]
    determination, 68–69
Mexico:
    certification status of colorants in, 94
    control of cosmetic product coloration in, 45
Milk, natural colorant for, 13
Mouth care products, 57–58
    association between product statements and colors for mouth wash, 5–6
Munsell color system in the U.S., 6

Nail polish, 58
National Color System in Sweden, 6
Natural colorants, 7
    naturally occurring food colorants, 13
New Zealand, certification status of colorants in, 94
Nicaragua, certification status of colorants in, 95
Nitro group ($-NO_2$), 8
Norway, certification status of colorants in, 95

Observed color, correlation between wavelength, light absorption and, 1, 2
Oil baths, 55
Oil-in-water emulsion (O/W cream), 56
Oil-soluble food and cosmetic colorants, identification of, 84–85
Optical whiteners, 2–3
Orange pigments, 86
Organic colorants, 7
Organic pigments (without lake), identification of, 87
Ostwald color system in Germany, 6

Paint lacquers, 7
Paints (coloring paints), processing of, 51–52
Pakistan, certification status of colorants in, 94
Panama, certification status of colorants in, 95
Paper chromatography for identification of water-soluble colorants, 81–82
Perception of color, 4–6
Peru, certification status of colorants in, 95
Philippines, control of cosmetic product coloration in, 45
Photometry, 64–67
    evaluation, 67
    principles of spectral photometry, 64–66
Pigments, 7–10

[Pigments]
   identification of, 85–87
      inorganic pigments, 86
      organic pigments (without lake), 87
   isolation in the finished product, 89
   processing of, 51–52
   test method for, 71, 75
Poland, control of cosmetic product coloration in, 45
Product development, 49–61
   cosmetic products, 54–58
      bathing salts, bathing tablets, 55
      eye makeup, 57
      hair dyeing and coloration products, 58
      lipstick, 57
      mouth and tooth care products, 57–58
      nail polish, 58
      oil and cream baths, 55
      oil-in-water emulsion, 56
      shading cream, makeup, 57
      shampoo, foam bath, shower gel, liquid soap, 54–55
      soap, 55–56
      water-in-oil emulsion 56
   drugs, 53–54
   food, 52–53
   processing indications, 50–52
      pigments and coloring paints, 51–52
      soluble colorants, 50–51
      special preparations, 52
   stability tests, 59–61
Public discussion of coloration of food, drugs, and cosmetics, 47–48
Purity requirements for cosmetic, drug, and food colorants, 77–80
   colorants for cosmetic products, 80
   colorants for food and drugs, 77–80
Pyrophyllite (data sheet), 362

Quality assurance, 63–64

RAL color register in Germany, 6
Red beet, natural colorant for, 13
Red beet pigment, 52
Red pigments, 86
Remission, determination of, 64
Riboflavin (natural food colorant), 13
   data sheet, 363–365
Riboflavin-5'-phosphate (data sheet), 363–365
Romania, certification status of colorants in, 95

Safety and quality, 63–75
   colorimetry and photometry, 64–67
      evaluation, 67
      principles of spectral photometry, 64–66
   measuring color, 68–75
      basics, 68
      calculation and evaluation, 70–75
      determination, 68–69
   quality assurance, 63–64
   technology and dermatology, 63
Salad, natural colorant for, 13
Saudi Arabia, certification status of colorants in, 95
Seeing colors, 1–3
   fluorescence and optical whiteners, 2–3
Shading cream, 57
   colorants for, 39
Shampoo, 54–55
   colorants for, 39
Shiny pigments, 86
Shower gel, 54–55
   colorants for, 39
Silver (data sheet), 336–337
Singapore, certification status of colorants in, 95
Soap, 55–56
   colorants for, 39
   liquid, 54–55
Soluble colorants:
   isolation in the finished product, 88–89
   oil-soluble colorants, identification of, 84–85
   processing of, 50–51
   water-soluble colorants, identification of, 80–83
Solvents for food colorants (EU guidelines), 20, 31
South Africa, certification status of colorants in, 95
Spectral photometry, 64
   for identification of water-soluble colorants, 82, 84–85
   principles of, 64–66
Spinach:
   natural colorant for, 13
   spray-dried, 52
Stability tests for colorants, 59–61
Standard color value, 68
Substractive color blending, 3, 4
Sudan blue B (data sheet), 365

Index

Sulfuric acid, concentrated, for identification of water-soluble colorants, 82, 83
Sweden, certification status of colorants in, 95
Switzerland, certification status of colorants in, 95
Synthetic colorants, 7, 10
Systematic of colorants, 11–12
    Color Index, 11–12
    EU number, 12

Tartrazine, 38
Thailand, control of cosmetic product coloration in, 45
Thin-layer chromatography for identification of oil-soluble colorants, 84
Thyric purple, 9
Tomatoes, natural colorant for, 13
Toothpaste (and gels), 57–58
Toxic metals contained in food, 77
Toxicology, 63
Trinidad and Tobago, certification status of colorants in, 95
Triple-beam colorimeter, 69
Turkey, certification status of colorants in, 95

United States (U.S.):
    certification status of colorants in, 95
    colorants requiring FDA certification, 32–33
    colorants requiring no FDA certification, 34–35
    control of cosmetic product coloration in, 45
    legal basis for food colorants in, 31–35

[United States (U.S.)]
    colorants for food, drugs and/or cosmetics, 32–35
    Munsell color system in, 6

Vacuum-dried blends of coloring food ingredients, 92
Vegetables, natural colorant for, 13
Venezuela, control of cosmetic product coloration in, 45
Violet pigments, 86
Vitrolan Rose BE (data sheet), 366

Water-dispersible pigments, 7, 8
Water-in-oil emulsion (W/O cream), 56
Water-soluble colorants, identification of, 80–83
    aluminum lakes, 85
    droplet reaction and solubility characteristics in concentrated sulfuric acid, 82, 83
    paper chromatography, 81–82
    spectral photometry, 82, 84–85
Water-soluble pigments, preparation of, 52
Wavelength, correlation between light absorption, observed color and, 1, 2
White pigments, 86
World Health Organization, 63, 92

Xanthophyll (data sheet), 367–368

Yellow pigments, 86

Zinc stearate (data sheet), 342–343